Famine, disease and the social order
in early modern society

*Cambridge Studies in Population, Economy and
Society in Past Time 10*

Series Editors:

PETER LASLETT, ROGER SCHOFIELD and E. A. WRIGLEY

ESRC Cambridge Group for the History of Population and Social Structure

and DANIEL SCOTT SMITH

University of Illinois at Chicago

Recent work, in social, economic and demographic history has revealed much that was previously obscure about societal stability and change in the past. It has also suggested that crossing the conventional boundaries between these branches of history can be very rewarding.

This series will exemplify the value of interdisciplinary work of this kind, and will include books on topics such as family, kinship and neighbourhood; welfare provision and social control; work and leisure; migration; urban growth; and legal structures and procedures, as well as more familiar matters. It will demonstrate that for example, anthropology and economics have become as close intellectual neighbours to history as have political philosophy or biography.

Famine, disease and the social order in early modern society

Edited by

JOHN WALTER

Lecturer in History, University of Essex

and

ROGER SCHOFIELD

Cambridge Group for the History of Population and Social Structure

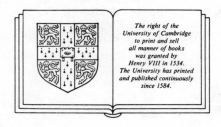

The right of the
University of Cambridge
to print and sell
all manner of books
was granted by
Henry VIII in 1534.
The University has printed
and published continuously
since 1584.

CAMBRIDGE UNIVERSITY PRESS

Cambridge
New York   New Rochelle
Melbourne   Sydney

Published by the Press Syndicate of the University of Cambridge
The Pitt Building, Trumpington Street, Cambridge CB2 1RP
32 East 57th Street, New York, NY 10022, USA
10 Stamford Road, Oakleigh, Melbourne 3166, Australia

© Cambridge University Press 1989

First published 1989

Printed in Great Britain at the University Press, Cambridge

British Library cataloguing in publication data

Famine, disease and the social order in
early modern society. – (Cambridge studies
in population, economy and society in past
time; 10)
1. Europe. Western Europe. Economic
conditions, 1453–1789. Demographic aspects
I. Walter, John II. Schofield, Roger S.
330.94'021

Library of Congress cataloging in publication data

Famine, disease and the social order in early modern society/edited
by John Walter and Roger Schofield.
p.   cm. – (Cambridge studies in population, economy, and
society in past time: 10)
Essays in honor of Andrew B. Appleby.
Bibliography.
Includes index.
ISBN 0-521-25906-1
1. Famines – England – History.   2. England – Economic conditions.
3. England – Population – History.   4. Famines – France – History.
5. France – Economic conditions.   6. France – Population – History.
7. Appleby, Andrew B.   I. Walter, John, 1948–   .   II. Schofield,
Roger. III. Appleby, Andrew B. IV. Series.
HC260.F3F36 1989
363.8'0942 – dc 19   88–30181 CIP

ISBN 0 521 25906 1

WV

This volume is dedicated to the memory of
Andy Appleby
friend and colleague

Contents

Contributors

Dr Jacques Dupâquier, *Directeur d'Etudes, Laboratoire de Démographie Historique, Paris*

Dr Peter Laslett, *Director of the Unit on Ageing at the Cambridge Group for the History of Population and Social Structure, and Fellow of Trinity College*

Professor David Levine, *Associate Professor, Department of History and Philosophy, Ontario Institute for Studies in Education, Toronto*

Dr Roger Schofield, *Director of the Cambridge Group for the History of Population and Social Structure, and Fellow of Clare College*

Dr Paul Slack, *Fellow and Tutor in Modern History, Exeter College, Oxford*

Mr John Walter, *Lecturer in History, and Director of the Local History Centre, University of Essex*

Dr David R. Weir, Associate Professor of Economics, Yale University

Dr Keith Wrightson, *Lecturer in History, University of Cambridge, and Fellow of Jesus College*

Professor E. A. Wrigley, *Co-Director of the Cambridge Group for the History of Population and Social Structure, and Senior Research Fellow of All Souls College, Oxford*

Figures

Tables

Andrew Appleby
A personal appreciation

PETER LASLETT

Andrew Appleby was a tall, quiet, judicious man – a large figure and a considerable presence. He came late to the writing of history, from a previous career helping to run a newspaper which his family owned in San Diego County, Southern California. The reasons why he changed were at bottom moral reasons, and the same could be said, I think, about his choice of a line of investigation. He felt a personal responsibility for the men and women of the past. He cared about what really weighed upon them much more than he cared about the traditional preoccupations of historians as he found them to be when he took up research.

Hence his settled concern with hunger, disease and death amongst our ancestors and predecessors in pre-industrial times, and his unwavering determination to get at the truth of these matters as far as that could possibly be done. The impression he gave to me was that he could afford to stand aside and wait until others saw things in the light in which he saw them himself. What a sad, sad thing that he should have died before that change had completely come about.

Nevertheless in the seven or eight years during which he cultivated his chosen territory, years when he was fulfilling the burdensome stint of teaching demanded by the State University of California, his output of books, articles and addresses was enormous. He must have worked at a pace and a pressure which his easy, equable bearing and his unwillingness to talk about himself concealed from his friends and associates.

For all his reserved manner – here was a man who was able to leave many things unsaid – Andrew Appleby had it in him to attract an audience and arouse an interest, an interest always more than ephemeral. I have it recorded in my diary that when he addressed the weekly seminar of the Cambridge Group for the History of Population

and Social Structure on 15 November 1977, our little library was
hysterically crowded. I reckon there were forty-two or forty-three
people, and in a space which is full when there are twenty. So great
was the press that we were fearful for the security of the wooden floor,
laid down in the 1840s and never designed for public meetings.

What he said on that occasion came out in a low tone and a rather
hesitant manner, but the discussion which succeeded was not like this
at all. Most of the issues, the paradoxes, the puzzlements, which have
become evident in the study of famine, pestilence and the social
structure in the succeeding ten years made their presence felt,
especially in Andy's answers and explanations.

Now these are not incidental questions, and they are not to be settled
by technical or specialist answers, important as it is that many
researchers now dig deeply where Appleby cleared the surface and
turned the first furrows. They have had to innovate for the purpose,
technically and otherwise. To know how far people did fear illness and
premature extinction is to know something of profound importance
about any society. Such knowledge is as significant to a society's
ideological and political life as it is to its economics, although far and
away its greatest significance is for the ordinary, everyday life of
ordinary people.

It is turning out to be very difficult to be quite certain whether the
peasants really starved, anywhere in Europe before industrial times. It
has become a nice problem as to how far famine ever was a direct result
of shortage of food and that alone. It is even questionable whether low
levels of nourishment do assist the spread of disease, or may actually in
some cases reduce its power to kill. Andrew Appleby would have had a
good deal to say about all this. It is not going to be easy to get it right
without him.

A bibliography of Andrew B. Appleby's principal works in chronological order

'Population crisis and economic change: Cumberland and Westmorland, 1570–1670', unpublished University of California doctoral dissertation, Los Angeles, 1973

'Disease or famine? Mortality in Cumberland and Westmorland, 1580–1640', *Economic History Review*, second series, 26 (August, 1973) 403–31

'Nutrition and disease: the case of London, 1550–1750', *Journal of Interdisciplinary History*, 6, no. 1 (Summer, 1975) 1–22

'Agrarian capitalism or seigneurial reaction? The north west of England, 1500–1700', *American Historical Review*, 80, no. 3 (June, 1975) 574–94

'Common land and peasant unrest in sixteenth-century England', *Peasant Studies Newsletter*, 4, no. 3 (July, 1975) 20–23

'Famine, mortality, and epidemic disease: a comment', *Economic History Review*, second series, 30, no. 3 (August, 1977) 508–12

Famine in Tudor and Stuart England, Liverpool University Press, Liverpool, 1978; Stanford University Press, Stanford, California, 1978

'Disease, diet, and history', *Journal of Interdisciplinary History*, 8, no. 4 (Spring, 1978) 725–35

'Grain prices and subsistence crises in England and France 1590–1740', *Journal of Economic History*, 39, no. 4 (December, 1979) 865–87

'Diet in sixteenth-century England: sources, problems, possibilities', in C. Webster (ed.), *Health, Medicine and Mortality in the Sixteenth Century*, Cambridge: Cambridge University Press, 1979, pp. 97–116

'Crises of mortality: periodicity, intensity, chronology and geographical extent', in H. Charbonneau and A. Larose (eds.), *The Great Mortalities: Methodologies Studies of Demographic Crises in the Past*, Liège, 1979, pp. 283–94

'Epidemics and famine in the Little Ice Age', *Journal of Interdisciplinary History*, 10, no. 4 (Spring, 1980) 643–63

'The disappearance of the plague: a continuing puzzle', *Economic History Review*, second series., 33 (May, 1980) 161–73

Abbreviations

AO	Archives Office
APC	*Acts of the Privy Council of England*
Bodl. Lib.	Bodleian Library
Brit. Lib. (BL)	British Library
Cal. S.P. Dom.	Calendar of State Papers, Domestic series
DPD	Durham University Department of Paleograpy and Diplomatic
DRO	Durham County Record Office
Hants	Hampshire
Harl. MS	Harleian Manuscript
HMC	Historical Manuscripts Commission
PRO	Public Record Office
RO	Record Office
Staffs	Staffordshire

1

Famine, disease and crisis mortality in early modern society

JOHN WALTER and ROGER SCHOFIELD

In 1965, when Peter Laslett first asked the question, 'Did the peasants really starve?', historical demography in England was scarcely in a position to provide him with an answer. Paradoxically, despite the interest of earlier demographers, with Malthus one of the foremost, the study of what has come to be known as 'crisis mortality' was still in its infancy. Apart from a seminal article by Drake based on the parish registers of south-west Yorkshire, there were few studies to match the work of French historical demographers on which Laslett drew. As he made clear, our knowledge of the critical issue of the reality of the threat of famine was rudimentary.[1] Such discussion as there was relied on the vivid impression of literary sources which, with their well-worn examples, carried a serious risk of exaggeration.[2] In the face of this uncertain knowledge, Laslett's conclusion was that, 'the relation between the amount and cost of food and the variations in the level of mortality, of men and women as well as children, must remain an open question for the time, along with that of whether crises of subsistence were a present possibility in the English town and countryside'.[3]

Eighteen years later, when he repeated his earlier question in *The World We Have Lost Further Explored*, he noted, 'Not one of these plaintive queries is as appropriate now in 1983.'[4] As his revised text made clear, we owe much of this gain in knowledge to the work of Andrew Appleby, an American scholar for whom Laslett's original

---

[1] Laslett, *World We Have Lost*, pp. 107–27; Drake, 'Elementary exercise in parish register demography'; Howson, 'Plague, poverty, population'; Goubert 'Problèmes démographiques', 'Mortalité en France', *Beauvais*, 'French population'; Meuvret, 'Demographic crisis in France'.
[2] As in Thirsk and Cooper, *Economic Documents*, p. 24. For an example of a generalisation from this source, see Watts, *Social History Western of Europe*, p. 102.
[3] Laslett, *World We Have Lost*, p. 127
[4] *Ibid.*, p. 151.

question had been the spur to begin research in this area. Through Appleby's untimely death in 1980 the scholarly world lost not only an innovative and penetrating mind, but also a warm and generous personality that left a deep and lasting impression on all who knew him. This volume is dedicated to his memory; its contents are intended as a further exploration of a significant domain in the 'world we have lost', in whose mapping Appleby played such a crucial and pioneering role. All who work in early modern social and economic history stand in his debt, and it is fitting that the first contribution to this volume should be a personal appreciation by Peter Laslett.

Not only was the theme of Appleby's research inspired by Laslett's original question, but his choice of area was influenced by the latter's citation of heightened mortality in 1623 in the parish register of Greystoke in Cumberland to suggest that it was perhaps here in the pastoral upland of the north-west that evidence might be found of a region vulnerable to famine.[5] First in a doctoral dissertation and later in articles and a book, Appleby focussed on the problems of demographic crises and economic change in the north-west.[6] Dearth and disease as the causes of crisis mortality lay at the centre of his work. In his first published article, an analysis of the demographic history of early modern Cumberland and Westmorland, he showed that the answer to Laslett's original was a sombre 'yes'.[7] Famine was a reality in this region in the late sixteenth and early seventeenth century. In *Famine in Tudor and Stuart England* he extended this analysis to offer a preliminary mapping of famine-prone and famine-free areas. A later article returned to the problem, this time in a comparative perspective, examining the reasons for England's eventual and, in European terms, early resistance to famine, highlighting the role of a mix of winter and spring cereals in destroying the fatal association between harvest failure, a symmetrical price structure, and famine. In the seventeenth century, he argued, England benefitted from a growing emphasis on spring-sown cereals which meant that all grains did not fail at the same time nor all rise in price to famine levels. In France the continuing stranglehold of winter cereals perpetuated the threat of dearth.[8]

In his work on famine in the north-west in the sixteenth and seventeenth centuries, Appleby had been anxious to restore to dearth

---

[5] Cambridge Group files: Andrew Appleby, letter to Roger Schofield, dated 27 July 1976: 'I only really chose the north-west because this region was hard hit by these famines.'

[6] The dissertation was entitled 'Population crisis and economic change: Cumberland and Westmorland, 1570–1670', and was submitted for the Ph.D. degree in the University of California, Los Angeles, in 1973.

[7] 'Disease or famine'.   [8] 'Grain prices'.

some responsibility for mortality, which historians had been inclined to attribute solely to disease, notably epidemics of plague. On the other hand, his strong interest in medical history led him to caution against any easy assumption of a universal and direct relationship between hunger and disease.[9] Taking advantage of the evidence of the London Bills of Mortality, which specified cause of death, and a series of bread prices, he was able to show a lack of correspondence between dearth and mortality from most forms of disease in early modern London, thereby providing evidence for fluctuations in disease independent of economic conditions.[10] Pursuing further the question of how far changes in mortality were autonomous, or mediated by economic or social institutions, in his last published article he tackled the problem of the disappearance of plague in the later seventeenth century, one of the great puzzles in English and European historical demography. Although he recognised that in the last resort the key to the disappearance of plague lay in the implementation of effective quarantine measures that would prevent its re-importation into England or Europe, he was sceptical of the effectiveness of such measures in the seventeenth century. Accordingly, he suggested that a biological process must also have been at work, in which the severe plague epidemics of the period resulted in the selection of rats with a higher resistance to the disease, thereby enabling infected rat fleas to remain on the rats, their preferred hosts.[11] Since the fleas no longer had to migrate to humans in search of new hosts, the latter obtained a breathing space during which administrative measures could be improved to a sufficient extent to prevent the re-importation of plague.

Appleby, therefore, combined detailed local and regional research with a wider interest in general and comparative historical issues. Within a short space of time, he went a considerable way, not simply to answering Laslett's call for research in this vital area, but in providing answers to some of the most important questions. A bibliography of his major writings is included in this book. In his work on famine, he established that in early modern England there was some vulnerability to famine, that it was confined to a particular type of region, and that in contrast to parts of the continent, England both escaped relatively lightly from harvest failure and saw the early disappearance of famine even on a regional level. His mapping of the geography and chronology of subsistence crises in England raised important questions about why some areas were vulnerable and others were not. In this

---

[9] See the draft prospectus for his intended volume, 'The Englishman's health: disease and nutrition 1500–1700', Longman Themes in Social History series.

[10] 'Nutrition and disease.'   [11] 'Disappearance of plague'.

work, as well as in related articles on diet, climate, and agrarian class relationships, he demonstrated the importance of understanding the inter-relationship of social, economic, and even political, factors in determining patterns of dearth and disease in the past. Appleby's work raised some important critical issues in the history of early modern societies, which are far from resolved. The contributors to this volume, all his friends and colleagues, take up the challenge, confirming some of his insights and findings, refining and extending others. As their contributions amply demonstrate, there is still plenty of life in the historical study of death.

Some basic concepts

Before we consider Appleby's contribution further, and take stock of the present state of our understanding of the issues that he raised, it may be helpful to discuss the biological and social processes that underlie the arguments he advanced, and to examine how far their operation in the past can be traced in the sources we have at our disposal.

Appleby was concerned with everyday matters of life and death, but his argument was about the frequency and severity of famine-related mortality, and involved concepts such as shortage of food, malnutrition, and starvation. Unfortunately, the latter are abstractions rather than events, so the information we can find about them in historical sources is necessarily indirect, at best the result of inferences drawn by contemporaries from their own experience. Valuable though such observations may be, they are sporadic, unsystematic, and subjective, and fall far short of a satisfactory basis on which to address the range of issues that Appleby raised. If we want to investigate questions such as how often people went so short of food that they were malnourished and starved to death, we need to find evidence recorded on a regular basis so that we can assess the typicality of our observations over time and space.

Unfortunately, the nutritional status of individuals was not regularly recorded in early modern England, nor was cause of death, so we are forced to draw inferences from such information as was given on a regular basis. For our purposes there are two elements in the story we are investigating which were recorded regularly in the past: grain prices in markets, and burials in parish registers. We shall need to consider the adequacy of the evidence for each of these elements. We shall also need to consider how far information on prices may be a reasonable indicator of the amount of food available to people in the past, and how far information about the frequency of deaths, when related to prices, gives us reasonable grounds for inferring the existence of malnutrition or starvation. The latter point will require us to examine the theoretical relationships linking insufficient food intake with death from hunger.

Questions and sources

It must be admitted at the outset that the evidence is far from satisfactory. While the burial registers kept by the Church of England recorded the overwhelming majority of deaths at least until the end of the eighteenth century, the absence of any regular statement of the cause means that the link between hunger and mortality has to be investigated at the crude level of deaths from all causes.[12] In examining this link Appleby and other historians have adopted two rather different approaches. In the first, fluctuations in the numbers of deaths are related to fluctuations in food prices of all magnitudes, so that the connection between low food prices and low mortality is taken into account as well as the level of mortality when food prices are high. With so general a procedure there is obviously a danger of drawing spurious inferences, so care needs to be taken in carrying out the statistical analysis. For example, in a pioneering study of the relationship between fluctuations in bread prices and deaths in seventeenth-century London, Appleby was unable to find any significant association between movements in London prices and deaths from various causes.[13] However, the method he used was unsatisfactory, and a recent and statistically more sophisticated study found that there was a positive association between fluctuations in wheat prices and deaths from epidemic disease (typhus, smallpox, and fevers) in the same calendar year.[14]

The second approach differs from the first in that attention is confined to outbreaks of exceptionally high mortality in specific localities, which historians have called mortality 'crises'. The temporal and geographical distributions of these crises are then examined in the light of fluctuations in food prices. Unfortunately, the identification of mortality crises also has its technical problems. First, there is the question of the definition of a 'crisis'; how high has mortality to rise

---

[12] For the adequacy of burial registration, see Wrigley and Schofield, *Population History*, table 5.27, p. 141.

[13] 'Nutrition and disease'.

[14] Galloway, 'Annual variations'. The results of this study are discussed more fully later in this chapter.

before it reaches a 'crisis' level? Historians, including Appleby, have traditionally identified local mortality crises by looking for periods in which the number of burials recorded exceeded the average frequency by some arbitrary factor, say a doubling.[15] Clearly, if this approach is adopted, care needs to be taken in identifying a suitably calm reference period for the calculation of the average burial frequency.[16] However, there is a further problem. Since 'crises' are typically short, sharp affairs, there are statistical difficulties in distinguishing them from random fluctuations in mortality especially in the case of small communities in which only a few burials normally occurred each year. The danger here is that random fluctuations will be mistakenly classified as mortality crises. It was to avoid this difficulty that an alternative method was devised in *The Population History of England* which took account of the amplitude of random fluctuations when identifying crises. In this approach a crisis was defined not as a fixed proportional increase in mortality above the average level, but in terms of the probability that an upward fluctuation in mortality was so great that it was unlikely to have arisen by chance.[17] While this approach avoids the problem of generating spurious crises in small parishes, it suffers from the opposite disadvantage of detecting more crises in large parishes, since they are more easily distinguished from random fluctuations than is the case in small parishes, even though the proportional increase in mortality is the same.

The identification of local crises, therefore, is beset by technical difficulties. But an even greater problem is that any definition of a crisis, whether based on a fixed or variable increase in the number of burials, is necessarily arbitrary, reducing the rich variety of fluctua-

---

[15] Unfortunately, historians have been unable to agree on the level of the 'crisis factor', thereby making it impossible to compare the incidence of crisis mortality in different historical contexts. For a systematic discussion of the strengths and weaknesses of different methods of defining a mortality 'crisis', see Charbonneau and Larose, *Great Mortalities*, pp. 21–9, 64–112, 153–6, 171–8, 283–94.

[16] Obviously crisis months or years should not form part of the reference period, nor should periods in which the number of burials recorded were unusually low. For example, Del Panta and Livi-Bacci recommend dropping the two highest and two lowest values from an eleven-year moving average, Charbonneau and Larose, *Great Mortalities*, p. 72. Unfortunately, some scholars have been rather careless about ensuring that the reference period does not contain extreme frequencies, thereby biassing downward, or upwards, the number of crises they detect.

[17] For a single month a probability of less than 1 in 10,000 that the burial total was a random fluctuation above the average monthly frequency of the reference period was taken to indicate a crisis. Periods of two or more successive months, in which each month had a probability of less than 1 in 100 of being a random fluctuation, were also classified as constituting a crisis. Wrigley and Schofield, *Population History*, pp. 646–9.

tions in mortality to a simple dichotomy between the presence or absence of a 'crisis'. Nonetheless, as Appleby found, the geographical distribution of local mortality crises in years of high food prices seems to make sense in the light of what we know about the social and economic history of early modern England, and promises to advance still further our understanding of important aspects of social and economic change.[18] But before we go on to consider the evidence, we first need to consider whether the historical data that we have on prices are an adequate guide to changes in the availability of food?

Ideally we should like to know the calorie and protein value of the food that families could command in England in the past, and how this varied over time and place. In practice, the evidence that we have on past diets is sparse and largely confined to aristocratic households and to institutions. We simply do not know in any detail the quantity and quality of the food of the people, how it varied over time, or what scope there was for substituting other foods in time of harvest deficiency.[19] However, such fragmentary evidence as is currently available indicates that while meat, fish, and dairy products constituted a significant element in many people's diet, for all except the rich, grain was the dominant form of food.[20] Moreover, the lower the income available to a household, the greater was the dependence on grain.

This relationship helps to explain changes in the proportions of expenditure on grain over time. For example, at the end of the seventeenth century Gregory King drew up a series of model food expenditure budgets for different levels of wealth.[21] According to King, 50 per cent of the food expenditure of the poorest 41 per cent of the population was on grain, 7 per cent on malt drinks (which contained a significant amount of grain), 19 per cent on dairy products, 11 per cent on meat, fish, and eggs, 9 per cent on fruit and vegetables, and 4 per cent on other items. By contrast, those who spent three times

---

[18] Appleby, *Famine*, chapters 9, 12; Wrigley and Schofield, *Population History*, pp. 670–85.

[19] Valuable earlier work on diet was for the most part anecdotal and impressionistic; Drummond and Wilbraham, *Englishman's Food*; Ashley, *Bread of our Forefathers*. For more recent work, see Appleby, 'Diet'; Dyer, 'Diet in the later Middle Ages'; Shammas, 'Food expenditure', 'Eighteenth-century English diet'; Anderson, 'Ethnography of yeoman foodways'; Walter, chapter 2, below.

[20] For food expenditures in a fifteenth-century priest's household and in sixty poor households in southern England in the 1790s, see Phelps Brown and Hopkins, 'Seven centuries of prices', pp. 180–1. Gregory King's model food expenditure budgets for the late seventeenth century are printed in facsimile in Laslett, *The Earliest Classics*, p. 210. Information for parishes in central Kent for the period 1793–1838 are tabulated in Richardson, 'Agricultural labourer's standard of living', p. 105. The Davies-Eden food budgets are analysed in Shammas, 'Eighteenth-century English diet'.   [21] See previous note.

as much on food, and whose expenditures were exceeded by only 10 per cent of the population, spent proportionately less on grain and dairy products (only 25 per cent and 13 per cent, respectively), and about the same on fruit and vegetables (8 per cent). Instead, they spent more on meat, fish, and eggs (23 per cent), malted drinks (17 per cent), and 15 per cent on other items such as spices, wines, and spirits. Even if we are generous and count the expenditure on malt drinks as attributable to grain, this group of rich consumers devoted 42 per cent of its expenditure to grain (25 per cent + 17 per cent) compared to the 57 per cent of expenditure devoted to grain (50 per cent + 7 per cent) by the poorest 41 per cent of the population. Thus, as people got richer they used their extra income on non-grain foodstuffs.[22]

At times of population pressure and high food prices, as in the century before the Black Death and at the end of the eighteenth century, about 50–70 per cent of food expenditure went on grain in the form of bread, flour and ale, and less than 20 per cent on meat and fish. However, in the century after the Black Death when population and food prices were low, expenditure on grain fell to 40–50 per cent (with one half of this in the form of ale), while expenditure on meat and fish rose to 35–40 per cent. According to Gregory King this late-medieval pattern of consumption was matched by only the richest 5 per cent of the population at the end of the seventeenth century.[23] For most of the period, however, grain-based food and drink comprised at least half of all food expenditures for all except the very rich. Consequently, we might reasonably expect that a significant fraction of the population, with the least financial resources, would have experienced substantial changes in the amount of food available from year to year as variations in the weather influenced the amount of grain that could be harvested. We might also reasonably expect that there were long-run changes in the amount of grain available per head as agricultural productivity either lagged behind, or outpaced, the demand for food generated by changing rates of population growth. Unfortunately, while these general surmises may be reasonable, we lack any information on total

[22] Total income and expenditure elasticities for the different types of food included in King's model tables have been calculated and shown to comprise a coherent and plausible set of relationships. Stone, 'Some seventeenth-century econometrics'. Expenditure elasticities for the Davies-Eden budgets for the period 1787–95 are calculated in Shammas, 'Eighteenth-century English diet', p. 259. A similar gradient in the proportion of expenditure on different kinds of food can be seen in the diets assigned to inmates and officials of different social statuses in the Sherborne almshouse in the period 1425–40. Dyer, 'Changes in nutrition', p. 40.

[23] Dyer, 'Changes in nutrition', p. 37; Phelps Brown and Hopkins, 'Seven centuries of prices', table 1; Richardson, 'Agricultural labourer's standard of living', p. 105. Laslett, Earliest Classics, p. 210.

food yields, and so cannot directly observe the amount by which the size of harvest, or the total quantity of food available per head, may have varied in either the short, or the long, run.[24] What we do have are series of food prices, especially grain prices. Can we use the fluctuations in these series as a measure of the scarcity or plenty of food in the past?

Prices, markets, and scarcity

The short answer is 'only to a limited extent'. The price series are drawn disproportionately from the south of England. The lack of regular local price series for other regions before the end of the eighteenth century would not matter if there had been an integrated national market in grains, because fluctuations in prices would have been common to all areas, even though the level of prices might have differed. Fortunately, local prices are available for several areas for a brief period of twelve years at the end of the seventeenth century, and in the case of wheat the regional price series show a remarkable degree of uniformity in their short-run fluctuations.[25] However, as Weir points out later in this volume, a correlation between the fluctuations in prices in different regions does not necessarily imply market integration, since it could be produced by a common pattern of weather affecting regions which in fact had independent markets.[26]

But in late seventeenth-century England, fluctuations in the regional prices of grains other than wheat were uncorrelated. This not only points to a lack of market integration for these grains, but also indicates that the weather conditions in the different regions were independent of each other. Thus in the case of wheat, which was the preferred food grain and the most common cash crop throughout most of England, it would seem reasonable to conclude that the common movement of regional prices indicates that a national market had indeed been achieved by the late seventeenth century, through which local shortages could be made good from surpluses accruing in other areas. Moreover, the lack of correlation between the movements in the prices of wheat and other grains suggests that by this date there was no longer any need for the demand to fall heavily on one of the alternative

---

[24] A national series of annual grain production in England begins only in 1884, but is available for France from 1815, and for Sweden from 1802. Mitchell, *European Historical Statistics*, table D2.

[25] Chartres, 'Marketing of agricultural produce', pp. 459–65, 828–31; Bowden, 'Agricultural prices', pp. 593–648, 815–21; Granger and Elliott, 'Fresh look at wheat prices'.

[26] See chapter 6, below.

cheaper grains as a result of local shortages of the preferred bread corn. Indeed the existence of a wider market network, integrating several climatic zones, is a necessary precondition for the geographical specialization in agricultural production that Appleby argued had emerged by the end of the seventeenth century. Although such a specialisation, in which each region grew the mix of grains most suited to local soil-types and climate would have the beneficial effect of increasing the total output of grain, such was the uncertainty of the weather that local specialisation would only be a viable strategy if local shortages and surpluses could be ironed out through a market network extending beyond the region and integrating several climatic zones. In developing a national market network, England was fortunate in that both weather and soil characteristics vary over quite small distances, and in being an island well endowed with navigable rivers, so that grain could be transported in bulk over long distances relatively easily.[27]

Although it may be reasonable to conclude that England enjoyed a national grain market by the end of the seventeenth century, we do not, however, know how long such a market had been in existence. For earlier periods, therefore, it must remain an open question whether or not it is reasonable to treat fluctuations in prices drawn from southern England as if they were representative of the country as a whole. The problem is particularly acute when examining local mortality crises in the north-west, Appleby's original area of interest. For example, in 1622/3 many upland parishes recorded mortality crises even though there was only a modest increase in the 'national' series of grain prices. However, prices in Scotland rose steeply in these years, and are likely to be a much better guide to harvest conditions in the north than the 'English' series, which are based on conditions in the south.[28]

In addition to doubts about their geographical representativeness, the English grain price series also suffer from the further drawback that they are drawn largely from the records of institutions, such as colleges.[29] The argument has been made that prices paid by bulk purchasers of this kind are likely to underestimate the degree of fluctuation that would have been experienced by individuals making small purchases for current consumption. On the other hand, it must

[27] As Weir notes in chapter 6, below, some of the French regional markets covered areas as large as England.

[28] That oats played an important part in Northern diets compounds the problem of using a southern-based 'national' index.

[29] Phelps Brown and Hopkins, *Perspective of Wages and Prices*; Beveridge et al., *Prices and Wages*; Rogers, *Agriculture and Prices*; Hoskins, 'Harvest fluctuations, 1480–1619', 'Harvest fluctuations, 1620–1759'; Bowden, 'Agricultural prices'.

be remembered that small purchasers are likely to have spent a higher proportion of their outlay on processed, or semi-processed, foods: on bread and beer, for example, rather than grain and hops. In the pre-industrial world the price of such commodities contained a significant labour component, the value of which did not fluctuate in the short run. Unfortunately, we do not know the extent to which people relied on purchasing processed foods rather than on preparing their own from raw materials; but it is likely to have varied between social groups and to have been greater in larger settlements, which could support a greater specialisation of occupation. Thus there is some doubt about which, if any, price series would give the best picture of the cost of food to the poor. In the light of this uncertainty it is fortunate that two series of sixteenth-century food prices representing rather different sets of consumers and degrees of processing of raw grain, namely the Bowden series of wheat prices and a London series of flour prices, exhibit more or less the same proportionate fluctuations from year to year.[30] The major wheat price series, therefore, are likely to provide a reasonable guide to the magnitude of the price variations that consumers of grain-based products will have faced. Over the long-run, however, the higher labour component in the price of flour compared to wheat does seem to have dampened the magnitude of the changes in the price series. For example, wheat prices increased 5.2 times between the 1490s and the decade 1600–9, while flour prices only rose 3.4 times. In reality, of course, consumers also purchased non-grain based foodstuffs which were subject to much less annual variation. Consequently, a price index of a basket of consumables, such as the well-known one constructed by Phelps Brown and Hopkins, has an annual coefficient of variation which is only about one-half that of the wheat and flour price series.[31]

But movements in prices do not on their own tell us much about changes in the availability of food over the long run. We also need to take into account changes in wages, which will influence the ability of households to afford the prices charged in the market. For convenience, the effects of changes in both wages and prices are combined by

---

[30] As measured by the coefficients of variation of the prices for each decade. The Bowden series is based largely on wheat prices in Exeter, adjusted by prices in other regional markets, when available. Bowden, 'Statistical appendix', pp. 816–20. The London series of flour prices, almost certainly referring to wheat flour, is taken from Rappaport, *Social Structure and Mobility*, table 5.4.

[31] Phelps Brown and Hopkins, 'Seven centuries of prices', appendix B. Over the long run the movement in the price of the composite basket of consumables was intermediate between that of the wheat and flour price series, increasing 4.7 times between the 1490s and 1600/9.

calculating a 'real wages' index, which represents the amount of food that can be purchased with the current level of wages. Although real wage series have been constructed for early modern England, there are considerable difficulties in interpreting them. First, the evidence for wages is even more restricted in scope than was the case for food prices; the most widely used real wage index, constructed by Phelps Brown and Hopkins, is based on wages of building craftsmen and labourers in the south of England.[32] Since conditions of employment and remuneration are likely to have varied widely between different occupations, the level of the resulting real wage cannot be expected to apply to everyone in the country. However, the purpose of calculating a real wage index is to track *changes* in the ability to purchase food over time. The index will only be misleading in this respect if *changes* in the wage levels of other occupations were different from those of the occupations used in constructing the index. This is more likely to be a problem over the long run: for example, it is known that during the eighteenth century wage rates in the urban north rose much faster than agricultural wages in the south. It is not yet known whether there were geographical, or urban–rural, differences in long-run rates of change in wages at earlier dates, but the possibility cannot be discounted, and cautions against an easy acceptance of the standard real wage series as an indicator of long-run changes in the availability of food.[33]

The problems of inference produced by hidden differences in wage movements would seem to be much less in the case of short-run fluctuations. Since the wage series changed slowly over time, the annual fluctuations in the real-wage index were almost entirely produced by variations in the price of grain in response to harvest conditions. This does not mean, though, that we can disregard short-run fluctuations in earnings as a factor affecting the ability to purchase food. The wage series are slow-moving because they are based on adult male wage *rates*, which remain at customary levels for long periods of time. The fact that the series are based on rates rather than earnings constitutes a second major difficulty in using them to determine changes in the ability to purchase food. Since consumption

[32] Phelps Brown and Hopkins, 'Seven centuries of building wages', 'Seven centuries of prices'. Series based on monetary payments of course ignore the important problem of what constituted the 'wage' in pre-industrial societies. For a discussion of the specific problems of calculating payments to building workers, see Woodward, 'Wage rates and living standards', pp. 28–45.

[33] For some evidence of earlier differences in regional wage-rates, see Foot, *Wages in England*, pp. 8–9; Roberts, 'Wages and wage-earners', p. 205. For the eighteenth and nineteenth centuries, see Lindert and Williamson, 'English workers' living standards'.

was organised by household, we need information on how total household income changed over time. This involves not just the wage rates of adult males, but the rates and, above all, the amount of work that all members of the household could obtain.[34] In pre-industrial societies, in which under-employment was rife, variations in the demand for labour are likely to have been much more significant than variations in wage rates. Moreover, the very conditions that determined the price of grain are likely to have produced an opposite effect on the demand for labour, and so have had a double impact, whether positive or negative, on the ability of individuals to afford food. For example, a deficient harvest both drives up grain prices and offers less work to agricultural labourers, while an abundant harvest does the reverse. Furthermore, in a society in which between a third and a half of the expenditure of ordinary families is directed towards grain-based food, any change in grain prices will have a more than proportionate impact on the income that is available for purchase of non-food articles.[35] This will reduce the demand for labour of families engaged in crafts and service trades precisely at the moment when they need to earn more to pay the higher food prices.

There are good reasons, therefore, for believing that movements in grain prices will have exerted a considerable influence on the ability of ordinary families to obtain food in early modern England. How great that influence may have been will depend on several factors, many of which, unfortunately, are still imperfectly known. First, not everyone will have been dependent on the market for grain. Subsistence farmers, living-in servants in husbandry, and agricultural labourers receiving payment in kind rather than money wages, will have been cushioned against movements in grain prices.[36] Although we do not know how large a fraction of the population was in such a sheltered position in early modern England, it is clear that there were always individuals who were not in so fortunate a position, and that their numbers increased over time. Even at the end of the thirteenth century a substantial proportion of landholdings in midland England (between 29 and 46 per cent) were below subsistence level, implying the

---

[34] For preliminary discussions of the contributions of women and children to family incomes, see Clark, *Working Life of Women*; Roberts, 'Sickles and scythes'; Charles and Duffin, eds., *Women and Work*.

[35] Approximately 70 per cent of expenditures are attributable to food: Shammas, 'Food expenditure', p. 91. Shammas estimates that 50–70 per cent of food expenditure went on grain-based products, but, for some upward revision of these figures (to 70 per cent), see Komlos, 'Food budget', p. 149.

[36] For further discussion, see Walter, chapter 2, below.

existence of local markets in both labour and food.[37] Furthermore, from the early sixteenth century, changes in the structure of landholding led to a polarisation of the distribution of farm sizes, with proportionatey fewer subsistence farms and more landless people selling their labour to large-scale farming units. For young unmarried adults, shelter from the market through employment in service in husbandry remained a possible option until the late eighteenth century in arable areas and well into the nineteenth century in pastoral zones. But many farm households, including those employing one or two servants, will have been forced on to the market in years of deficient harvest. And outside the agricultural sector there was a growing proportion of the population engaged in crafts and services that was dependent on the market for food.[38]

For all those who were in such a position it was not just a question of the physical availability of food, but also their ability to pay the going prices. This point has been recognised by economists who refer to an individual's *entitlement* to food.[39] Clearly, an entitlement might be jeopardized by a fall in income consequent upon unemployment or short-time working, regardless of the movement of food prices. Similarly, the entitlements of some members of a society would be reduced if the price of a commodity a person produced failed to keep pace with food prices, as happened with handicraft goods in the sixteenth century. This distinction between the amount of food available for consumption and the ability of people to afford it is also important, because it alerts us to the possibility that changes may occur in the quantity of food available without there necessarily being a change in price, and vice versa. For example, if the purchasing power of most of the population were severely limited, prices could not rise substantially even if grain were in very short supply. In these circumstances, movements in prices would fail to indicate the extent to which people were going hungry.[40] And, if the rich people used their

---

[37] The figures in the text refer to the percentages of villein and free holdings, respectively, that were recorded in the Hundred Rolls of 1279 as being less than five acres. It is estimated that subsistence required a plot of nearly ten acres. Kosminsky, *Studies in Agrarian History*, pp. 240, 253–4.

[38] For a recent summary of developments see, Clay, *Economic Expansion*, chapter 3–4. For service in husbandry, see Kussmaul, *Servants in Husbandry*; and for changes in occupational structure, see Wrigley, 'Urban growth'.

[39] Especially by Sen, *Poverty and Famines*.

[40] Appleby, 'Diet', pp. 112–13. Malthus made the same argument to explain the observation that in 1799 food prices rose much less than in England even though the distress occasioned by the harvest shortfall was far more severe. *Investigation*, pp. 5–6. For a contemporary awareness that 'scarcity of money and scarcity of corn [maketh] the price indifferent', see Thirsk and Cooper, eds., *Economic Documents*, p. 25.

purchasing power to hoard grain beyond their immediate consumption needs, prices could rise, even though there was no shortfall in the total amount of food available for consumption.

Prices, yields, and food availability

Price movements, therefore, may not necessarily provide a good guide to variations in the quantity of grain available; in some circumstances they may exaggerate, while in others they may underestimate them. Wrigley examines the relationship between grain prices and the size of the harvest in some detail in his contribution to this volume.[41] He makes an important distinction between gross yields, and the net yields available for human consumption once the 'overheads' have been met of retaining seed-corn for the next harvest and for feeding the livestock and draught animals. Since these overheads could only be modified to a limited extent without endangering the continued operation of the farm, the net amount of food available for human consumption is likely to have varied much more violently than variations in the gross yield of crops as determined by the weather. This helps to explain the observation made by Davenant at the end of the seventeenth century that grain prices rose to a far greater extent than the shortfall in harvest yields would seem to warrant.[42] Wrigley also shows that the 'runs' of successive years of high and low grain prices, that are a feature of pre-industrial societies, probably do not reflect runs of deficient or abundant harvests, caused either by runs of good or bad weather, or by a 'knock-on' effect on the amount of seed-corn available for the next harvest. In fact, both the size of each harvest, and the amount of grain set aside as seed, seem to have been independent of the size of the previous harvest. The runs of prices, therefore, seem rather to indicate the existence of a carry-over of grain stocks from one year to the next, the size of which varied with the abundance of the harvest, so that the supply of grain on the market each year, and hence the price, was not independent of what had happened in previous years.

Wrigley's arguments about the greater variation in net yields bring out the vulnerability of the small farmer to what may appear to be quite modest variations in gross yields. The closer, on average, the farmer is to the level of subsistence, the larger the number of years in which he will have no surplus to sell and must enter the market as a buyer at high prices. Conversely, the greater on average the margin of production

---

[41] See chapter 7, below.   [42] Davenant, *Essay*, p. 83.

over subsistence, the higher the price at which the farmer will still have surplus to sell. The inescapable variation in harvest yields, therefore, builds in an economic advantage to the large-scale farmer. But Wrigley also makes the point that, as yield per acre increases, the variations in net yields available for consumption become proportionately less violent. Since by the late eighteenth century yields per acre were at least double what they had been in the Middle Ages, farmers on the margins of subsistence would have become progressively less likely to have been driven by harvest variations into the market as buyers of food.[43]

Wrigley's distinction between variation in harvest yields and variation in grain prices, especially the greater volatility of the latter and their tendency to occur in runs, brings out the importance of prices in determining short-run changes in the availability of food. While the productivity of English agriculture may have increased greatly during the early modern period, prices still occasionally rocketed upwards. In these circumstances, the critical issue for the increasing proportion of the population that did not have the means to grow its own food was whether its income would buy sufficient for survival. One strategy in high-price years was to 'trade down' and buy cheaper grains; but this would become self-defeating if large numbers did so, or if the yield of the substitute grains were equally deficient. In such cases the prices of all grains would rise, as Appleby noted was the case in the 1590s in England. But he also pointed out that by the end of the seventeenth century prices of different grains no longer peaked simultaneously in England, though the earlier pattern could still be found in French markets as late as the eighteenth century. As we have noted Appleby attributed the change in the behaviour of grain prices to a greater geographical specialisation in production in which winter- and spring-sown grains were more effectively matched to local soils and climates.[44] Providing transport and market networks were adequate, this would provide both higher yields and greater protection against fluctuations in the weather. Interestingly, Wrigley cites figures from Davenant which show that by the end of the seventeenth century the crop mix in England was indeed well spread between wheat, barley, oats, and rye. He also points out that the parallel movements of all grain prices that Appleby noted was still a feature of the French market of Pontoise in the mid eighteenth century was associated with a heavy domination of a single grain, wheat. In these circumstances, any trading-down to cheaper grains in years of high wheat prices would

[43] Overton, 'Estimating crop yields', pp. 363–78.
[44] Appleby, 'Grain prices'.

indeed become self-defeating, since the increase in the demand would be so much greater than the available supply of alternative grains that prices would be driven up to very high levels.

Thus the evidence of grain prices in England appears to suggest that at least by the end of the seventeenth century developments in agricultural practice, and in transport and market networks, resulted in a high-yielding and varied production of grain, which prevented the occurrence of simultaneous catastrophic increases in the prices of all grains that still afflicted other parts of Europe. Unfortunately, it is not clear when England achieved this state; against Appleby's citation of the 1590s, when grain prices moved together, Wrigley points to other years in the same period, when the prices of some grains were high, but others were not. Further research into the co-variation of different grain prices before the late seventeenth century would be valuable in helping to identify the period in which changes in the economy made it less likely that prices of all grains would reach famine levels.

Nevertheless, there were years in which grain prices did rise sharply, well into the nineteenth century. Depending on the magnitude of the rise a greater or lesser proportion of the poor would have found difficulty in purchasing sufficient food to safeguard their health. And for those who found their income reduced by a fall in the demand for their labour, the question of how their entitlement to food could be supported became a matter of critical concern. If such support was not forthcoming, malnutrition would follow and, *in extremis*, death might supervene. Appleby was interested in the whole network of relationships that we have outlined here, but especially in the frequency of the ultimate and fatal outcome, since the latter provides a measure of the adequacy of the economic and social arrangements of a pre-industrial society in achieving its basic function of ensuring the survival of its members. Before we go on to consider these relationships, and how they may be modified by social intervention, we need to consider the biological mechanisms that can be involved in the interplay between famine, disease, and death.

Nutrition and mortality

While the link between prolonged starvation and death may appear to be unproblematical, the connection between malnutrition, whether chronic or acute, and the ability to combat infection is far from clear-cut. To avoid misunderstanding it must be emphasised that malnutrition needs to be considered in a relative, rather than an absolute, sense. What is at issue is not the volume of food that is eaten, or its nutritional composition, but whether it is adequate for the energy demands that the body has to meet. Apart from supplying the needs of basic metabolic functioning, sufficient energy needs to be available to meet the demands of work, to feed parasites, and to resist infection. The balance that is struck between nutritional intake and energy outputs is known as *nutritional status*. Thus individuals who eat very little may have high nutritional status, if they do not have to work and are not exposed to parasites or disease. Conversely, a person who has to work hard in a cold and disease-ridden environment may have a low nutritional status despite a large intake of food.[45]

The situation, therefore, is much more complicated than the way in which historians have been accustomed to picture it. It is not just a matter of a simple causal step from insufficient food to a greater probability of dying from infectious disease. Since the incidence of disease is itself a factor in determining nutritional status, some scholars have argued that a mutually re-inforcing interaction, or *synergy*, can occur, in which the presence or absence of disease affects the level of nutritional status, which in turn affects susceptibility to disease.[46] There are, therefore, two variables in play which can disturb the normal balance of nutritional status in a population: fluctuations in the availability of food, and variations in energy demands, such as work, climate, or the incidence of disease. While the former may be inferred from prices, subject to the qualifications outlined above, fluctuations in climate can only be observed systematically from the mid seventeenth century, and variations in work and disease cannot be observed directly in the historical record.[47] Thus if nutritional status were to deteriorate to such an extent that the mortality rate increased, we should have no way of telling how far this was due to food shortage, and how far to independent fluctuations in other factors, such as climate or the incidence of disease.

The difficulties, however, go even further than this. Despite confident statements on the effect of nutritional status in lowering immunological competence and thereby increasing the chance of dying from disease, it is in practice very difficult to demonstrate the connection.[48] Indeed it now seems to be well-established not only that

[45] The literature on nutritional status is conveniently summarised in Fogel, 'Changes in stature and nutrition', in Rotberg and Rabb, *Hunger and History*, pp. 252–3. See also Scrimshaw, 'Functional consequences of malnutrition', for biological adaptation to low food intake; and a graphical presentation of the links between nutrition, disease and environment in Rotberg and Rabb, *Hunger and History*, p. 306.

[46] See, for example, Taylor, 'Synergy among mass infections'.

[47] Monthly mean temperatures are available for England from 1659. Manley, 'Central England temperatures'.

[48] The large and contentious literature on this subject is conveniently summarised in

the immune system fails only in conditions of extreme malnutrition, but also that moderately malnourished individuals actually have a slight advantage in overcoming infection.[49] Moreover, a number of infections that were prevalent in the past, such as bubonic plague, smallpox, malaria, and typhoid, are so virulent that death or survival does not appear to depend upon nutritional status.[50]

Further problems arise from the complexity of the interaction between nutritional status and infection, which makes it hard to distinguish in real life between the effects of nutritional status and those that might be due to economic circumstances or living conditions. For example, high case fatality rates may be found amongst individuals of low nutritional status, but such people are likely to be poor, they are also more likely to live in crowded conditions and so be more exposed to infectious disease. Consequently, it is very difficult to design an experiment so that the effects of the different factors involved can be properly separated and assessed. Many of the nutritional studies carried out in the Third World, which are frequently cited as evidence of the link between nutritional status and mortality, fail to achieve such a separation, and so cannot be taken as unambiguous evidence of the link they purport to establish. For example, measles is often cited as a clear case of a disease for which nutritional status plays a significant role in determining the outcome, yet recent research suggests that the connection may be spurious, and that the critical factor is the dosage an individual receives.[51] The original mis-attribution to nutritional status was easy to make, because the malnourished tended to live in the most crowded circumstances where the chances of repeated infection were higher. Moreover, the situation is further complicated by a direct synergy between infections, in which each infection increases susceptibility to a further one, over and above any effects involving nutritional status. Finally, the difficulty in making simple inferences from food intake, or even nutritional status, to disease or mortality is underlined by the fact that in the case of the one carefully controlled experiment in starvation, carried out in Minnesota in the 1950s, no greater susceptibility to infection was observed.[52]

Livi-Bacci, *Population and Nutrition*, chapter 2 and in Carmichael, 'Infection, hidden hunger'.
[49] They have less free iron to make available to invading micro-organisms. The biological literature is summarised in Carmichael, 'Infection, hidden hunger', pp. 52–3.
[50] See table of 'Nutritional influence on outcome of infection', Rotberg and Rabb, *Hunger and History*, p. 308.   [51] Aaby, 'Overcrowding'.
[52] Keys, *et al.*, *Biology of Human Starvation*, chapter 46.

Thus the belief in a causal link between an insufficient intake of food and death, which used to inform discussion of famine in the past, is far too simple a representation of the processes involved, and may well also be seriously misleading. Even if nutritional status were to be accepted as being a significant element in the outcome of disease, and we have seen that this is far from firmly established, the logic of synergy suggests that changes in exposure to disease are just as important as changes in the intake of food, as are changes in other energy demands, such as climate or work-load. At best, therefore, famine-related mortality is only partly a story of an inadequate intake of food. At the limit, of course, if extreme privation were to occur for a long period of time, or recourse were had to polluted or poisonous substitute foods, then disorders of the digestive tract might well prove fatal. But most famine-related mortality occurs in less extreme circumstances, and from infectious disease. In these circumstances, the unresolved question is how far the increased mortality is due to a lowering of nutritional status as a result of a reduction in the intake of food, and how far to a greater exposure to infectious disease as a result of the dislocation of normal behaviour that famine conditions entailed. If the former is the case, then the synergy between nutritional status and infection would be involved, and nutritional status would have a direct causal role. But if the nutritional synergy model is wrong, and the real reason for a rise of mortality in famine conditions is due to an increasing exposure to disease, then the critical mechanisms in increasing mortality would include increases in dosage and a synergy between infections. In this alternative perspective, nutritional status should be viewed as a consequence of the level of infection, rather than as its cause.

Doubt over the biological mechanisms involved in the interaction between nutrition, disease, and death, together with difficulties in interpreting the available evidence on deaths and prices, counsel caution in pursuing the questions that Appleby raised. For example, it has been asserted that mortality crises due to famine can be distinguished from those due to disease by the presence of a fall in births, which produces a characteristic 'scissors-effect' on a graph.[53] But disease can also result in a contemporaneous shortfall of births, by increasing the number of miscarriages and stillbirths; the 'scissors-effect' can be found on graphs of mortality crises due to epidemic disease in years of plenty.[54] Clearly, when several different circum-

---

[53] Appleby, 'Disease or famine?', 423; Rogers, *Lancashire Population Crisis*, p. 26.
[54] In sixteen of the twenty years of the most extreme upward fluctuations in mortality in England, birth rates were below average; but in half of these cases food prices were

stances can produce the same pattern in the visible data, inferences need to be drawn with great care.

Above all, the complexity of the way in which the concepts of food shortage, nutritional status, disease, and death are linked in the real world, together with the imperfection of our understanding of those links , makes it exceptionally difficult to unravel the causal chain that lies behind the events recorded in the historical record. Yet the questions that Appleby raised touch upon so much that is of interest in the social and economic history of the past that the attempt must be made. Fortunately, although imperfections in the data may cloak our observations in a haze of imprecision, some of the patterns and trends are so bold that we are unlikely to mistake their outlines. In interpreting what we find, however, we shall need to be aware that since Appleby wrote, our understanding of the network of interaction linking famine and death has become both more subtle and less certain. In the remainder of this chapter we shall use the phrase 'famine-related mortality' as a shorthand expression to denote unusually high mortality that occurs at the same time as high-food prices. But, as the preceding pages will have made plain, we are in no position to claim a direct causal relationship between high prices, food shortage, and death from malnutrition. Yet a consideration of the patterns of coincidence of high food prices and high mortality across both time and space may reveal some significant dimensions of changing conditions of life in the past. It is, therefore, in a spirit of wary adventurousness that we take up the issues that Appleby raised, and reconsider his findings in the light of the contributions that other scholars have made.

The ecology of famine

One of Appleby's most suggestive ideas was his 'thesis of the two Englands', the one vulnerable to famine, the other resistant to it. His work on the demographic history of Cumberland and Westmorland was always more than an exercise in local and regional history. In *Famine in Tudor and Stuart England* he made it clear that his interest was not solely in the experience of the north-west, but in the more general problem of the variable demographic impact of harvest failure on different regions. For dearths that saw a doubling or trebling in background levels of mortality in the north-west in 1596/7 and 1622/3

below average too. Wrigley and Schofield, *Population History*, pp. 321–2. (Note that in the original 1981 edition the column headings for 'Real Wage' and 'Death Rate' on p. 322 were erroneously transposed.)

failed to register a similar seismic impact in the lowland south. As Appleby concluded in his first article, 'Apparently there were two Englands, one subject to trade depression and harvest failure but able to avoid widespread starvation, the other pushed past the edge of subsistence by the same dislocations.' The economy of the north, he suggested, was more like that of Scotland, Ireland, and parts of the Continent, than lowland England.[55] In this widely quoted conclusion can be seen the basis for subsequent research on what might be termed 'the ecology of famine'.

The originality of Appleby's work lay in his marrying of the approaches of two important schools in early modern historiography – the Leicester School of Local History's interest in the relationship between local agrarian and social structures and the historical demography of the Cambridge Group – to determine and to explain the pattern of famine. He argued that in the north-west population growth, promoted in places by partible inheritance and the enclosure of minute holdings out of the waste, created a large, but marginal, smallholding sector. In a region of limited agricultural diversity where poor soils and upland location favoured pastoral farming, and in a century in which demand rewarded cereal production, prospects were not good for this growing body of smallholders. Poor grain yields were further depressed as increasingly marginal land was forced under the plough. The demand for labour was low in a largely pastoral economy and in Westmorland the situation was made worse by a long-term decline in the cloth industry, punctuated in the short term by depressions which reflected the industry's sensitivity to fluctuations in effective demand for its products following a bad harvest. Seigneurial appetite for a greater share of the surplus nudged the smallholders closer to disaster. It was weaknesses in the ecology of the north-west, therefore, which left it vulnerable to harvest failure.[56]

Appleby's thesis of the 'two Englands' was based on the regional contrasts he had noted in the local incidence of mortality crises in years of major dearth amongst the parish register data being assembled at the Cambridge Group. A year after his death, when national maps based on data for 404 parishes were published in *The Population History of England*, his thesis was spectacularly confirmed.[57] Subsistence crises were largely absent from the south-east and, while the north was clearly vulnerable, this ceased to be the case after the mid seventeenth century. However, the maps also revealed that in the pre-1650 era the

[55] Appleby, 'Disease or famine', p. 430.
[56] The argument is summarised in Appleby, *Famine*, chapter 12.
[57] Wrigley and Schofield, *Population History*, pp. 670–85.

picture was considerably more complex than that suggested by a simple north–south dichotomy. Not only did some northern parishes escape mortality crises in years of dearth, as Appleby himself realised, but there were also clusters of communities that were affected in an otherwise immune south. Unfortunately, the geographical distribution of the 404 parishes was too sparse in some parts of the country to take the matter further, but some intensive local studies of crisis mortality have provided evidence which suggests that there may have been systematic ecological differences between regions which experienced subsistence crises and those which did not.

For example, Rogers' study of the subsistence crisis in Lancashire in 1623 found a clear contrast between a crisis-free lowlands and a crisis-prone upland zone; and the same contrast emerged from Slack's analysis of crisis mortality in Devon and Essex over a longer period.[58] Both within the north-west and elsewhere subsistence crises seem to have been more likely in upland areas where soil and climate were hostile to arable agriculture. Other pre-disposing ecological characteristics suggested by the marked vulnerability of the north-west would include a specialisation in pastoral farming involving a dependence on imported grain, and a social structure marked by a rapidly growing and marginal small-holding population. Vulnerability was especially marked where, as in Westmorland or the West Riding of Yorkshire, these populations were also dependent for employment on the vagaries of a rural industry, itself notoriously sensitive to demand dictated by the quality of the harvest.[59]

Thus, despite the attractive simplicity of a simple geographical contrast between north and south, the historical reality was more complex. As Professor Everitt, one of the pioneers of an ecological analysis, cautions: 'One of the features of seventeenth-century England was the sudden change of scenery and society to be met with even in the same shire.'[60] For example, even within Appleby's 'north' there were extensive areas of arable land in the Vales of York and Pickering, and on the coastal plains, which were not 'pushed past the edge of subsistence'. However, in 1623 Appleby found that some parishes in the Vale of York experienced a crisis of mortality, striking testimony to the severity of harvest failure in the north in that year.[61] Similarly, there was a scattering of communities in southern England, for example in the predominantly pastoral and densely populated

---

[58] Rogers, *Lancashire Population Crisis*, p. 11; Slack, 'Mortality crises', pp. 34–5.
[59] Drake, 'Elementary exercise', especially p. 437, and *Historical Demography*, unit 7; Palliser, 'Dearth and disease', pp. 54–75.
[60] Everitt, *Change in the Provinces*, p. 7.   [61] Appleby, *Famine*, p. 151.

Sussex High Weald, that shared common ecological features with famine-prone 'northern' communities and also experienced mortality crises in high food-price years.[62] Significantly, most of the Essex parishes that registered a doubling or trebling of mortality in the crisis of 1596–98 were located in the north or west of the county where there was less emphasis on arable farming and poor access to grain markets.[63] For example, in 1595 Essex villages like Toppesfield were described as 'pasture towns and [with] little or no tillage used by them', and in the harvest failure of 1630 magistrates for the region reported that even in plentiful years markets in the area received hardly any corn and lacked dealers in grain. Moreover, this was one of the most densely populated areas of the county with a large rural proletariat many of whom depended on the notoriously unstable cloth industry.[64] Factors such as geographical location, ecological type, employment opportunities, and the degree and nature of market integration may each help explain why some communities or regions suffered from famine while others escaped. But no single factor was fatal; dependence on a pastoral economy or entanglement with rural industries did not of themselves doom communities to the threat of famine. What made them vulnerable was a combination of unfavourable factors. For example, while the presence of the textile industry in north-east Norfolk was associated with poverty, it was not associated with famine. Both the integration of the industry into the family economies of the poor and the integration of the regional economy into the national market were different from those to be found in the north-west. In Norfolk the industry played a supplementary role, providing additional rural employment for women and children in an area of arable farming that was producing an agricultural surplus.[65]

In this way communities which may have had some ecological characteristics in common with famine-prone communities, but which were located in the predominantly mixed or arable regions of East Anglia or the south-east, were insulated from famine by greater market integration and easier access to grain.[66] Here geography counted, and

---

[62] On the Kentish Weald, see Brent, 'Devastating epidemics', pp. 42–8; for the possibility of famine-related mortality in the Cambridgeshire fen in 1596 but not in other years, see Spufford, Contrasting Communities, p. 152.

[63] Slack, 'Mortality crises', p. 35. The apparently high frequency of crises in Essex that Slack reports is largely due to his method of identifying crises, which is less demanding than that used by other scholars. In fact, crises were much less frequent in Essex in these years than in the north-west. Wrigley and Schofield, Population History, p. 672.

[64] Hull, 'Agriculture and rural society', pp. 327–66.

[65] Wales, 'Poverty, poor relief', p. 387.

[66] Chartres, 'Marketing of agricultural produce', pp. 469–95.

counted against those north-western communities whose geographical isolation and poor, or unfavourable, market integration made them especially vulnerable. But lowland arable areas not only enjoyed the advantage of easier access to grain surpluses even in years of harvest failure, they were also more likely to have local social structures and administrative institutions capable of ensuring that surpluses would be made available to those who lacked the purchasing power to command them in the market place. Indeed an important element in the ability of the textile region of north-east Norfolk to escape famine was the existence of a social and political structure that provided both informal charity and organised formal relief of the poor.[67]

In contrast, the problems of those grain-deficient pastoral woodland areas, which were unable to feed populations swelled by employment in the textile industries without importing grain, were likely to have been compounded by a weak parochial administration and by the absence of a resident gentry or magistracy.[68] Consequently, if the large populations of marginal smallholders, cottagers, and squatters of these communities were to escape famine, they would not only need to be located in close proximity to arable areas, but also to be situated in regions where there was an active tradition of policing the grain markets at the level of the county magistracy. Even then, as the experience of the south-western forest communities suggests, it may have needed the threat or reality of riot to set this policy in motion.[69] Whether the disadvantageous circumstances of woodland communities in fact resulted in a significantly greater vulnerability to subsistence crises remains to be discovered through further research. However, in the case of the north-west the problems of this grain-deficient region do seem to have been exacerbated by an absence of a tradition of political intervention in support of the poor.[70]

The sociology of famine

The identification of communities that were vulnerable to subsistence crises might also be revised by research which pays greater attention to social differentiation. We have already emphasised that the criteria that are adopted to identify mortality crises will to a large extent determine the results, but one particular aspect of this problem merits

---

[67] Wales, 'Poverty, poor relief'.

[68] For a good discussion of marketing practices in forest areas, see Kingsman, 'Markets in Forest of Arden'.

[69] Walter, 'Geography of food riots', p. 79.

[70] Watts, *Northumberland*, pp. 202–3; Fletcher, *Reform in the Provinces*, pp. 185–238.

further discussion. There is always the danger that a definition of crisis based on an increase in the mortality of the overall population may distort or disguise the demographic response to harvest failure of particular social groups. As Ron Lee notes, 'a strong reaction to prices by part of the population appears as if it were a weak or moderate reaction by the whole population'.[71] Famine is a collective problem, starvation an individual fate. The problem of adequately capturing the mortality experience of particular social groups may be especially acute in regions that overall measures of crisis mortality would designate as famine-free. Moreover, the absence of any severe shortage in such areas might well have resulted in such famine-related deaths as may have occurred amongst the poor being spread over a longer period of time, thereby making it even less likely that communities in these areas would register mortality crises. Furthermore, defining crisis mortality as some arbitrary increase over background levels of mortality presupposes that the proportion of the population that was harvest-sensitive was large enough to raise the mortality of the whole population to a sufficiently high level to be designated a crisis. It is, however, possible to envisage communities in which some individuals were highly vulnerable to harvest failure, but insufficiently numerous for an overall mortality crisis to be visible.

For example, as modern studies of famine suggest, it might be the case that it was only the very young and the very old that were likely to die in years of high food prices.[72] Unfortunately, it is difficult to discover whether this was the case in the past, both because of the scarcity of information on age at death, and because mortality at young and old ages was in any case highly variable from year to year due to fluctuations in infectious disease. Adequate data, however, exist for London and Sweden in the eighteenth century, and an analysis of the covariation between fluctuations in deaths by age and fluctuations in grain prices found that the strongest relationships between annual fluctuations in prices and deaths in the same year occurred among the very young and the very old. But the links were weaker in London, where background mortality was higher, than in Sweden, and they were immediately offset by a counter-fluctuation in the number of deaths in the following year.[73]

---

[71] Lee, 'Short-term variations', p. 357.
[72] Watkins and Menken, 'Famine in historical perspective', p. 654; Bongaarts and Cain, 'Demographic responses', pp. 4–5.
[73] Galloway, 'Population, prices and weather', pp. 141–2, 152. However, it should be noted that these results may not be robust. In another analysis of the same Swedish data the link between fluctuations in prices and mortality was only visible for the age range 20–65, and not amongst the very young and very old. Bengtsson and Ohlsson,

More significant differences in the incidence of famine-related mortality are likely to have occurred between social groups, which could well be missed by measures of crisis mortality which relate to the experience of the whole population. For example, Slack's work on the social geography of urban crisis mortality in the 1590s found evidence of higher mortality in the poorer quarters of cities such as Bristol.[74] On the other hand, Galloway found no difference between rich and poor areas in eighteenth-century Rouen in the size of the mortality response to fluctuations in food prices.[75] Though of great importance, the social dimension of famine-related mortality is difficult to capture, since English registers rarely record status or occupation, or the simple, but valuable, designation 'poor' to be found in Scottish registers.[76] In principle, this information could be obtained by linking other local sources to the register entries, but in practice, as Wrightson and Levine show in their study of the mining community of Whickham later in this volume, communities which may have been most vulnerable to harvest failure are likely to have contained an exceptionally high proportion of transient members, whose life-course events were imperfectly recorded in the parish registers or other local documents.[77]

If harvest failure resulted in the most vulnerable leaving a community, then their deaths would have been registered elsewhere, either in the parish through which they were travelling, as those anonymous 'poor wanderers', or in the towns and cities into which subsistence migrants crowded in years of harvest failure. Evidence from urban areas suggests that in sixteenth- and seventeenth-century England, as in other societies, enforced migration was a common response to harvest failure, though it is impossible to say whether it was on a sufficient scale to ensure that the burial registers in the communities of origin thereby failed to reflect their real vulnerability.[78] More generally, however, the urban evidence does reveal a significant pattern of movement out of the marginal communities of the north and

'Age-specific mortality', p. 317. Moreover, in an another analysis of London data, Galloway confirmed the link between prices and mortality for the elderly, but found a stronger link in the case of the 20–39 year-olds than for the very young. 'Annual variations', pp. 496–7.

[74] Slack, 'Mortality crises', p. 38. See also the argument for the differential impact of poor harvests of the early seventeenth century on the poor in the woodland area of the Warwickshire Arden. Skipp, *Crisis and Development*.

[75] Galloway, 'Differentials in demographic processes'.

[76] Flinn *et al.*, *Scottish Population History*, p. 177.

[77] See chapter 3 below.

[78] Slack, 'Vagrancy', pp. 369–70; Clark and Slack, *English Towns*, p. 93; Watts, *Northumberland*, p. 203; Kent, 'Population mobility', pp. 37, 48–50; Beier, *Masterless Men*, p. 77.

west into the towns of the lowland south-east.[79] Indeed the location in the south-east of London, the greatest urban magnet of them all, may have been a factor contributing to the scarcity of crises of subsistence in those communities in the lowland south whose disadvantageous ecological position might otherwise have made them vulnerable to harvest failure. On the other hand, the migrants would have been exposed to a more intense environment of disease in the metropolis, and it is significant that some of the greatest increases in mortality in London in high-price years occurred amongst the age group 20–39, which contained a high proportion of the migrants.[80]

The evident variation in vulnerability by social group, and the possible variation by age, means that any map of the 'two Englands', based on famine-related 'crisis' mortality, however subtly drawn its contours, should not be misread as meaning that everyone in the apparently famine-free 'southern' communities was able to avoid a higher risk of mortality. More detailed research into the experience of 'southern' pastoral–woodland or rural–industrial parishes, whose ecologies suggest similarities with vulnerable 'northern' communities, may yet reveal high levels of mortality among particular social groups. However this may be, such groups were clearly in a minority in the south; and in this respect Appleby's map of the 'two Englands' indicates important differences in the social, as well as the geographical, distribution of famine-related mortality in the past.

The chronology of famine: mortality crises

If there is scope for further work on the geography of famine, then the same is even more true of the incidence of crises of subsistence through time. This is especially the case with what we might term the pre-history of early modern famines. Does the geography of famine mapped out by early modern historians represent a fundamental pattern of ecological weaknesses which can be read back into the demographic history of medieval England? Or was the pattern of early modern famines formed out of the collision between weaknesses in regional ecologies and the economic and demographic pressures of the sixteenth century? Appleby himself thought it 'unlikely that Cumberland and Westmorland suffered famine in the first half of the sixteenth century', but admitted that parish records were too few and unreliable for analysis before 1570.[81]

---

[79] Patten, *Rural–urban migration*.
[80] Galloway, 'Annual variations', pp. 496–7.
[81] Appleby, *Famine*, p. 185, but *cf.* p. 95.

Despite remarkable advances in medieval demographic history, hard evidence about the extent of crisis mortality in that period remains sketchy. The demographic impact of the Great Famine of 1315 and 1316, let alone possible regional patterns in its impact, remains uncertain. Communities in many regions appear to have been hard hit, but there is some evidence to suggest that its effects may have been particularly severe in the highland zone.[82] If further evidence could be found to confirm that this was indeed the case, then the situation in the first two decades of the fourteenth century would provide an interesting parallel with the later sixteenth century, though with a significant difference. Both were periods of rising population in which the severity of the regional impact of harvest failure reflected ecological weaknesses, but in the earlier period the effects of famine would seem to have been felt much more widely.[83]

After the savage mid-fourteenth-century losses of population associated with the Black Death and subsequent plagues, the general economic context would suggest that famine should not have been a problem, at least on a national scale. Indeed, Gottfried's study of fifteenth-century mortality, based on the less satisfactory evidence of wills for London, East Anglia and Hertfordshire, confirms that, 'with the possible exceptions of the 1430s and some years in the 1470s, deaths due directly or even indirectly to famine must have been rare indeed'. Unfortunately, there are severe problems in identifying famine-related mortality from estimates based on the numbers of wills proved in the ecclesiastical courts, or from the experiences of particularly well-recorded groups like the clergy. But if Gottfried is right that there may have been famine in this region in 1438/9 and again in 1473, then once more there would be a suggestion that famine was not a problem restricted to the 'highland', 'northern' zone, as was the case by the late sixteenth century.[84] John Hatcher, writing of demographic trends in later medieval England, similarly argues that mortality in the period was not determined by the state of the harvest, but he goes on to add that 'this is not to say that there were not

---

[82] Kershaw, 'Great famine', pp. 37–46. That, in a period of generally rapid population growth, the north may well have 'recorded the highest rates of growth in England' (Miller and Hatcher, *Medieval England*, p. 32) must have contributed to its vulnerability.

[83] For examples of heavy famine-related mortality in areas in the midlands and the south, see Poos, 'Rural population of Essex', p. 521; Razi, *Halesowen*, pp. 25, 39–40. For a counter-example of an East Anglian manor less obviously hit by the 'great famine', see Campbell, 'Population pressure', pp. 98–9. Smith, 'Human resources' provides a helpful summary of the as yet inconclusive early fourteenth-century map of famine-free and famine-prone regions.

[84] Gottfried, *Epidemic Disease*, pp. 39, 76, 101–2.

innumerable local subsistence crises during which the death rate rose sharply'.[85] Whether Hatcher in this passage is discussing the situation in pre-industrial societies in general or is referring to the experience of late medieval England is not clear. But there remains the possibility that the local ecologies of corn-poor and remote pastoral–highland communities may have exposed some communities to the threat of famine in a society in which markets were less well integrated, and which lacked later forms of market intervention or provisions for ensuring collective welfare. Indeed, following a suggestion made by Wrigley in his contribution to this volume, it might be possible to argue that when population growth was negligible there may have been some retreat from arable cultivation in areas of marginal productivity, which would have left the communities there more vulnerable to the effects of harvest failure.[86] Nevertheless, it seems more likely that in the later fourteenth and fifteenth centuries the reduction in the size of local populations brought about by plague and epidemic disease resulted in an improved balance with local resources, so that, over much of the country, the problems arising from shortfalls in the harvest stopped short of famine.

In the light of the highly unsatisfactory state of the medieval evidence, it can only be a supposition that famine is unlikely to have been a serious problem after the mid fourteenth century, even in the highland zone. Furthermore, the relative paucity of evidence before the inception of parish registration in the late 1530s makes it very difficult to trace the emergence of the pattern of famine-related mortality that can be observed by the end of the sixteenth century. When population growth again quickened in the early sixteenth century, a comparison of fluctuations in deaths, as indicated by collections of wills for six midlands and southern dioceses, with fluctuations in grain prices, together with contemporary comments, suggest that famine may again have become a possibility, especially in 1521 and 1527–29. However, the rôle of famine in these mortality crises is ambiguous, since plague was also present.[87]

Again, when direct measures of mortality crises become available from parish registers in the mid sixteenth century, the evidence would seem at most to point to 'mixed' crises, in which high food prices coincide with apparently independent fluctuations in diseases, so that

---

[85] Hatcher, *Plague, Population*, p. 72.

[86] For a similar argument that after the mid fourteenth century there was abandonment of arable for pastoral agriculture over much of the marginal and under-populated Scottish Lowlands, see Smout, 'Diet and Scottish history', pp. 9–10.

[87] Slack, 'Mortality crises', pp. 15, 54; Faraday, 'Mortality in Hereford', pp. 163–74.

the rôle of famine is far from certain. For example, despite serious harvest deficiencies in 1555 and 1556 the proportion of the parishes in the Cambridge Group's sample registering mortality crises did not rise above 7 per cent until August 1557. Then an unusually plentiful harvest was gathered in, yet the proportion of parishes experiencing mortality crises each month rose, rather than fell, to reach a maximum of 20 per cent in November 1557 before falling back to normal levels in January 1558. Another surge in crisis mortality occurred in the following August, and this time the high frequency of crises continued throughout the autumn and following winter, with normal levels being regained only in the late spring of 1559. Thus there were two periods of crisis mortality separated by seven months of calm. The timing of the first period indicates that if there were any link with the deficient harvest of the previous two years, it only became operative after a delay of at least eight months. Thus the first crisis period may well have been due to infectious disease quite independent of the scarcity of food. This is almost certain to have been the case in the second crisis period, which began in the summer of 1558, after a second abundant harvest. The persistence of crises throughout the following winter, coupled with a high proportion of parishes experiencing recurrent crises, suggests that this period may have witnessed a synergy of diseases in which a succession of infections took their toll of a progressively weakened population.[88] The connection between harvest deficiency and crisis mortality in the mid sixteenth century seems tenuous at best. However, the fact that only a limited number of parishes were in observation at that date, and none for areas later known to be vulnerable, prevents us from concluding that the pattern of the 'two Englands' was not yet already in existence. There is clearly a need for further work on the regional pattern of crisis mortality in the mid sixteenth century, exploiting all extant registers, including those rejected as unsuitable for the analysis of longer-term trends.

When crises of subsistence become visible in the late sixteenth century, they coincide with a period of rapid population growth. One might, therefore, be tempted to see them as a classic symptom of a Malthusian crisis in which population pressure inexorably drove up food prices, and caused exceptionally violent price fluctuations in years of harvest failure. The temptation should be resisted. First, rising food prices did not cause the general level of mortality to rise to a high level in the late sixteenth century: expectation of life at birth was generally above thirty-five years, which corresponds to a low level of

[88] Wrigley and Schofield, *Population History*, pp. 664–6.

mortality by the standards of pre-industrial societies.[89] Secondly, the occurrence of mortality crises in high food-price years was far from universal: in 1596/7, which witnessed the most severe increase in food prices for the entire period 1541–1871, only 18 per cent of the parishes in observation in the Cambridge Group sample experienced a crisis of mortality.[90] As Appleby has shown, even in the worst period of population pressure on food supplies, the impact in terms of mortality was largely confined to a remote and agriculturally backward region in the north-west.

However, on closer inspection, the problem afflicting the north-west may not have been so much the region's backwardness as its premature specialisation in pastoral agriculture. In the sixteenth century smallholders in the north-west shifted the emphasis from subsistence farming to a greater specialization in dairying and livestock rearing, and so became dependent on purchasing grain brought into the region, especially when the harvest failed. Appleby argued that the rise in the price of grain relative to the price of pastoral products in the later sixteenth century

disrupted the theoretical advantages of specialization and . . . [led] to the relative impoverishment of the region specializing in crops with low relative prices.[91]

In terms of Sen's concept of exchange entitlements, pastoral farmers suffered from declining 'endowments'.[92] In this perspective, the famines of the later sixteenth century appear as the penalty to be paid by communities that had engaged in a form of agricultural specialisation in circumstances in which not only had the market failed to reward them adequately, but the degree of specialisation had also been insufficient to ensure either a sufficient surplus of grain or an effective means of distribution from areas of surplus to areas of shortage. Although the absence of hard information for the earlier period makes any conclusion more than usually speculative, it might be suggested that the map of the 'two Englands', visible in the late sixteenth century, reflects not a pattern etched deep into the medieval past, but one drawn more recently by the economic changes of the sixteenth century, changes which lifted famine from the south but imposed it more firmly on the north.[93]

---

[89] *Ibid.*, pp. 230–1.
[90] In the following year, which witnessed the ninth most extreme upward fluctuation in prices, 28 per cent of parishes experienced a mortality crisis. *Ibid.*, pp. 321, 653.
[91] Appleby, *Famine*, p. 186.   [92] Sen, *Poverty and Famines*, chapters 1, 5, 10.
[93] For a similar argument about economic specialisation adding economic risk to natural risk and creating famine, see Watts, *Food, Famine and Peasantry*.

A similar argument for the penalties of specialisation in pastoral agriculture in conditions of population growth within the context of an immature market economy could also explain the vulnerability at a later date of those neighbouring countries with whom the north-west shared the experience of famine, namely Scotland and Ireland. Though there is also evidence of regional vulnerability to famine (in Ireland the poor coastal lands of the west and south-west, in Scotland, the Highlands), the threat of famine in those areas seems to have been increased as they were drawn into specialisation. In the case of the Scottish Highlands the increasing possibilities of supplying livestock to the English market after 1700 and buying in grain with the profits of that trade promoted population growth and a switch of diet, from meat to grain, that left the region more vulnerable to harvest failure. It is this that helps to explain the persistence of famine in the Highlands into the later eighteenth century.[94]

In Ireland, exploitation of parish registers has only recently begun and knowledge of demographic trends before the eighteenth century is both limited and subject to controversy.[95] But despite evidence of famines in the late sixteenth and early seventeenth century, some of which, however, were a product of war, it is thought that Ireland, despite very rapid population growth between 1600 and 1712, escaped the famines of the 1690s and 1710s that wreaked havoc elsewhere in Europe.[96] But over the seventeenth century the Irish economy became heavily export-oriented. The rapid commercialisation of food surpluses promoted food substitution – bread and potatoes for the more resilient 'butter' diet of dairy products and oats – for home consumption. As the population grew, holdings became more parcellised, landlessness increased, and ownership of cattle became even more restricted. There was a vital loss of flexibility in food supply whose consequences for many was fatal. The absence of dairy products left the population vulnerable to failure in its staples of grain and potatoes. Once again, there was, at least for the first half of the eighteenth century, a strong link between famine and depression in the textile industry in the 1720s and 1740s. The result of the growing commer-

---

[94] Smout, 'Diet and Scottish history', pp. 9–11; and 'Famine'; Mitchinson, 'Control of famine'; Flinn *et al.*, *Scottish Population History*.

[95] We have drawn on the following works in the discussion of Ireland's experience: Butlin, 'Land and people'; Cullen, *Emergence*, 'Population growth and diet', *Economic History*, and 'Population trends'; Daultrey *et al.*, 'New perspectives'; Drake, 'Irish demographic crisis'; Gillespie, 'Harvest crises'; Lee, 'Irish economic history'; Mokyr and Ó Gráda, 'New developments'; Ó Gráda, 'Pre-famine economy', and 'Population of Ireland'.

[96] Wrigley and Schofield, *Population History*, p. 341.

cialisation of the Irish economy was, then, a vulnerability to famine that was both regional and socially specific and, in the case of the famine of 1740/1, probably far worse than the better known 'Great Famine' of the nineteenth century.

In England, the concentration of famine-related crisis mortality in pastoral areas, visible in the sixteenth century, persisted into the seventeenth. Communities within the highland zone of the north and west again suffered crises of subsistence in 1623; but the evidence suggests that the underlying trend was such as to draw the contours more narrowly and to make famine almost exclusively a problem of the northern uplands. The Cambridge Group's analysis suggests that overall mortality in 1623/4 was a little less pronounced. In the two worst crisis years of the last decade of the sixteenth century – 1596/7 and 1597/8 – mortality rates were 21 and 26 per cent above trend. The figure for 1623/4 was 18 per cent. There had also been a slight fall in the proportion of parishes registering at least one month of crisis-level mortality, from 19 per cent in 1597/8 to 16 per cent in 1623/4.[97] But far more impressive than these figures is the map showing the change in the geographical distribution of the affected communities. Figure 1.1 shows how those who experienced a crisis at the earlier date fared during the second period of November 1622 to December 1623: they either succumbed a second time and were asterisked, or they were immune and awarded an 'E', indicating that they were vulnerable only in the early period. The communities who escaped crises in the earlier period but did succumb during the later period were awarded an 'L', while those that escaped altogether are shown on the map by a dot. The figure shows how the parishes awarded an 'L' in this year of high prices became confined to the northern section of the highland zone. Local studies of other previously vulnerable regions also confirm their new immunity.[98]

Thereafter, despite continuing harvest failures, there was a further, sharp decline in the incidence of crises of subsistence. Even in the heartland of the previously famine-prone northern highland zone there was little response in mortality levels to the harvest failure of 1630. As Appleby wrote of the north-west

a different pattern of mortality was emerging as early as 1649 and was clearly evident in later periods of dearth: mortality began to be limited in both intensity and extent. . . . The region as a whole was overcoming famine.[99]

[97] *Ibid.*, p. 653.
[98] For an example of the lifting of famine from a region exhibiting famine-related mortality in earlier crises, see Davies, 'Death and disease in Herefordshire', pp. 307–14.   [99] Appleby, Famine, p. 156.

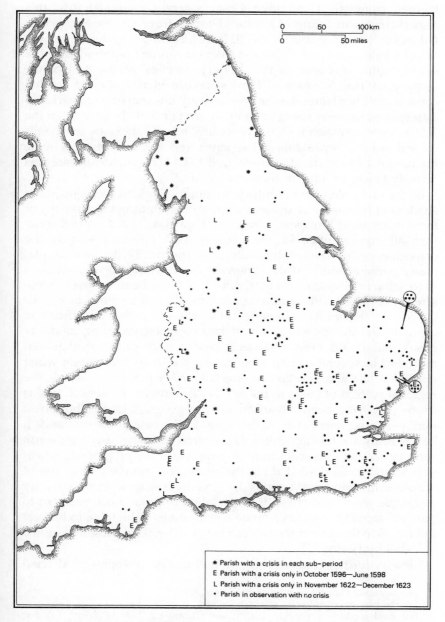

Figure 1.1 Geographical distribution of local crises in October 1596–June 1598
and November 1622–December 1623

Figures from the Cambridge Group's larger study confirm this remarkably swift lifting of famine. Despite three successive harvest failures in the mid century – 1647/8, 1648/9, 1649/50 – the death rate was actually below average.[100] But the sharpest contrast is provided by the demographic response to the 'hungry nineties' at the end of the century. A run of years of harvest failure in that decade created considerable hardship. But the annual death rate remained remarkably unresponsive, never rising by more than 6 per cent above trend in the 1690s. Moreover, although the years 1697/8 and 1698/9 saw sharp falls in real wages, representing the tenth and thirteen most extreme fluctuations below trend in the period 1541–1871, the death rate was actually below average in those two years.[101]

By the mid seventeenth century, therefore, England had slipped the shadow of famine, in sharp contrast to the continuing vulnerability of most other west European countries. However, this does not mean that all communities in the country had entirely escaped the consequences of harvest fluctuations. In the late 1720s, for example, many parishes suffered exceptionally heavy mortality caused by a succession of diseases, two of which – typhus and enteric fever – were often associated with famine conditions. The occurrence of a poor harvest in the midst of a series of epidemics makes it difficult to evaluate the independent rôle of famine in engendering mortality crises, but it has been cited as a contributory cause of increased mortality in several communities in the midlands, the region worst affected.[102] If the suggestion is correct, it may be possible to explain the regional pattern of crises in the late 1720s in much the same terms as those that have been advanced for the geographic distribution of famine-related crises at an earlier date. In the case of the midlands it has been argued that agricultural specialisation in the early eighteenth century had led some communities to an emphasis on growing wheat that would have denied them the protection afforded by a mix of winter- and spring-sown grains. In other areas without access to easily navigable rivers and cheap transportation of grain a commitment to pastoral farming may have made communities vulnerable to harvest failure, as in the case of the Leicestershire village of Bottesford studied in detail by Levine.[103]

Clearly, further local work is needed on the ecologies of affected

[100] Wrigley and Schofield, *Population History*, p. 321.
[101] For the national distribution of crises see *Ibid.*, p. 682.
[102] For local studies of variable quality, see Chambers, 'Vale of Trent'; Gooder, 'Population crisis in Warwickshire'; Johnston, 'Epidemics of 1727–30'; Jackson, 'Somerset and Wiltshire'; Skinner, 'Crisis mortality in Buckinghamshire'.
[103] Levine, 'Demographic implications' pp. 146–8.

communities, but in some parts of the midlands the harvest failure of 1728/9 may have seen prices rise to a point that made existing levels of poor relief inadequate for a population already weakened by disease. Moreover, the consequences may have been especially serious in areas where poor communications continued to hinder the ready transportation of bulky foodstuffs. In the late 1720s the combination of a succession of infections and a deficient harvest put a considerable strain on the nutritional status of the English population. These years saw some of the largest increases in the national death rate and some of the highest percentages of parishes experiencing crisis mortality during the entire period from 1540 to 1840.[104] That so many of these crises were located in midland communities provides a reminder of the need for more detailed local studies of the ecology of famine-related mortality before we can adequately explain changes in its incidence through time and space. In general, however, a study of the incidence of mortality crises suggests that by the late seventeenth century famine was no longer a serious problem, even in regions that previously had been vulnerable.

Systematic relationships between fluctuations in prices and mortality

As we have already emphasised, the incidence of crises only provides information on the more extreme consequences of famine in the form of exceptionally high mortality. There may also have been a less obvious, yet systematic, relationship between the availability of food and death operating across the whole range of fluctuations in prices and mortality. Such a relationship would be difficult to detect by scanning long series of data with the naked eye, especially if the effects of fluctuations in food prices on mortality were spread over several years. Its investigation, therefore, requires a careful statistical analysis of the covariation of food prices and series of vital events.

In such analyses a calculation is usually made of the magnitude of the association between a fluctuation in one of the series (say food prices) and fluctuations in a second series (say mortality), not only in the year in which the fluctuation in the first series occurred; but also in the four subsequent years, so that lagged relationships between the series can also be examined.[105] The analysis takes account of fluctuations of all sizes both above and below trend, and so probes far

---

[104] Wrigley and Schofield, *Population History*, pp. 652–3.
[105] Since population size and age structure do not change much in the short run, fluctuations in death rates are essentially driven by fluctuations in the numbers of deaths, so a series of the latter can be used directly in the analysis without the need to calculate a mortality rate.

deeper into the relationship between the series than is possible in a study based only on extreme fluctuations. However, there are some complications. For example, each series may both carry within it echoes of previous fluctuations: for example, fewer people surviving to die in subsequent years. And the demographic series may be affected by fluctuations in other demographic series quite independent of prices: for example, a fluctuation in the birth series will change the proportion of infants in the population who have a higher than average risk of dying. Consequently, care needs to be taken to remove both internal echoes and external contamination when calculating the strength of the association between any pair of series. The latter, summed across fluctuations of all magnitudes in each direction, is usually reported as the percentage change in the second series (say mortality) that would be associated with a doubling (or halving) of the current average value of the first series (say prices), net of the effects of earlier fluctuations in the series concerned and of fluctuations of other series included in the analysis.[106] It should be noted that when results of studies of this kind are reported in the literature the assumption is usually made that independent fluctuations in one of the series in some sense cause the fluctuations in the other series. Thus, for example, investigators report the magnitude of a mortality 'response' to a price 'shock'. Although we shall adopt the same manner of speaking, we cannot emphasise too strongly that analyses of this kind only measure the statistical association between fluctuations in the series. The sense in which it is proper to interpret such an association as indicating a causal relationship depends upon the plausibility of the theoretical model being invoked, and its relevance to the historical context. Fortunately, the patterns of the presence or absence of such statistical associations between the series, and their strengths in different historical circumstances, often provide valuable information from which one can draw some reasonable inferences about the nature of the substantive causal relationships that are likely to have obtained in the past.

Lee has carried out a pioneering analysis of this kind on English data on vital events and prices during the period 1541 to 1871. He found that there was indeed a systematic relationship between fluctuations in

---

[106] Note that the estimation procedure requires the association between the series to be proportional across the whole range of values that the series may assume. Some investigators have checked whether this is in fact so, and in some cases have found non-linearities in the relationships, typically that mortality fluctuations are strongly associated with extreme upward fluctuations in prices, but only weakly associated with modest price fluctuations, or those in a downward direction.

wheat prices and mortality; but that it was weak.[107] Only 16 per cent of the short-run variation in mortality was associated with price changes, and much of that was due to the effect of a small number of extreme upward fluctuations in prices. Mortality fluctuations, therefore, were overwhelmingly determined by other factors, such as the prevalence of epidemic disease. However, the pattern of the lag between fluctuations in prices and mortality was suggestive: only when prices were high did mortality rise in the same year, otherwise mortality fluctuated sympathetically after a delay of one or two years.[108] One interpretation of this result would be that it was only in years of exceptional shortage that the dislocation was such as to provoke life-threatening actions, such as recourse to contaminated food. Otherwise, the normal effect of harvest fluctuations would have been to vary the proportion of the population that could maintain its accustomed standard of living at home, driving the rest to seek food and work elsewhere, thereby more effectively spreading disease through the countryside. Furthermore, Lee also found that the sympathetic response to prices was followed by a compensating negative echo, so that the net effect of price fluctuations on mortality, cumulated over five years, was essentially zero. Only in the case of the nine years with the greatest upward fluctuation in wheat prices was there any net increase in the number of deaths over a five-year period. This suggests that most variations in scarcity or plenty merely advanced, or delayed, by a few years the normal pacing of deaths.[109]

Similar analyses were carried out on the relationships between fluctuations in prices, on the one hand, and fluctuations in nuptiality and fertility on the other. In both cases the associations between fluctuations in the demographic series with fluctuations in prices were more pronounced: 41 per cent of the annual fluctuations in marriage, and 64 per cent of fluctuations in fertility, could be associated with annual variations in prices, compared with 16 per cent in the case of mortality. Moreover, in both cases the main effects occurred both in the same year as the price fluctuation and in the year after, and were followed by compensatory echoes.[110] Cumulated over five years the effects of price fluctuations were more substantial than in the case of mortality. A doubling (or halving) of prices was associated with a 22 per cent loss (or gain) of marriages and a 14 per cent loss (or gain) in fertility.[111] A more finely-grained analysis also showed that the

---

[107] Lee, 'Short-term variations', pp. 371–84, 392–401.   [108] *Ibid.*, pp. 379–80.
[109] Nor did runs of consecutive years with high prices have any significant additional effects on mortality beyond the sum of the effects of the years involved. *Ibid.*, p. 377.
[110] *Ibid.*, p. 375.   [111] *Ibid.*, pp. 368–70.

negative response of fertility to fluctuations in prices peaked after a lag of three to eighteen months. Thus variations in prices would seem to have affected foetal mortality during the first two trimesters of pregnancy, and to have influenced the number of conceptions that occurred during the following nine months. The latter may have been due to the effect of fluctuations in the level of nutrition on fecundity, or to the physiological or psychological effect of food shortage on the intensity of sexual activity.[112]

Lee's econometric analysis of the English data on the whole confirmed Appleby's conclusion that while variations in food prices might be significant in a regional context, they were not an important element in determining national fluctuations in mortality in England in the past. But his analysis also revealed many other aspects of the relationships between short-run changes in demographic behaviour and fluctuations in the environment. We have seen how both nuptiality and fertility were more affected in the short run by fluctuations in food prices than was the case with mortality. But fluctuations in fertility were also even more strongly affected by fluctuations in mortality, the cumulative negative effect after five years being more than twice as great as the response to price fluctuations.[113] It would seem, therefore, that fluctuations in the prevalence of disease had a double effect, increasing mortality and depressing fertility; their combined demographic effect far outdistancing that of fluctuations in food prices.

Lee also estimated the strength of the short-run relationships for three sub-periods (1548–1640, 1641–1745, and 1746–1834) to examine how far they changed over time. Briefly, the cumulative five-year response of fertility to food price fluctuations showed no change, while the response of nuptiality to prices approximately halved between the first and third periods. The most dramatic decline was in the cumulative response of mortality to food price fluctuations. Before 1640 this was at quite a high level, higher than the comparable figures for nuptiality and fertility. In the period 1641–1745 the cumulative response of mortality to prices fell to a third of its previous level, while from the mid eighteenth century the response weakened to vanishing point.[114] Unfortunately, a later analysis of the same data by Galloway has somewhat upset this neat progression. If the second period is begun in 1675 rather than 1641, the response of mortality to price fluctuations remains close to the level it was during the period before this date. This result arises because there was an unexpected *negative*

---

[112] *Ibid.*, pp. 370–1.   [113] *Ibid.*, pp. 363–6, 372.   [114] *Ibid.*, pp. 373–7.

association between price and mortality fluctuations in the years 1641–74, which depressed the overall figure that Lee obtained for the second period when these years were included in it.[115] Clearly there is some difficulty in this kind of analysis in dealing with periods in which relationships are temporarily inverted. Perhaps the safest conclusion to be drawn at present is that there was an association between fluctuations in prices and mortality in England up to the mid eighteenth century, after which fluctuations in prices found no echo at all in movements in the death rate.

This is an interesting result, which somewhat modifies the picture of the chronology of famines that emerged from a study of the incidence of mortality crises. While the latter suggested that high food prices were not a significant cause of catastrophic mortality after the mid seventeenth century, and in some areas not even in the sixteenth century, a more subtle analysis of the association between mortality and food price fluctuations of all magnitudes reveals that, although the connection between food price fluctuations and mortality was always very weak, it was not until the mid eighteenth century that it was entirely broken.

The disappearance of famine: explanations

In accounting for England's early escape from famine-related mortality it is natural to appeal to the well-established improvement in the productivity of English agriculture during the early modern period. It is generally accepted that the growing demand for food in the sixteenth century brought about a gain in agricultural output, not only through an increase in the cultivated area, but also through the adoption of improved agricultural techniques. The latter were cumulative rather than revolutionary in their impact, and in many areas were accompanied by a significant polarisation in the distribution of sizes of landholdings leading to an increase in the number of landless labourers and to more land being farmed in self-contained large units free from the constraints of communal open-field agriculture.[116] With the lifting of population pressure after the mid seventeenth century, agricultural output outstripped demand, so that by the late seventeenth century England had become an exporter of grain. The improvements in real wages brought about by these changes had a greater impact in a society which now had a much larger proportion of

---

[115] Galloway, 'Basic patterns', p. 291, note 37.
[116] For recent summaries of English agricultural developments see, Clay, *Economic Expansion*, chapters 3–4; Overton, 'Agricultural revolution?'

wage labourers and town dwellers.[117] Increased consumer demand for non-cereal foodstuffs and non-agricultural products promoted mixed farming and a diversification of occupations in the countryside, leading to a better balance between cereal-growing and animal husbandry, and, more generally, to a strengthening of marketing networks.[118] In addition, the increase in both the acreage and yield of oats and barley created a more advantageous mix between spring and winter-sown crops, which of itself, as Appleby argued, helped to mitigate the impact of harvest failure by preventing the simultaneous failure of all crops. Improvements in transport and better market integration made it easier to iron out regional deficiencies. The ability to carry over more grain between harvests coupled with the ability to move grain more easily between regions had the effect of giving greater protection against harvest failure by temporal and geographical risk-spreading.[119]

Appleby provided a model study of how these changes benefited the north-west and freed it from famine.[120] The fall in population and cereal prices, a more favourable price structure for the region's pastoral economy and some economic diversification brought significant improvement in the region's 'exchange entitlements'. Greater incorporation into the national economy brought not only better returns for the region's products but also easier access to grain. Although harvest failure remained a problem, this was now a regional economy better able to cope with its consequences.[121] With modifications to take account of local variations, this model can also explain the improved position of other parts of the previously vulnerable 'highland zone'. For example, in their paper in this volume Wrightson and Levine show how for one County Durham community, Whickham, the expansion of the coal trade brought rapid social change and, initially, a greater vulnerability to famine.[122] Eventually, however, greater market integration with London and the ports of East Anglia enabled the community to escape the threat of famine. But in this case there was a price to pay: in avoiding the consequences of local harvest failure Whickham became more vulnerable to the more devastating threat of plague. The example of Whickham underlines the inadequacy of a

---

[117] Wrigley, 'Urban growth'.
[118] See works cited above in note 116, and Kussmaul, 'Agrarian change'.
[119] Chartres, 'Marketing of agricultural produce'.
[120] Appleby, *Famine*, pp. 155–81.
[121] It should be noted, however, that if 1623 was indeed the last serious year of famine-related crisis mortality in the north-west, then the region's escape must have ante-dated many of these changes.
[122] See chapter 3, below.

simple north/south division and the appropriateness of a 'topological' mapping of crisis mortality. It is to be hoped that further detailed local studies on the lines laid down by Wrightson and Levine will make possible a more accurate picture of the changing incidence of crises of mortality through space and time.

Despite the general consensus on the gains in agricultural output that freed England from famine, there has been less agreement on the timing and extent of those changes in land use and agricultural technique that have been held responsible for those gains.[123] The distinction that Wrigley makes in his contribution to this volume between gross and net yields offers a potential resolution of this debate.[124] If gross yields rise, and deductions for seed and fodder remain constant, net yields available for human consumption will rise even faster. For example, Hoskins estimated that between the early sixteenth and mid seventeenth centuries, when the size of the population doubled, gross yield ratios also doubled, apparently keeping pace with population growth.[125] However, Wrigley's calculations would suggest that net yields available for consumption would have risen by 33 per cent more than this, comfortably outstripping the rate of population growth.[126] Consequently, less land would be required at the end of the period to provide the population with the same amount of grain per head. The land that was surplus to meeting this requirement could either be used to generate a surplus of grain, enabling consumption per head to be increased or exports to be generated, or it could be released for planting with other crops or for use in animal husbandry, options which were indeed taken up to varying extents in the course of the seventeenth century.[127]

Wrigley's distinction between gross and net yields also helps to explain why harvest failure had a diminishing demographic impact over time as grain yields increased: the higher the yield, the lower the penalty to be paid in the form of a greater proportionate shortfall in food available for consumption in years of deficient harvests, once fixed deductions for seed and fodder had been made. In the light of this effect, it is also easy to appreciate why regions in the highland zone, where grain yields were among the lowest, should have continued longer than most to be vulnerable to harvest failure.[128] The model

---

[123] Outhwaite, 'Progress and backwardness', paints a somewhat less optimistic picture, at least for the period up to the mid seventeenth century.

[124] See chapter 7, below.

[125] Hoskins, 'Harvest fluctuations, 1620–1759', p. 27.

[126] See below, p. 257.

[127] For a convenient summary see Clay, *Economic Expansion*, chapter 4; and Kussmaul, 'Agrarian change'.   [128] Appleby, *Famine*, pp. 64–6.

advanced by Wrigley offers considerable scope for development or modification by further research, especially since it would appear to provide important clues for understanding an essential aspect of England's increasing resistance to famine.

But while an increase in agricultural productivity would raise the amount of food available per head, if it were achieved by changes in the structure of landholding and employment, it might at the same time increase the vulnerability of part of the population to famine. In early modern England, as we have noted above, gains in agricultural productivity were in fact accompanied by the growth of a land-poor and labouring sector, dependent on the market both for employment and food, and highly vulnerable to falls in the demand for labour and sudden sharp increase in grain prices. In such circumstances harvest failure could have a dramatic effect on the ability of labourers and cottagers, as well as smallholders forced on to the market by loss of their own small surpluses, to buy grain. While pushing food prices sharply upwards, harvest failure could also seriously lower earnings. It could directly reduce the seasonal demand for agricultural labour, a savage blow given the importance high earnings at harvest time had in the incomes of rural families. Furthermore, a poor harvest might cause farmers to hire fewer servants in husbandry, and could seriously intensify the problems of under- and un-employment amongst rural textile workers and urban artisans. Not only would there be less demand for their labour in producing non-food goods and services, but there would be less opportunity to supplement their earnings by harvest labour. For all these groups therefore, harvest failure meant not only high prices, but also diminished earnings, reducing their 'exchange entitlements' to grain. In the sixteenth century the threat was all the greater, since the underlying trends of a decline in real wages and the lack of employment for the surplus population left such groups with few, if any, reserves with which to face such a disaster. If we are to explain the absence of famine over many areas of England and the muted response of mortality to high prices, then we need to explain how harvest-sensitive groups survived the collapse in their exchange entitlements.

As Walter argues in this volume, a partial answer to this problem may be found in a critical re-examination of the economic indices used to measure the extent and impact of harvest failure. As we have already pointed out, both the construction and the applicability of the indices need questioning. The existing price series for grain are mainly southern and based on wholesale transactions. As such, they not only ignore the problems of regional differences, but may also provide a misleading guide to the impact of harvest failure on smaller consumers, and, where based on a single crop such as wheat, fail to reflect the ability of consumers to trade down to cheaper grains at times of scarcity. Moreover, the attempt to read off the size of the harvest from grain prices may be fraught with difficulties, since the operation of the market stands between the harvest and the subsequent price of grain. As Wrigley suggests, under conditions of low average yields, grain prices towards the end of the harvest year may have underestimated the shortfall since the purchasing power of poorer consumers would have been exhausted. And, as we have seen, wage rates are dogged by similar problems of representativeness and interpretation. Finally, there is the larger problem that the use of these measurements assumes that individuals were dependent upon the market for grain or employment, but the proportion of the population for whom this was the case at different times in the past remains uncertain.

To the need for further research on the history of prices and wages, might be added the need to re-assess estimates of the level of poverty in early modern society. Work in progress suggests the need to look more critically at measurements of the poor derived from taxation records. These measure relative inequalities and should not be used without support from other sources as a measure of destitution. A proper appreciation of the meaning of poverty involves going beyond such summary abstract measures and locating the poor in the local social and economic context, as Walter discusses more fully below.[129] However, while a critical scrutiny of the indices used to measure the level of poverty and the impact of harvest failure might modify our appreciation of the scale of the problems faced in some areas and by some sections of the poor, it cannot do more than qualify that growth in poverty which rendered an increasing proportion of the population even in lowland arable communities vulnerable to harvest failure. Censuses of the poor drawn up in years of dearth are one of the most sensitive measurements of potential indigency. Their long lists of those 'destitute of grain', easily dwarfing the recipients of regular poor relief, graphically reveal the consequences of a collapse in the 'exchange entitlements' of these otherwise independent families. For these groups we need to move beyond economic explanations which put the emphasis on the presence of markets and improvements in transport networks to confront the problem of how those groups without the ability to purchase grain in the market place survived.

The dominance of the nuclear-family household and the low kinship

---

[129] See chapter 2, below.

densities that prevailed in early modern England meant that the destitute had to look for support from the collectivity, in the form of the local community or the State, rather than from family and kin.[130] Protection against dearth and the provision of grain came publicly and formally through the system of communally organised and funded welfare provision represented by the poor law. It is this aspect of crisis relief that has received most attention from historians, but insulation against harvest failure could also be found in the set of social and economic relationships that linked the harvest sensitive with other groups in the local community. In analysing the protection afforded those at risk by their relationships with the collectivity it is possible to see another factor shaping the map of famine-free and famine-prone communities. In terms of communal protection, more is known of the formal relief offered by the poor law. If, however, it is true to say that more is known of the poor law's provisions than of its practice, then this is even more the case with crisis relief. In normal circumstances, the parochial administration of the poor law under the late Elizabethan statutes offered support to a relatively small proportion of individuals and families that found themselves at a stage of dependency within the cycle of family formation and dissolution, as in the case of the widowed and families temporarily overburdened with small children. To cope with the crisis of harvest failure, relief was needed in much larger amounts and for much greater numbers. The State's provisions for harvest failure, codified in the first Book of Orders of 1586/7, were designed to ensure a sufficient stock of grain to which the poor should be given priority of access, if necessary with financial assistance. With a more generous definition of eligibility, this policy offered the possibility of relief to a much larger number of the poor. The practice of selling grain on a sliding scale of prices carefully adjusted to reflect the varying degrees of poverty of its recipients was well-designed to cope with the collapse in the 'exchange entitlements' of the labouring poor. It offered, therefore, valuable relief – where it was successfully implemented. But we need to know much more about the implementation of this aspect of crisis relief than we do at present. In particular, the geography and chronology of its implementation awaits detailed research. The rhythm of its increasing enforcement, and its seemingly subsequent abandonment in the later seventeenth century, seem to march in step with demographic pressures in the later

---

[130] Although relations with kin might offer some protection against dearth, the high level of migration that led to low kinship densities suggests that this would always have been limited. For a contrary argument stressing the importance of kinship ties in a northern community see Chaytor, 'Household and kinship'.

sixteenth and early seventeenth centuries and their subsequent lifting.

If the successful implementation of the Book of Orders reflected the favourable degree of political and economic integration in early modern England, its successful local implementation required the existence of a local administrative and tax base to organise and fund the provisioning of grain. While there is considerable evidence for the successful provisioning of the poor in south-eastern counties like Essex, Kent, and Norfolk, evidence is thinner and sometimes altogether lacking for the famine-prone regions like Cumberland and Westmorland. Here, then, may be an additional reason for their vulnerability. Not only were these areas corn-poor; they may also have lacked the necessary administrative and financial structures to remedy this weakness.

The poor in the famine-prone communities of the highland zone may also have been denied the protection afforded against harvest failure by more informal relationships within the collectivity. Because the latter lacked an institutional framework, they have escaped systematic historical investigation. But, as Walter argues, insulation against harvest failure may have come for some sections of the poor not solely from the parish or the state, but also from the relationship of servant and master, tenant and landlord or labourer and employer. All of these could include the valuable perquisite of access to food independently of the market. Where such perquisites were customary rather than contractual, and withstood the impact of harvest failure, they too could offer some insulation from the threat to 'exchange entitlements', at least in the short term. For others, the provision of relief may have been entailed in relationships with neighbours or with members of the local elite. As in many other societies, there is considerable evidence to suggest that such relief was an accepted part of the relationship between superiors and inferiors, playing an important part in the legitimation of the social order.

Because evidence of the protection afforded within these relationships is necessarily diffuse, it is difficult to gauge or to quantify their importance in combating dearth. Like crisis relief they may have provided valuable access to grain and, when combined with parish relief, tided those otherwise vulnerable over the months of greatest difficulty. But such support was socially selective. At minimum it presupposed membership of a community. It may also have been geographically selective, requiring membership of a community which not only had a surplus to transfer but also patterns of settlement and employment that encouraged relationships of which the provision of relief was an integral part. Although there was undoubtedly considerable variety in the degree of isolation between hamlets or households in the highland zone, it seems likely that corn-poor highland communities, with a pattern of dispersed settlements and no greater presence of kin, would have been less able to offer such informal protection. Indeed, this may help to explain why migration as a response to harvest failure was more common in these areas.

Though England and the north-west had escaped from mortality crises in the wake of famine by the mid seventeenth century, harvest failure continued to impose severe penalties. In the last analysis, mortality rates are too crude an indicator by which to judge the problems that harvest failure continued to create. That this was a society that escaped the demographic disaster of famine did not mean that all escaped the distress that dearth occasioned. As Walter argues, it was the continuing reality of the threat of harvest failure that underlined the value to the poor of their unequal relationships with their superiors. In accepting these, they escaped vulnerability to crises of subsistence but became further enmeshed in a web of deference and dependence.

England and Europe

Appleby's awareness of the importance of local and regional differences in the patterns of famine-related mortality extended across the Channel to include France. Indeed it was in France that the notion of a 'subsistence crisis' was first formulated by Meuvret in 1946, and greatly popularised by Goubert in 1960 through his influential study of Beauvais and the Beauvaisis.[131] It is, therefore, especially appropriate that this volume contains two contributions that reconsider the relationship between mortality crises and fluctuations in food prices in France, and draw explicit parallels with the situation in England.

Dupâquier analyses the frequency and timing of mortality crises in the two countries during the period 1650–1725.[132] He finds a similar overall incidence of mortality crises in France and England, but the timing of the crises was very different in the two countries in the seventeenth century. As reported in *The Population History of England*, the chronology of mortality crises in England in this period was closer to that of north Holland than to those of France or Scotland.[133] However, Dupâquier shows that in the early eighteenth century there are some years in which crises occurred simultaneously, or in close

[131] Meuvret, 'Crises de subsistances'; Goubert, *Beauvais*.
[132] See chapter 5, below.
[133] Wrigley and Schofield, *Population History*, pp. 340–2.

succession, in England and France. While this may indicate increased contact between the two countries, Dupâquier emphasises that it was not the case that crises became more widely diffused during the period, since at the same time there was considerable regional variation in their incidence within France, as indeed was the case in England.

In his contribution Dupâquier also confronts the important issue of the role of famine in provoking mortality crises in France in the late seventeenth and early eighteenth centuries. This is the classic period of subsistence crises in French historical writing, but Dupâquier's analysis of the geographical and temporal pattern of local mortality crises leads him to be sceptical of the importance of famine in provoking crises independent of epidemic disease. He finds a poor match between mortality crises and high food-price years: many serious crises occurred in years of low food prices, and in several years with high food prices there was little upward movement in mortality. Moreover, even when crises did coincide with high food prices, as in 1691–94, the pattern of their diffusion from the east and south-east, through the centre to the north, and finally to the west of the country, suggests the spread of epidemic disease rather than a direct impact of harvest failure on mortality through malnutrition. In Dupâquier's view mortality crises are primarily generated by the independent dynamics of epidemic disease and fungal infections. So far as famine is concerned, Dupâquier makes the important suggestion that it played an indirect role, increasing exposure to infection through the dislocation and migration that it entailed.

The lack of coherence between years of high prices and high mortality that Dupâquier reports for France has turned out to be a feature of several countries. For example, in England, the twenty years with the greatest proportional increases in food prices during the period 1541–1871 were by no means all years in which mortality rose. In fact, in ten of them mortality rates were actually below normal, as one might expect to occur by chance if there were no association between famine and mortality.[134] Dearth on the grand scale, therefore, does not seem to have been either a sufficient, or a necessary, cause of mortality on the grand scale.[135]

None the less, there remains the possibility that there was a less dramatic, yet systematic relationship between fluctuations in food prices and mortality of all magnitudes. We have discussed how the

---

[134] *Ibid.*, p. 321.

[135] For a recent summary of the position in several European countries, which comes to the same conclusion, see Livi-Bacci, *Population and Nutrition*, chapter 3. For Japan, see Janetta, *Epidemics and Mortality*, chapter 7.

existence of such a relationship can be demonstrated in the case of England before the mid eighteenth century. Since similar analyses have been made for other countries, it is now possible to put the English experience into a European perspective.[136] In the light of Dupâquier's comparative analysis of crises, a point of particular interest is how France compared with England. We have seen how France continued to experience the occasional mortality crises associated with high food prices, as in the 1690s, when crises were conspicuously absent from England. Was mortality in France also more responsive to fluctuations in food prices of all magnitudes? Unfortunately, it is not possible to make an exact comparison because data are available for France only from 1677, and in the case of mortality only for deaths over age five. However, Galloway has recently investigated data for several European countries, including France and England, according to a standard and uniform procedure.[137] Applying a method similar to the one that Lee used on the English data, as described above, Galloway found that 46 per cent fluctuations of deaths over age five in France in the period 1677–1734 were associated with fluctuations in grain prices. In England in the period 1675–1755 the figure was much lower: only 24 per cent of the fluctuations in the non-infant death rate were associated with grain price fluctuations.[138] Moreover, the magnitude of the mortality response in the year of a price shock, and in the subsequent year, was considerably greater in France (30 per cent, 29 per cent) than in England (11 per cent, 19 per cent).[139] Furthermore, in France, but not in England, runs of years of high prices had an extra effect in raising mortality.[140] Thus in the late seventeenth and early eighteenth centuries not only was France more subject to *crises de subsistence*, but price fluctuations of all kinds had a more consistently and greater effect on mortality than was the case in England.

In the circumstances it is especially interesting that when the

---

[136] The literature is conveniently reviewed in Galloway, 'Basic patterns', with references cited on p. 276, note 4, and p. 279, note 15.

[137] The method is described briefly in Galloway, 'Basic patterns', pp. 282–5. Other scholars have occasionally used other methods, which makes it difficult to compare results. The main differences in approach are discussed in Galloway, 'Population, prices and weather', pp. 16–18, 258; in unpublished papers by Bengtsson and Broström, and by Schultz, cited in Galloway, 'Basic patterns', p. 279, note 15.

[138] Galloway, 'Basic patterns', appendix, table 1, column headed 'R-Sq'.

[139] *Ibid.*, columns headed 'Lag 0' and 'Lag 1'.

[140] Taking runs of prices into account increases the measure of association between the mortality and price series (r-square) from 46 to 69 per cent in France, while in England including runs of prices only increases r-square from 25 to 28 per cent. Galloway, 'Population, prices and weather', table 2.5 on p. 37; column headed 'Eq K' and 'Eq M'.

analysis is performed for France in the period after 1750, the relationship between prices and mortality is much reduced, with the main response occurring two years after the price shock.[141] Clearly important changes had occurred in the structure of French economic and social life. In his contribution to this volume Weir throws new light on the nature of these changes by working with regional, and even more local, data.[142] He uses regional price and mortality series not only to make separate estimates of the relationship between prices and mortality for each region, but also to examine the extent to which French grain markets became more integrated over time. France emerges from the analysis as a country with largely independent regional grain markets, though Weir notes that the area they covered was quite as extensive as national grain markets in England and some other countries. Both the volatility of prices and the response of mortality to price fluctuations varied considerably between regions, reflecting differences in social structure and in economic factors such as the strength of price controls, the availability of credit facilities, and the possibility of consuming alternative grains in high-price years. Weir confirms that both the volatility of prices and the responsiveness of mortality fell considerably between the first and second half of the eighteenth century. But the scale of the change varied a great deal between the regions. For example, in the north and north-east the relationship between price fluctuations collapsed, as in England, while in the south and centre the responsiveness of mortality to prices fell to about one half its earlier level, and in the east there was almost no change at all.

Weir's analysis not only adds regional detail to the national picture for France, he also reports findings which raise important questions for our understanding of the mechanisms by which food-price fluctuations may have provoked sympathetic movements in mortality in the past. First, he notes a relationship between the strength of the association between food prices and mortality, and the lag at which the greatest response occurred: in general, the weaker the response, the longer the lag. This is similar to the result found for England, where it was only years when prices were extremely high that mortality also rose sharply, and in the same year as the price fluctuation. We have argued in connection with the latter observation that strong and instantaneous mortality responses may be evidence that death occurred mainly through extreme privation, or through eating contaminated substitute food, while mortality responses at longer

---

[141] Galloway, 'Basic patterns', appendix, table 1.
[142] See chapter 6, below.

lags, without intervening runs of high-price years, are more consistent with a social mechanism whereby variations in the size of the harvest influenced the amount of migration in search of work and food, and so varied the intensity of exposure to infectious disease.[143]

Weir provides further evidence which suggests that the dislocation effects of harvest variation may indeed have become the dominant cause of famine-related mortality in France by the second half of the eighteenth century. For example, he notes that although local price series became less inter-correlated during the eighteenth century, mortality variations in the individual regions corresponded more closely with the price series from St Etienne than with the price series for the region concerned. He also finds that the lag between the price variation in St Etienne and the regional mortality response varied according to the distance of the region from that town, and suggests that some diffusion process was occurring, such as would be the case if the volume of outmigration, and hence the intensity of the inter-regional spread of disease, depended on the level of food prices. The importance of the rôle of migration in spreading disease is also suggested by Weir's analysis of differences in the responsiveness of mortality to food prices variation by social class and as between town and countryside. Although there were some regional differences in the ability of towns to insulate themselves from their hinterland, there were cases in which the price-mortality relation was stronger in the towns; indeed in Toulouse it even increased over time while weakening in the surrounding villages. Moreover, Weir uses data from Rouen to show that within a town there was no difference in the price-mortality relation as between rich and poor districts, implying that it was the prevalence of disease rather than the ability to buy food that was the critical factor.[144] Weir's evidence strongly suggests that while towns might be able to secure adequate supplies of food in high price years, they also attracted migrants who brought disease with them.

A similar conclusion is suggested by some of the results that

---

[143] Alternative explanations seem less plausible. For example, if one were to assume a direct causal link between nutritional status and mortality, one would have to explain why a fluctuation in the availability of food would have a lagged effect despite the fact that harvest fluctuations would have occurred during the lag period and so nutritional status would not have remained constant. It also needs to be remembered that the price–mortality relation is symmetrical. So an explanation of lagged effects must also be able to provide a plausible account of why a year of *increased* availability of food should mean *fewer* deaths some years later, regardless of subsequent fluctuations in prices.

[144] Galloway reports a similar result. 'Differentials in demographic responses', pp. 292–6.

emerged from Galloway's analysis of the relation between grain-price fluctuations and mortality from various causes of death in London in the period 1670–1830. Briefly, he found that deaths from typhus responded quite markedly to price fluctuations with a lag of one year. Since typhus is usually associated with crowding and filth, he concluded that the lag pattern was consistent with the epidemiological consequences of variations in the number of rural poor crowding into London following annual variations in dearth or plenty. He also found that the only other causes of death that varied significantly in response to grain prices were smallpox (in the same year) and a miscellaneous category of 'fevers' (in both the same and the subsequent year). Neither deaths from tuberculosis nor mortality associated with endemic diseases responded to grain-price fluctuations.[145] Interestingly, Landers has shown that smallpox and 'fevers' stand out from other causes of death in London in this period in having an age distribution which points to a heavy contribution from recent migrants. He argues that this arises because immigrants from the countryside would not have had the same exposure to infections such as smallpox that were endemic in London at the period, and so would not have acquired immunity to them. Consequently, it is highly likely that the association between price fluctuations and smallpox mortality in London reflected rural stress in periods of high prices, and that in so far as urban mortality responded to price movements it was because of the immigration of adolescents and young adults who lacked immunological protection against specific infections.[146]

Both Weir's findings for France, and those of Galloway and Landers for London support Dupâquier's conclusions based on an analysis of mortality crises, and strongly suggest that the major impact on mortality of variations in food availability, as indicated by price movements, was an indirect one, through the effect of harvest variation on migration and exposure to disease, rather than directly through changes in susceptibility to infection.[147] Thus, in so far as mortality was related to famine, the critical link was not a biological one through nutritional status, but rather a social structural one which determined how the impact of food shortage would be distributed

---

[145] Galloway, 'Annual variations', pp. 498–500.

[146] Landers, 'Mortality and metropolis', pp. 72–5; 'Mortality, weather and prices', pp. 356–61.

[147] It is interesting to note that when Meuvret, one of the pioneers of the study of subsistence crises, reconsidered the subject in 1965 he argued that 'the connexion between disease and dearth seems to be mainly due to the spread of infection consequent upon movement undertaken to escape regions experiencing food shortage'. 'Demographic crisis in France', p. 511.

between individuals and the range of actions, including migration, that they might take in response.

However, as Weir points out, the size of the harvest is produced by fluctuations in climate, which may well also have had a direct influence on the incidence of disease. For example, colder than usual winters have not only been found to be associated with more deficient harvests in the past, but even today are associated with increased mortality from respiratory infections, heart malfunctions, and intestinal disease. In conditions of extreme cold the normal mechanisms for maintaining body temperature can become impaired, and deaths can occur from hypothermia, especially among the very young and very old. In earlier times with inadequately insulated housing, more extreme winters would not only have put greater strain on each individual's energy resources in maintaining basic body temperature, but also encouraged people to spend longer in close proximity in badly ventilated conditions indoors, thereby increasing the chance of infection from airborne disease.[148] Similarly, in summer high temperatures can increase the number of bacterial, insect, and animal vectors and so promote the spread of infectious disease, especially those affecting the digestive system. For example, an increase in soil temperature in summer increases the rate at which flies' eggs are hatched. In pre-industrial conditions, with food often left uncovered indoors, and human and animal excrement left lying on open ground, variations in the density of flies could well influence the risk of infection from contaminated food.[149]

Not surprisingly, the seasonality of deaths from airborne infections peaked in late winter in Europe in the past, while the peak season for intestinal infections was the late summer.[150] We might, therefore, expect that climatic fluctuations from year to year would increase the chance of infection, and so have an independent and direct effect on variations in mortality, over and above any influence they might have indirectly through variations in harvests and food prices. Indeed, if we do not take climatic fluctuations into account we might mistakenly conclude that there was a direct link between fluctuations in prices and mortality, when in fact both were responding to a common

[148] The energy requirements for maintaining body temperature are high, accounting for up to 80–90 per cent of oxidative energy. Curtis, *Biology*, p. 685.

[149] These, and other connections between climate and mortality are discussed in Howe, *Man, Environment and Disease*.

[150] See, for example, the analysis of seasonality by cause of death in London in the period 1845–75 in Buchan and Mitchell, 'Influence of weather'. For differences in the patterns of burial seasonality in northern and southern Europe, see Wrigley and Schofield, *Population History*, pp. 296–8.

meteorological stimulus. Ideally, therefore, we need to study the associations between fluctuations in prices and mortality net of the effects of climatic variation. In practice, data on monthly temperatures are only available on a systematic basis in England from the mid seventeenth century, and usually only from the mid eighteenth century in the case of other European countries.[151] Several scholars have investigated the effects of climatic variation on mortality in England, France, Sweden, and Italy. In general, the results were as expected: fluctuations involving more extreme temperatures (cold in winter, hot in summer) were associated with higher mortality.[152] Recently Galloway has reported the results of a study in which he estimated the independent net effects of fluctuations in both climate and prices on mortality for England in the period 1675–1755, and for England and nine other countries from the mid eighteenth century until 1870.[153] Since the prices and seasonal temperature varied greatly in the range over which they fluctuated, Galloway measured the responsiveness of mortality in terms of the percentage change over a period of five years associated with a fluctuation of one standard deviation in each of the meteorological and price variables.

Taking all countries together, fluctuations in both seasonal temperatures and prices were independently associated with fluctuations in mortality, net of the effect of fluctuations in the other series. Higher summer and autumn temperatures were accompanied by increases in mortality of 4 and 6 per cent, respectively; while lower winter and spring temperatures were in each case also accompanied by a rise in mortality of 8 per cent. The response of mortality to fluctuations in prices was slightly higher at 10 per cent.[154] In England and France the magnitudes of the mortality responses were somewhat lower than these figures. In England in the period 1675–1755 the response to a fluctuation of one standard deviation in grain prices was 6 per cent, the same as for winter temperature, with lower figures for other seasonal variations in temperature (2 per cent for spring and summer, 4 per cent for autumn). As we have seen, in England there was no longer any

---

[151] Lamb, *Climate*, vol. 2, pp. 24–5.

[152] There were, however, exceptions. Fluctuations in summer and winter temperatures were not associated with variations in mortality in France. Richards, 'Weather, nutrition and the economy', p. 380. In Sweden only fluctuations in winter temperatures had an impact on mortality (Eckstein *et al.*, 'Short-run fluctuations', p. 306), while in Italy such fluctuations particularly affected young infants (Breschi and Livi-Bacci, 'Saison et climat', p. 35).

[153] Galloway, 'Population, prices and weather', chapter 3, using data for France, Denmark, Sweden, and Prussia from 1756; for Belgium and the Netherlands from 1811; for Tuscany from 1820; and for Austria from 1827.

[154] *Ibid.*, p. 70.

response in mortality to grain price fluctuations after the mid eighteenth century; but the response to winter temperature variations also disappeared, while that to temperature fluctuations in the three other seasons remained the same. In France from the mid eighteenth century, there was a similar response to temperature variation, ranging from a low figure of 1 per cent in winter to a high of 5 per cent in autumn. And a standard-deviation fluctuation in grain prices was still accompanied by a 4 per cent variation in mortality.[155]

Galloway's analysis, therefore, confirms earlier findings that fluctuations in both climate and grain prices were independently associated with variations in mortality. His results also confirm that both the disappearance of the link between prices and mortality in England by the mid eighteenth century, and the continued, though weak, presence of such a link in France, were genuine, and not artefacts of changes in climatic variation. Although the latter played an undoubted role, it is noteworthy that if the strength of the link between mortality and grain prices is calculated without taking fluctuations in temperature into account, almost exactly the same figures are obtained. This should increase our confidence both in the calculations of the price-mortality relation that Weir has made for France in the absence of climatic data, and in his conclusions about change over time in France and the differences between France and England.

Pre-industrial European societies, therefore, were evidently vulnerable to the vagaries of the climate, whether operating directly through variations in the prevalence of infectious disease, or indirectly through variations in harvest yield and food prices. Occasionally, as in 1740–42, the climatic variation was extreme over a large part of Europe, providing an opportunity for a comparative investigation of the interplay between weather, food availability and mortality in crisis conditions in societies with a wide range of political and economic circumstances. Although many areas experienced extreme weather conditions in these years, with cold winters and dry springs and summers, there were marked regional differences in the severity of the increases both of food prices and of mortality. Post has made an exhaustive study of conditions in thirteen countries in 1740–42, and concluded that the primary impact of the extreme climatic variation was through epidemic disease: respiratory infections and louse-borne typhus during the long winters, and fever and dysentery during the drought-ridden summers.[156] Climate also affected the harvest, but there was no relation between the amplitude of the rises in grain prices

[155] *Ibid.*, tables 3.13–3.14, pp. 85–6.   [156] Post, *Food Shortage*.

and the severity of the mortality crises. England, for example, experienced severe epidemics of fever and dysentery with only moderate dearth and little increase in vagrancy. In contrast, in Prussia where food prices increased more sharply and military activities complicated the situation, increases in mortality were more modest. The severity of the mortality crises in these years of climatic stress was determined not so much by the availability of food, as indicated by increases in grain prices, as by the amount of dislocation that occurred as a result of climatic stress and deficient harvests, leading to crime, disturbances, and migration in search of work and food. Significantly, Post concludes that the connecting link between subsistence crises and epidemic mortality

proved to be more social than physiological; that is to say that the rising incidence of infectious disease derived more from social disarray and dysfunctional behavior than from dangerously lowered human resistance to pathogenic microorganisms.[157]

Mortality: the role of human intervention

As Appleby insisted: 'famine can only be understood properly when it is solidly placed in its social and economic context'.[158] Subsequent studies of famine-related mortality, whether in the context of mortality crises, or through a statistical analysis of the relation between fluctuations in food prices and mortality of all magnitudes, have confirmed the justice of Appleby's observation. They have also revealed the interconnectedness of death from various causes, and shown that patterns of mortality as a whole were profoundly mediated by the social and economic order. This, in turn, raises the important question of how far patterns of death in the past were autonomously determined, being produced by the operation of chance factors within a fixed biological framework, or whether they should rather be seen as having been substantially determined by human ecology, and so capable of modification by conscious, or unconscious human action.

In approaching this question it may be helpful to consider some of the main features of the evolution of mortality in England and Europe in the past. First, in the case of England, for which it is possible to estimate levels of mortality back to the sixteenth century, it is evident that there were long-term swings in the level of mortality. Indeed, one of the most striking features of English mortality history is a long oscillation in death rates lasting three centuries. After a marked

[157] *Ibid.*, p. 28. [158] Appleby, *Famine*, p. 3.

improvement during the second half of the sixteenth century, expectation of life then deteriorated during the seventeenth century, losing all the ground that had previously been gained. Then, after an uncertain period around 1700, there was a long period of improvement over the eighteenth and early nineteenth centuries, during which expectation of life at birth regained its late sixteenth-century level around 1800.[159] The improvement in mortality during the eighteenth century can be observed in several European countries, as data become available. Unfortunately, it is only in Geneva that mortality estimates have been extended back to the sixteenth century. In fact, Geneva, like England, suffered a rise in mortality during the seventeenth century; but there is no way at present of knowing how far this was a general European experience.[160]

Superimposed on these long-run swings in mortality was an intense short-run variation, many aspects of which have been discussed already. However, as Flinn observed in data from local studies in various parts of Europe, the intensity of the short-run variation in mortality diminished from the seventeenth century onwards.[161] In England this process of 'stabilisation' of mortality, as Flinn termed it, can be observed to be occurring from the mid sixteenth century, and at different levels of aggregation. For example, at the national level the mean percentage deviation of the series of annual crude death rates fell from 17.7 in 1550–74 to 12.0 in 1650–74, continuing downward to reach 6.1 in 1750–74 and 4.0 in 1850–70. The same downward trend over time is visible if one considers the frequency of years, or months, of exceptionally high mortality. Although short spurts of mortality occurred even in the late eighteenth and nineteenth centuries, their frequency declined over time as did the amplitude of the fluctuations. Indeed, with the exception of a particularly unstable period in the late 1720s, almost all the largest upward fluctuations in mortality occurred before the last quarter of the seventeenth century.[162]

A similar picture emerges if one considers the distribution of mortality crises over time at the parish level. Taking all parishes together the percentage of months in which mortality reached a 'crisis' level fell from 1.46 in 1550–74 to 1.08 in 1650–74, then further to 0.98 in 1750–74 and 0.60 in 1800–24.[163] However, if one looks instead at the

---

[159] Wrigley and Schofield, *Population History*, pp. 230–1, 234–6.
[160] Schofield, 'Population growth'; Perrenoud, 'Mortality decline'.
[161] Flinn, 'Stabilization of mortality'.
[162] Wrigley and Schofield, *Population History*, table 8.7, p. 317; tables 8.11–8.13, pp. 333–4, 338–9.
[163] 1800–24 was the last twenty-five period in observation at the parish level. *Ibid.*, table A10.1, p. 650.

number of parishes experiencing a crisis in any year, it becomes clear that crisis mortality was always present somewhere in England in the past. Even in years in which the national death rate was well below normal, there were always 2–3 per cent of parishes experiencing a local crisis.[164] At the local level, therefore, crisis mortality was never absent. Potentially lethal micro-organisms were always present, and environmental circumstances might change in one locality, but not in others, to produce a burst of mortality in epidemic form. Moreover, micro-organisms could also be carried between communities either by individuals in the normal course of daily life, or by insect or animal vectors. In this way, infections could assume a peripatetic character, striking individual communities infrequently, while remaining continuously present at the regional or national level. If the proportion of localities experiencing local epidemics were roughly constant, even though the identity of the communities concerned might change, regional or national mortality levels would remain at a fairly even level, despite the existence of local crises. Thus local epidemic mortality need not necessarily entail epidemic mortality at a higher level of geographical aggregation.

But if crisis mortality was never absent, it was also never universal, for even in the years or months of most severe crisis on a national scale only a minority of parishes were affected.[165] For example, in the two worst national crisis years, 1557/8 and 1558/9, only 33 and 39 per cent of parishes, respectively, were affected. The only other years which approached these figures were 1727/8 and 1728/9 in which 28 per cent of the parishes recorded crisis level mortality. In other years of high mortality on the national scale, in which the death rate was more more than 20 per cent above trend, only between 15 and 20 per cent of parishes were affected.[166] National crises, therefore, were far from universal in their incidence; they were the outcome of a synchrony of local crises affecting only a small fraction of the country.

The changing patterns of mortality pose a challenging problem of explanation. If all elements had moved in the same direction, it would be possible to tell a fairly straightforward story. For example, if the decline in the incidence of national and local crises that occurred in England since the sixteenth century had been accompanied by a continuous fall in the general level of mortality, one might plausibly

---

[164] *Ibid.*, fig. A10.1, p. 652.

[165] The figures quoted below refer to the percentage of parishes experiencing at least one month with crisis-level mortality during the year running from July to June. The percentage of parishes experiencing a crisis in any specific month during these years is, naturally, lower. [166] *Ibid.*, pp. 652–3.

infer that there had been a decline in the incidence of exogenous shocks, such as extreme weather conditions, which would have reduced the occurrence of epidemic disease or harvest failure and so lowered mortality. Unfortunately, an explanation of the course of mortality based on changes in the weather is unlikely to be correct. First, there were no significant changes in the variability of seasonal temperatures at least since the mid seventeenth century.[167] Secondly, and more importantly, different aspects of mortality did not always move in step. While the incidence of crisis mortality declined from the mid sixteenth century, and the level of mortality also fell at the same time; paradoxically, during the seventeenth century mortality rose, even though the incidence of crises continued to decline.

Upon closer inspection, however, the movements in the different elements of mortality are not so paradoxical. Throughout this period one of the most important factors in determining the exposure of individual communities to crisis mortality was their distance from the nearest market town.[168] Thus the continuing urbanisation and development of market networks, that were such marked features of early modern England, are likely to have increased contacts between communities, and so have entailed a more effective distribution of diseases as well as goods and services. In this way infections would become more effectively endemic on a regional or national scale, increasing the total exposure to disease and the general level of mortality. Moreover, in accordance with the argument outlined above, a more effective 'endemicisation' of specific diseases would diminish the probability of an *epidemic* outbreak at the national level, since at any one time many localities would already have suffered a local outbreak in the recent past and lack sufficient susceptible individuals for a recurrence. Thus changes in the patterns of social and economic life that increased contact between previously isolated communities could both raise the general level of mortality, and lessen the intensity of national epidemics.

However, there are two further features of English mortality patterns in the past which are not well accounted for by this argument. First, the incidence of local, as well as national, crises fell during the seventeenth century when a more effective distribution of infections might be expected to have caused local crises to become more frequent.

---

[167] Galloway, 'Population, prices and weather', table 3.1, p. 72. There were *long-run* changes in temperature, which fell in the later seventeenth century and then rose again in the early eighteenth century. Manley, 'Central England temperatures', p. 402. Despite these changes the incidence of crisis mortality continued inexorably downward.

[168] Wrigley and Schofield, *Population History*, pp. 685–93.

And during the eighteenth century, when urbanisation and market integration were even more advanced, not only did the incidence of local crises continue to fall, but the general level of mortality also declined. Evidently, other factors were involved which changed the relationship between the incidence of mortality crises, and the general level of mortality. Furthermore, since the decline in both aspects of mortality occurred throughout much of Europe, any explanation for such a change must have a wider field of application than England alone.[169]

In discussing the stabilisation of mortality in Europe during this period Flinn pointed to two areas in which human intervention may have had a significant impact on the incidence of crisis mortality. First, he noted that from the end of the seventeenth century military movements no longer caused outbreaks of epidemic disease on the scale that had been common in the past. Some of this difference may have been due to a greater exposure of local populations to a wider range of infections and hence a greater probability that they would already have acquired immunity to any micro-organisms imported into the area by troops.[170] Typically, however, military movements also brought with them diseases such as typhus and dysentery, products of crowding and poor hygiene. Part of the reduction in the impact of military dislocation on mortality, therefore, is likely to reflect better management and control of the conditions of military life.[171] The second area in which Flinn noticed a fall in the incidence of crisis mortality was harvest failure. We have argued above that the evidence now available suggests that this was due not only to improved methods of agricultural production and distribution, but above all to advances in devising methods of social intervention to limit the dislocation, and potential spread of disease, that harvest failure could entail. Here, too, human agency had a significant role to play.

Plague

The early modern period also saw some important changes in the structure of diseases, of which the most striking feature was the disappearance of bubonic plague as a significant cause of death.

---

[169] Flinn, 'Stabilization of mortality'; Schofield, 'Population growth'; Perrenoud, 'Mortality decline'.

[170] For example during the English civil war mortality crises were more frequent in areas where there were military movements by non-local troops. Wrigley and Schofield, *Population History*, pp. 680–1.

[171] Flinn, 'Stabilization of mortality', pp. 296–8; Kunitz, 'Speculations on the European mortality decline', p. 354.

Strictly speaking, the general lack of information about cause of death means that we can only observe the disappearance of plague directly in London, and in one or two other towns which kept records detailing cause of death. However, plague was distinguished by an unusually high case fatality rate (between 60 and 85 per cent), and by a marked seasonality of deaths which typically bunched in the late summer and early autumn.[172] Consequently, epidemics of bubonic plague in which there was any significant exposure to the disease in a community leave clear traces in the records which are difficult to overlook. Furthermore, the lethal nature of the disease, the lurid character of its symptoms, and the apparent arbitrariness of the way it spread, made it a matter of comment in registers which were otherwise silent as to cause of death, no less than in records of local government authorities struggling to contain the disease. However, mortality crises of a seasonality and intensity characteristic of a significant exposure to bubonic plague are signally lacking in English parish registers after the 1670s, as are comments about its presence either in the registers or in local government records.[173] Thus, despite the lack of direct evidence, it is highly probable that plague did in fact cease to be a significant cause of death in England, as in most of western Europe, in the late seventeenth century.

The disappearance of plague as a major component of mortality remains one of the great puzzles of history. It was a question which exercised Appleby, and formed the subject of his last published paper.[174] Part of the difficulty of the issue lies in the complicated way in which plague is spread, for it is primarily a disease of small mammals such as rats, and man is an accidental host. The first question, therefore, relates to the underlying level of risk: was plague endemic in England in the early modern period? Or was it periodically re-imported from abroad? A second set of questions relates to the circumstances in which plague, once present in a locality, might flare up into an epidemic amongst a rat population. Relevant factors here are the predominant species of fleas infesting the rats, which affects the efficacy of transmission of the plague bacillus from rat to rat, and the levels of temperature and humidity, which govern the activity and rate of reproduction of the fleas. A third set of questions relate to the probability with which a plague epidemic amongst rats might be

---

[172] Biraben, *Les Hommes et la Peste*, chapter 1; Shrewsbury, *History of Bubonic Plague*, esp. pp. 1–6; Slack, *Impact of Plague*, chapter 1.

[173] Cambridge Group's unpublished calculations of severity indices of mortality crises. According to Shrewsbury, the last burial entry attributed to plague was in 1671, in Redruth, Cornwall. *History of Bubonic Plague*, p. 537.

[174] 'Disappearance of plague'.

transferred to humans. Here the critical question is the proximity of humans and rats, so relevant factors include the predominant rat species and the construction and density of human habitation. Finally, there is the question of whether in certain circumstances in the past, plague may have been transmitted directly between humans without the intervention of rats and their fleas.

In his contribution to this volume Slack provides an excellent summary of the present state of knowledge on these issues, and critically reviews the various theories about how changes in one or more of these factors in the complex chain of transmission may have resulted in the disappearance of plague as a human epidemic disease.[175] He starts from the observation that in the sixteenth and seventeenth centuries plague epidemics originated in ports and spread to market centres with only sporadic outbreaks in the adjoining countryside. Like Appleby and most other scholars, he infers that plague was not endemic in the rat population, but continually re-imported as a result of overseas trade contacts. Consequently, any effective method of preventing re-importation would remove the threat of plague, and any effective method of preventing its spread from ports would limit its impact.[176]

Appleby had recognised that by the mid seventeenth century local government authorities in England, and elsewhere in Europe, had devised progressively severe quarantine requirements; but he felt that the low level of administrative efficiency, together with the prevalence of smuggling, would frequently have allowed the re-importation of infected rats and fleas. He therefore proposed an alternative explanation for the sudden disappearance of plague in the form of an hypothesis that the last round of epidemics had resulted in the selection of rats with higher resistance to the plague bacillus. This allowed a breathing space during which quarantine regulations could be improved sufficiently to provide a permanent protection against plague. Slack demurs, pointing out that rat populations soon lose their immunity, and that earlier plague visitations did not seem to have provided a breathing space for more than a few years. He also points out that human epidemics of plague occurred at the end of a long chain of transmission, beginning with the re-importation of infected rats and fleas. The processes involved in the early links in the chain, namely the initial importation into the country and the spread to market centres, were the result of human agency, in which rats and fleas were innocent

---

[175] See chapter 4, below.
[176] For a comprehensive recent review of evidence of morbidity patterns of plague, see Benedictow, 'Morbidity in historical plague epidemics'.

passengers. Once plague had arrived in a community, it might well fail to become established in the local rat population. And once established, it might fail to flare up in an epidemic form amongst the rats, so that their fleas would have no need to migrate and infect humans. Finally, even if plague were present in an epidemic form in a rat population, the chance of transmission to humans would depend critically on how far the life-styles of the human and rat populations brought them into contact with each other.

Slack argues that with a chain of transmission as long as this, several factors need to be present in order to produce a human plague epidemic. Consequently, any change in circumstances which reduces the probability of transmission across any link in the chain will significantly reduce the overall probability of the final outcome. In this perspective, collective action to control the passive movement of rats and fleas, such as quarantine, does not have to be wholly effective in order to reduce the *probability* of the occurrence of a plague epidemic amongst rats or humans in a specific locality to a low level. Slack sees the introduction of progressively more effective, if imperfect, quarantine control in England and Europe as the critical factor that provided the 'breathing space' of relief from plague in an epidemic form. Later developments, such as the replacement of the more adventurous black rat by the timid and unsociable brown rat, and changes in the construction of housing, made it even less likely that humans would be exposed to rats and their fleas, even if plague had inadvertently been introduced into a locality.

Slack's argument leaves open the possibility that plague may still have been present in England after the 1670s, re-imported from time to time, but lying dormant and endemic in the rat population. For example, in a small area of Suffolk in 1906–18 during the third pandemic, when plague-infected rats are thought to have swum ashore from grain ships from Argentina that were lying in a river estuary, the rat populations of several villages became infected. In this case, however, not only was the geographical spread of plague amongst the rats confined to a relatively small area, but there were very few cases of human deaths from plague. Moreover, the latter lacked the classic symptoms of bubonic plague, and were only correctly diagnosed after laboratory analysis.[177] Thus if plague had occasionally been re-imported into the English countryside after the end of the seventeenth century, the lack of characteristic symptoms such as buboes would have made it appear to contemporaries that people were

---

[177] Van Zwanenberg, 'The last epidemic of plague'.

dying from a particularly lethal fever. And since its incidence would have been sporadic, and the number of cases small, it would have excited little attention. Although the possibility that plague may have been re-imported into England or others parts of western Europe after the end of the seventeenth century cannot wholly be ruled out, it was evidently no longer a major threat to large numbers of people. Confined to the hedgerows and byeways, plague was no longer in a position to make a significant contribution to mortality.

Conclusion: mortality and human ecology

Taken together, the reduction in mortality from plague, typhus and the consequences of harvest failure help to explain the decline in crisis mortality that occurred in England in the early modern period. However, one of the features of local crises in England, even in the eighteenth century, was their late-summer seasonality, which suggests that diseases which were spread through contaminated food and water continued to play an important role.[178] Again, the lack of information on cause of death in England prevents clear conclusions being drawn, but where such information is available, as in Sweden in the late eighteenth century, intestinal infections emerge as the fourth most important cause of death, after bronchitis/pneumonia, tuberculosis and smallpox. And both the seasonality of urban mortality, and information of cause of death in the bills of mortality show that death from intestinal infection was a continuing problem in cities with high population densities such as London.[179] Although the mechanisms of transmission were not properly understood, current theories of disease stressed the role of unhealthy vapours given off from ill-drained areas such as swamps, and from corpses and refuse.[180] Consequently, action was taken to treat pathogenic sites by improving drainage, and by removing excrement and rotting matter from the streets. Though not intended, these actions had the consequence of reducing the density of insects, notably flies, thereby diminishing the

[178] Wrigley and Schofield, *Population History*, pp. 657–9.
[179] Basic data in Marshall, *Mortality in the Metropolis*. Calculations in Finlay, *Population of London*, p. 138; Landers and Mouzas, 'Burial seasonality', table 1, who show that the typical burial summer peak disappears in the middle of the eighteenth century. The summer peak can also be found in Geneva in the same period, being caused by a high summer level of mortality amongst children. Perrenoud, *Population de Genève*, pp. 429–31.
[180] For an example of an explanation of differences in mortality patterns in terms of the healthiness of soil and air, see Short, *New Observations*. Even Creighton in his *History of Epidemics*, published in 1891 held that miasmata rising from the ground were an important cause of mortality. Eversley, 'Epidemiology as social history', pp. 7–17.

probability that the latter would spread disease by contaminating food.[181] Although urban death rates continued to be higher than rural ones until well into the nineteenth century, there was a marked decline in infant and child mortality in London beginning at the end of the eighteenth century.[182] The improvement occurred well before the major public health measures of the mid nineteenth century, but after a sustained campaign to improve the urban environment by paving and washing streets, and by removing excrement.[183] Thus with intestinal diseases, as with plague, human intervention by public authorities, even though based on an incomplete, and sometimes erroneous, understanding of the causal mechanisms of the transmission of disease, none the less resulted in the attenuation, if not the interruption, of the chains of transmission, and so contributed to a reduction in mortality.

One consequence of the ability of public authorities in early modern Europe to reduce mortality transmitted by insect or animal vectors was that mortality became more dominated by airborne infections, such as tuberculosis, smallpox, measles, and whooping cough.[184] This change had important consequences for both the level and the pattern of mortality. We have argued that the same process of market integration that permitted a more effective distribution of food also brought a more effective distribution of these infections. Thus a reduction in vulnerability to famine was accompanied by a greater exposure to disease, as is illustrated by the case of the north-east mining community of Whickham, discussed by Wrightson and Levine in this volume. Moreover, since several of the airborne infections involved (with the important exception of tuberculosis) confer life-time immunity, and can only take hold if there are a sufficient number of susceptible individuals to which they can spread, small local populations could escape re-infection on an epidemic scale for several years after an earlier outbreak.

Initially, therefore, the result of a more effective distribution of airborne infections amongst local populations would have been to increase the prevalence of local pockets of temporary immunity, thereby replacing infrequent national epidemics, which used to spread through a population of individuals with no previous exposure, with a pattern of peripatetic local epidemics. Since the latter would involve a greater total exposure to infection, we have argued that background

---

[181] Riley, *Eighteenth-Century Campaign*.
[182] Landers, 'Mortality and metropolis', pp. 63–8.
[183] Porter, 'Cleaning up the Great Wen'.
[184] Kunitz, 'Speculations on the European mortality decline'.

death rates would rise. However, the greater the mobility and degree of market integration, the wider the geographical area that would effectively be integrated into a common pool of susceptibles, and the larger the population within which airborne infections would have an effective endemic presence. In such circumstances individuals would be more likely to become infected for the first time by a specific disease in infancy or childhood, rather than later in life. Moreover, since the very young are protected by maternal antibodies we should expect that children above the age of weaning would be affected relatively more severely than those who were still fed at the breast.[185] Interestingly, we can observe just such a change occurring in the age-structure of mortality amongst the young between the later sixteenth and early seventeenth centuries, when childhood death rates rose, while infant rates hardly changed.[186] Furthermore, Kunitz has pointed out that infection in childhood is usually less severe than later in life. This raises the possibility that the long-term effect of increased mobility and integration may have been to ensure that the exposure of a higher proportion of the population to airborne infections was in the more benign form of endemic childhood diseases.

If this line of argument is correct, it suggests that the changing patterns of mortality in early modern societies were structurally influenced by changes in the social and economic context that altered the degree of the exposure of the population to airborne infection. Evidently what is at issue here is not the occasional mobility caused by desperation, as we have noted occurring in high food-price years, but rather the intensity of everyday mobility as individuals go about their daily business. The degree of urbanisation and market integration are likely to have played a key role in determining the overall level of mobility, and since by European standards the pace of urbanisation and market integration in England in the seventeenth and eighteenth centuries was particularly high, the structural impact on mortality patterns of economic change in this country is likely to have been especially powerful.[187] In England, therefore, while greater mobility is likely to have progressively reduced the intensity of both national and local epidemics over a longer period of time, its *initial* effect, already visible in the seventeenth century, would have been to increase exposure to airborne infections and raise the general level of mortality, offsetting any gains from a reduction in mortality connected with plague and typhus. But in the *long run* increasing mobility, although

[185] *Ibid.*, p. 352.
[186] Schofield and Wrigley, 'Infant and child mortality', pp. 67–9.
[187] Wrigley, 'Urban growth', pp. 145–52.

further increasing exposure, would have changed the age profile of morbidity of the most important diseases, and so produced a lower overall case-fatality rate and a lower general level of mortality.

However, unlike diseases spread through insect vectors or poor sanitation, airborne infections were more difficult to control. Despite some attempts, such as inoculation in the case of smallpox, effective intervention had to wait upon the discovery of improved procedures and the emergence of the political will to implement them, developments which probably only began to make a significant impact in the nineteenth century.[188] Thus in the important area of airborne infections, it would appear that the influence of human agency on the evolution of mortality in England in the past occurred as the indirect result of structural changes in economic life, rather than through direct intervention by public authorities.

In the case of mortality from other causes, however, no less than in the management of the consequences of harvest failure, political action to control movement and hence the spread of disease is likely to have played a critical role. Both epidemics and harvest failure were experienced as exogenous shocks that were an inescapable part of the early modern world. Although pre-industrial societies had neither the ability to influence the magnitude or intensity of the shocks themselves, nor an adequate understanding of the processes by which they resulted in disease and death, they were far from being helpless victims of the vagaries of a malign fate. As recent work on early modern *mentalités* has shown, men and women evolved attitudes and rituals that, by seeking to tame death, enabled them to cope with the emotional trauma and social disturbance it brought: a 'corporate culture of death explored for Whickham by Wrightson and Levine in this volume.[189] They were also capable of using simple observation and commonsense in their experience of death as a basis for effective intervention to mitigate the consequence of exogenous shocks, even though the theoretical reasoning they used in justification might be incomplete or faulty.

What was critical was the degree to which the prevailing ideology of the social order allowed, or even required, the magistracy to intervene in the normal processes of social and economic life on behalf of the community at large. The contributions to this volume by Slack and Walter make it clear that in England in conditions of plague and dearth

---

[188] Mercer, 'Smallpox and epidemiological–demographic change'.

[189] See chapter 3 below; also Aries, *Hour of our Death*; Gittings, *Death, Burial and the Individual*; Whaley, *Mirrors of Mortality*.

not only were public authorities expected to intervene, but they might be forcibly reminded of their duties by an apprehensive public. Furthermore, in conditions of dearth the English magistracy was under a double obligation. As social leaders and employers they were expected to recognise a personal responsibility to help the poorer members of the community, an obligation that was reciprocated by the deference and obedience expected of the latter in the social ideology of the day. And, as magistrates, they not only possessed powers to police the marketing of grain and so prevent a price-driven collapse of 'exchange entitlements', but from the end of the sixteenth century they also presided over a statutory system of local poor relief. Since entitlement to relief was tied to the parish of settlement, it was counter-productive for individuals to leave their locality to seek relief elsewhere. In principle, therefore, the poor law in England provided an institutional barrier against migration in times of dearth, thereby limiting the dislocation occasioned by harvest failure and inhibiting the consequent spread of disease. In practice, however, in some areas the full implementation of the Elizabethan poor law was delayed until well into the seventeenth century. But although both the chronology and the geography of the implementation of famine-relief measures of the poor law need much more research, it seems evident that over time an important institutional constraint to subsistence migration gathered strength and affected a growing proportion of the country. The lack of any rise of mortality in England in the high food-price years of the mid 1690s, in contrast to the situation in Scotland, France, and other parts of Europe, suggests that England may already have had an effective system of local entitlement-support by this date. The growing effectiveness of the poor law in this domain may help explain why there was so little concern in government circles in London about the possibility of social dislocation due to famine in the 1690s, in contrast with the extreme anxiety shown during the high food-price years in the last decade of the previous century.[190]

Although the support of food entitlements, along with other forms of social intervention, were of critical importance in coping with the consequences of dearth, the magnitude of the problem depended upon the ability of a society to expand its agricultural production in step with the growth of its population. With most land already under cultivation and without the technology to raise yields per acre continuously, pre-industrial societies sooner or later faced a problem of

[190] Outhwaite, 'Dearth and government intervention', pp. 389–406; Clark, 'Migration in England', pp. 81–90.

diminishing marginal returns to agriculture.[191] Consequently, rapid population growth was likely not only to mean less food per head but also, by driving up food prices, to threaten economic differentiation and expansion by reducing the purchasing power available for non-food goods and services. To avoid a downward spiral in which population growth reduced everyone to penury until mortality rose and Malthus' positive check supervened, it was essential that fertility should be responsive to changing economic conditions so that population growth rates could be checked, or even reversed.

In his contribution to this volume Schofield argues that pre-industrial European societies were able to achieve this goal because they had evolved a pattern of family formation which stressed the desirability of residential independence at marriage, in contrast to the situation in most other parts of the world, where most married couples continued to co-reside with their parents as part of the same economic unit.[192] Since each new household in Europe was expected to be economically independent, marriage, and thus fertility, were open to the influence of changing economic conditions.

However, Schofield goes on to distinguish between two stylised variants of the European pattern of marriage, and argues that they not only have different demographic and economic consequences, but are themselves associated with wider differences in the ideology of family relations. In a relatively simple economy dominated by peasants and craftsmen, in which the basis for economic viability lay in obtaining access to a restricted number of units of physical capital such as a farmstead or a craft workshop, the opportunity to marry was closely related to the rate at which economic niches were vacated, so that nuptiality was closely linked to mortality. In more differentiated societies such as early modern England, on the other hand, a significant proportion of the population had insufficient access to capital or land to ensure survival, and so was dependent on selling its labour. In these circumstances, the link between marriage and economic conditions was more indirect, operating through changes in the standard of living as it affected the wage economy.

Schofield argues that not only are undifferentiated economies and familistic ideologies of social relations likely to be found together, but

---

[191] The classic formulation is in Malthus, *Essay*, chapters 1–2. A traditional response to population pressure is the adoption of more labour intensive farming techniques. Boserup, *Conditions of Agricultural Growth*, and *Population and Technology*, chapter 3 and 8. But there were limits to which yields could be increased in this way. See, for example, Campbell, 'Agricultural progress'.

[192] See chapter 8, below.

the latter also tend to evolve political and legal structures which favour stability, resisting change in the distribution of property and constraining individual independence and mobility. Familistic ideologies, in short, are likely to inhibit economic development in the form of improvements in agricultural organisation, economic differentiation and urbanisation, and the emergence of markets in labour and goods. The less the power of the family as an organising principle in social relations, the greater the mobility and the more flexible the property relations, with beneficial consequences for increasing agricultural output, providing a wider range of goods and services, and the development of markets and distribution networks, Moreover, the necessity of finding an alternative means of support for the elderly when family obligations are weak, strengthens the notion of the indispensibility of the role of collective action, in which officials and magistrates are seen to be acting for the public good, rather than in the interest of some arbitrary political power.

Schofield characterises England as lying towards the individualist–collectivist end of the spectrum of family structures, and suggests that it was no coincidence that a differentiated market economy and productive commercial agriculture emerged there at an early date. In this perspective a more diversified and mature 'traditional' economy, and a higher standard of living, can be seen as the economic rewards of a system of social values and power-relations that responded to changes in the demand for food generated by changing population growth rates, not by a hardening of the arteries of a family-based subsistence economy, but by market-induced changes in agricultural practice and landholding structure. This is not to deny that in the dynamic process of interaction between population growth, food prices, and agricultural production there were not periods in which a growing proportion of the population became proletarianised and suffered declining exchange entitlements for their labour, thereby becoming more vulnerable to harvest deficiencies. But the critical point is that the same set of social values and power-relations not only included an awareness by both governors and governed of the necessity of supplementing individual freedom of action by collective intervention in the common good, but also produced both the economic basis and the political institutions through which such intervention could be made effective.[193]

---

[193] Disputes and negotiation over the extent of rights and obligations within the 'paternalism–deference equilibrium' of power-relations in early modern England are discussed in Thompson, 'Eighteenth-century English society', and Walter, chapter 2 below.

England, therefore, may well have been unusually well placed socially, economically, and politically to deal with the consequences of harvest failure and other exogenous shocks. Whatever the merits of the particular arguments in relation to England, by the mid eighteenth century there does seem to have been a clear association in pre-industrial Europe between the responsiveness of mortality to fluctuations in food prices and the level of economic development. In a study of nine countries in the period 1756–1870 Galloway found that the magnitude of the mortality response to food price fluctuations was positively related to the proportions of the populations still employed in agriculture, and negatively related to the percentage of the population in an urban environment and the level of income per head.[194] In this period by far the highest scores for economic development were to be found in England, where there was no association between mortality and food-price fluctuations. Galloway's finding of a consistent relation between the magnitude of the mortality response to price fluctuations and the level of economic development is all the more remarkable because in the case of fertility the response to food-price fluctuations was uniform across all countries, and bore no relation to indicators of economic development. There are many reasons why fertility in the past may have fluctuated in response to food-price fluctuations; but since the major association between price and fertility fluctuations occurred after a lag of one year, Galloway pointed to

a reduction in the number of conceptions resulting from increased famine or stress amenorrhea, a greater frequency of induced and spontaneous abortions, more use of contraceptives or reduced coital frequency.[195]

If the fertility response could be so uniform across societies when so many different biological and behavioural mechanisms may have been involved, it may be reasonable to conclude that the large differences between societies in the case of mortality owed little to biological or behavioural mechanisms linking the availability of food directly with death, but were largely created by the differential operation of social, economic, and political factors that were systematically related to the level of economic development.

When Laslett first posed the question 'Did the peasants really starve?', scholarly attention was directed towards questions of

---

[194] Galloway, 'Basic patterns', pp. 295–7. For the countries studied and the periods for which data are available, see above note 153. Data on urban percentages and per capita incomes are only available for five countries, viz. England, France, Prussia, Denmark, and Sweden.   [195] *Ibid.*, p. 285.

quantity such as the amount of food available per head, and much was made of the powerlessness of that world in the face of autonomous fluctuations in climate and disease. Early modern societies were seen as victims of natural variation caught in an inexorable web of unalterable biological processes. Following in Appleby's footsteps, many scholars, especially those who have contributed to this volume, have led us to appreciate the extent to which the world that past societies inhabited was in fact of their own making: their family patterns and economic practices determined not only the food available to them, but also the nature of their symbiosis with a myriad of micro-organisms. The system of economic and political interaction that they evolved determined not only the amount of food at their disposal and how it was distributed amongst them, but also both the incidence and distribution of disease. Furthermore, their ability to monitor changes in their circumstances and formulate effective evasive action enabled them to exercise a considerable measure of control over their own fate. The social order mattered: as a critical determinant of demographic change, and as the basis of political as well as economic institutions, it fashioned the conditions of death, no less than those of life.

2

The social economy of dearth in early modern England

JOHN WALTER

The impoverished repertory of English folk tales lacks those tales, common in other early modern European societies, in which peasant culture confronts the dilemma of too many mouths to feed and in which supernatural salvation so often took the form of a super-abundance of food.[1] This hitherto largely unnoticed absence of English Hansels and Gretels wandering through a Malthusian world takes on added meaning in the light of recent work on the demography of early modern England. This work has challenged the central role accorded harvest failure as a cause of crisis mortality. By the period at which parochial registration begins, crises of subsistence were absent from the demographic record of many regions. Even those areas scarred by crises of subsistence were free of such crises after the mid seventeenth century. In contrast to the experience of most of continental Europe and her Scottish and Irish neighbours, England had slipped the shadow of famine at an early date.[2] If crises of subsistence were largely

I am grateful for comments on earlier drafts of this chapter to Roger Schofield and to members of the following seminars: the ESRC Cambridge Group, the Economic and Social History of Pre-Industrial England Seminar, Institute of Historical Research, Comparative Political Economy of Development, Queen Elizabeth House, Oxford, Professor S. J. Woolf's Poverty in Early Modern Europe Research Group, European University Institute and History of Poverty Seminar, All Souls, Oxford.

[1] I am grateful to Ben and Angharad Walter for first giving me the opportunity to realise this. The absence of references to famine is based on an examination of the following sources: Aarne and Thompson, *Types of the Folktale*; *Collection of Seventy-Nine Black Letter Ballads*, ed. Halliwell and Wright; Rollins, *Pepys Ballads*, 8 vols.; Rollins, *Pack of Autolycus*; Rollins, 'Analytical index to ballad-entries'; Chappell and Ebsworth, eds., *Roxburghe Ballads*, 9 vols.; Ebsworth, ed., *Bagford Ballads*; Briggs, *Dictionary of British Folk-Tales*, 4 vols. Dearth, rather than famine, is the focus of English popular literature. For the importance of famine as a motif in French folk-tales, see Darnton, *Great Cat Massacre*, pp. 9–72.

[2] Flinn, *European Demographic System*; Flinn et al., *Scottish Population History*; Wrigley and Schofield, *Population History*.

76 JOHN WALTER

absent from early modern England, so were crises of disorder. Despite the predictions of contemporaries and presumptions of historians, years of harvest failure were not marked by widespread and frequent food riots.[3] This chapter takes as its focus the series of discrepancies between the dominant and widely accepted model of socio-economic change which suggests a sharp growth in the proportion of the early modern population 'harvest-sensitive' and the more muted record of death and disorder that has emerged from recent studies.

A plethora of contemporary comment and practices point to the central importance of the harvest and to the sharp threat its failure posed to early modern society. Diaries and personal correspondence record with uneasy alarm the uncertain weather, most usually cold springs or wet summers, that threatened the harvest.[4] The terse comments that break through the orthodox formulae of parochial registration and the recording therein of anonymous burials of 'poore wandering folk' found starved bear witness to the shock of harvest failure on a society for which bread was still literally the staff of life.[5] That harvest time was normally a period of higher wages, better food, and gargantuan celebration made the inversion of harvest failure all the harder to bear. The dating of past events in contemporary recollections and urban annals by reference to past dearths reflects the psychic hold harvest failure had on contemporaries. While urban annalists ordered their accounts by reference to past dearths, almanacs (and proverbial lore) reflected their readers' anxieties about future harvests. (The claim to be able to offer means of determining and influencing the quality of the harvest was yet another important area of overlap between the church and popular culture.)[6] The febrile correspondence between central and local authorities in years of dearth testifies to the fears of those in authority that harvest failure threatened the fabric of the social order. 'Nothing will sooner lead men to sedition than dearth of victuals', noted William Cecil, and others chorused their agreement.[7] There is

[3] Walter, 'Geography of food riots'.
[4] Many of the diaries listed in Matthews, *British Diaries*, show this concern: see, for example, 'Diary of Philip Wyot', in Chanter, *Sketches Literary History Barnstaple*; Roberts, ed., *Diary of Walter Yonge*; Macfarlane, ed., *Diary of Ralph Josselin*.
[5] For some examples see, Laslett, *World We Have Lost Further Explored*, p. 131; Beier, *Masterless Men*, p. 46; Bodl. Lib., Oxford, MSS. D. D. Par. Wendlebury d. 1, fo. 43.
[6] Coventry RO, Acc. 4, City Annals F; Leighton, 'Chronicles of Shrewsbury', pp. 239–352; Capp, *Astrology*, pp. 64, 114; Thomas, *Religion and Decline of Magic*, pp. 74, 284, 368, 396, 404–5; Campbell, *English Yeoman*, p. 369; Hutchinson, ed., *Works of G. Herbert*, pp. 321–55 (proverbs 516, 749).
[7] Fletcher, *Tudor Rebellions*, p. 112; cf. Bacon, 'Of seditions and troubles', in *Works*, pp. 406–12; Gouge, *God's Three Arrowes*, p. 136; Ling, *Politeuphia*, p. 114; Cornwall, *Revolt of the Peasantry*, p. 106.

perhaps no better illustration of the central importance of the harvest to the maintenance of early modern society than the temporary suspension of social rules otherwise held sacrosanct. The urgent need to gather in the harvest set aside traditional divisions of labour between men and women, industry and agriculture; it suspended the laws against vagrancy to secure a labour force, and sanctioned work on the sabbath.[8]

Despite this welter of evidence, we lack as yet a systematic survey of the full consequences of harvest failure for early modern society and economy.[9] Its economic consequences were extensive in a society where agriculture was the major source of income for the majority of the population and the harvest the major factor dictating levels of demand for non-agricultural production. Both directly and indirectly, the harvest determined levels of prosperity and poverty. Directly, its failure has been seen as playing a major role in the restructuring of landholding, accelerating the decline of the smallholder in the last decade of the sixteenth century and contributing to the growth of the great estates in the later seventeenth century.[10] For those without land, the potential loss of the high harvest wages, accounting for a disproportionate slice of their annual income, combined with often savage price rises to send them spiralling into poverty. Harvest failure led to sharp increases in vagrancy and in rural–urban migration.[11] Indirectly, harvest failure, by cutting purchasing power, was a major cause of the depressions that afflicted both rural industrial and urban manufacturing and service sectors.[12] Attempts to relieve the sharp increases in poverty that dearth brought compounded this problem. Years of harvest failure brought a sharp rise in the cost of poor relief

[8] Trotter, *Seventeenth Century Life*, pp. 143–4, 190; Thomas, 'Work and leisure', pp. 52–3; Noake, *Worcester in Olden Times*, p. 21; Hudson and Tingey, eds., *Records of the City of Norwich*, 2, pp. 134–5, 377; Ashton, *Economic Fluctuations*, p. 7; Jones ed., *Agriculture and Economic Growth*, p. 25; PRO, SP 16/173/11; Hill, 'Sabbatarianism', p. 150.

[9] Ashton, *Economic Fluctuations*, chapter 1 provides the basis for such a study in the eighteenth century, while Barry Supple provides a short, but highly valuable discussion of the economic consequences of harvest failure for the seventeenth century in his *Commercial Crisis and Change*, pp. 14–19. For an interesting attempt to reconstruct the impact of the dearths of the 1590s in a specific locality, see Clark, *Provincial Society*, chapters 7–8.

[10] Spufford, *Contrasting Communities*, chapters 2–4 and pp. 165–6; Beckett, 'English landownership', pp. 567–81.

[11] Beier, *Masterless Men*, pp. 15–16, 77; Slack, 'Vagrants and vagrancy', pp. 369–70; Clark, 'Migrant in Kentish towns', pp. 143, 160n.; Souden, 'Indentured servant', p. 34; Kent, 'Population mobility and alms', pp. 37, 48–50.

[12] Roberts, 'Wages and wage-earners', pp. 260–1; Hull, 'Agriculture and rural society', p. 500; Supple, *Commercial Crisis*, p. 111; Ashton, *Economic Fluctuations*, p. 44; Bowden, 'Agricultural prices', pp. 636–8.

and, where foreign grain had to be imported, could have an adverse effect on the terms of trade. Directly, harvest failure might cause a drop in the state's revenues while indirectly, where harvest failure coincided with attempts to extend the tax base (as in the 1590s and later 1640s) it could provoke opposition to the state's fiscal demands.[13] Directly, it led to riots over food supply while, indirectly, it might synchronise other forms of opposition, for example to enclosure, in both major rebellions and minor riots. Everywhere, lengthening court rolls provide evidence of the direct impact of harvest failure on levels of appropriation and of its indirect impact, complex and contradictory, on the presentment and prosecution of theft.[14]

The harvest also dictated the demographic rhythms of early modern society. Its timing helped to determine the seasonality of marriage; its failure frustrated marriage. In a society where marriage was a process rather than an event, dearth's disruption of this process has been invoked to explain an increase in illegitimacy (as in the decade of the 1590s) and a consequent intensification in local social regulation.[15] Indeed, it might be argued, that it was the knowledge of the possibility of frequent harvest failure that helped to drive up the age at which couples considered themselves to have attained the economic independence permitting marriage in this society. The economic stress that harvest failure brought led on the one hand to the break-up of marriages and, on the other, to the formation of family groupings whose hybrid character belies the simple nuclear form under which they were listed.[16] But, above all, it is the mute testimony of the demographic record which has been held to provide historians with the most graphic confirmation of the serious consequences of harvest failure for early modern society: the failure of the fields being thought to have been followed by a rich crop of burial in the churchyard.

Years of harvest failure in modern England were years of heightened

---

[13] Ashton, *Economic Fluctuations*, p. 47; Thirsk and Cooper, eds., *Economic Document*, p. 59.

[14] Amongst an extensive literature see, Walter and Wrightson, 'Dearth and the social order', pp. 24–5; Cockburn, 'Nature and incidence of crime', pp. 49, 67; Sharpe, *Crime in Early Modern England*, p. 62. For a particularly sensitive discussion of the relationship between harvest failure, appropriation and prosecuted crime see King, 'Crime, law and society', pp. 59–64, 125, 135, 147–8.

[15] Kussmaul, 'Agrarian change', pp. 1–30; Bradley, 'Seasonality in baptisms, marriages and burials', p. 39; Wrigley and Schofield, *Population History*, pp. 421–2; Wrightson, 'Nadir of illegitimacy', pp. 176–91; Wrightson and Levine, *Poverty and Piety*, chapter 7; Ingram, 'Ecclesiastical justice', p. 152; Ingram, 'Religion, communities and moral discipline'; Smith, 'Marriage processes', pp. 43–99.

[16] Chaytor, 'Household and kinship'; Houston and Smith, 'New approach to family history?'.

mortality. Harvest failures did bring increases in burial figures that were both local, regional, and national. More strictly (though still variously) defined as crises of subsistence which saw at least a doubling of background levels of mortality, such crises have been identified by Appleby for Cumberland and Westmorland, by Palliser for Staffordshire, and for parts of Devon by Paul Slack. Other work has added to the map of subsistence crises.[17] In the later sixteenth and early seventeenth centuries especially, harvest failure took its toll of the population. But the most recent work on the demographic history of early modern England, notably Wrigley and Schofield's *Population History of England*, has suggested a more restricted incidence through space and time for harvest-related crisis mortality than these essentially regional examples might suggest.

Wrigley and Schofield argue that conspicuous but isolated examples have led some historians to suggest that there was a close and determined relationship between years of high prices and high mortality. While there were years in which the two did coincide, there are also striking exceptions. In some years real wages fell savagely but the death rate scarcely rose above trend. For example, in 1586/7, when harvest failure prompted the government first to issue the Book of Orders designed to cope with the consequences of dearth, there was no great recorded increase in mortality, while in the later crisis of 1649/50, coming after several years of harvest failure and in the midst of civil and military strife, the death rate was actually below trend. Years of harvest failure might be years of heightened, but not necessarily heavy, mortality. Even crisis years on which much attention has been focussed, for example the 1590s, assume less significance in their impact on 'national' mortality trends. Famine was above all a regional problem. In the crisis of 1597/8 when mortality was 25.6 per cent above trend, little over a quarter (28 per cent) of the parishes under observation in the Cambridge Group sample registered crises of subsistence. This regional (as well as age-specific) pattern to famine meant that unless the rise in prices was exceptionally high, the cumulative effect of crises of subsistence on 'national' population

---

[17] Appleby, *Famine*; Palliser, 'Dearth and disease'; Slack, 'Mortality crises'; Drake, 'Elementary exercise in parish register demography'; Drake, *Historical Demography*, pp. 89–118 (Yorkshire West Riding); Rogers, *Lancashire Population Crisis*; Cox, *Parish Registers*, p. 173 (Minehead, Somerset, 1597); Foster, 'Demography in the north-west'; Martin, 'Parish register and history', pp. 3–15; Davies, 'Plague, death and disease in Herefordshire', pp. 310–11; Taylor, 'Population, disease in early modern Hampshire', pp. 352–7, 378, 641ff. The lack of a common definition of crises of subsistence makes comparisons between these studies (some of which employ statistical measures which perhaps favour the finding of crises) difficult.

trends was after five years essentially zero. While the earlier period saw individual years in which there was a marked increase in famine-related mortality, by the 'hungry 1690s' the relationship between high food prices and mortality was muted. In a decade that saw some of the sharpest falls in the index of real wages the death rate was unusually stable and even fell below trend in those years registering the lowest real wage rates. Even on a regional basis the impact of crises of subsistence was becoming less great at the point when the dominant model of social change suggested that they should be at their peak. By the difficult years of the 1640s (and perhaps even earlier) even the previously vulnerable north-west was no longer registering crises of subsistence.[18]

If crises of subsistence were less severe than has been supposed, absent by and large from many areas at an early date and no longer even a regional problem after the mid seventeenth century, then this raises the problem of why. For the chronology of this growing immunity to crises of subsistence seems to contradict expectations based on the widely accepted model of social and economic change in the period. This, which sees there having been a sharp growth in the size of the landless, labouring population matched by a steep decline in real wages, would suggest a growing vulnerability to periodic harvest failure. But, as we have seen, the reality was very different. The climacteric of the later 1640s, coming at the peak of these changes and marked by a succession of bad harvests in the midst of civil war (classic conditions for continental crises of subsistence), witnessed no sharp increase in mortality rates.

Why was this? Clearly, in the longer term, England's relative immunity, and early escape from famine is to be explained by important economic changes. To these should be added the controls on unrestrained population growth afforded by the nature of England's 'low-pressure' demographic regime. By far the most important economic changes were those in agriculture. An improvement in agricultural techniques (cumulative, rather than revolutionary) perhaps doubled gross yields between the early sixteenth and mid seventeenth centuries and, as Professor Wrigley argues elsewhere in this volume, brought even greater gains in net yields. By the mid seventeenth century this had lifted population pressure on food resources; by the late seventeenth century, England had become a net

[18] Wrigley and Schofield, *Population History*, especially pp. 319–35 and appendix 10, pp. 645–93; Schofield, 'Impact of scarcity and plenty', pp. 67–93; Watkins and Menken, 'Famine in historical perspective', pp. 155–6.

exporter of grain.[19] In the longer term, therefore, it would be possible to explain the disappearance of famine in terms of economic change. While the weaknesses of local ecologies, fragile surpluses, poor and unfavourable market integration explain the pattern of famine, agrarian change and better market integration explain its disappearance. Access to grain in southern communities allowed them to escape famine; increased agricultural output and better communications later extended this immunity to the highland zone. These gains in agricultural productivity combined with the favourable nature of England's low-pressure demographic regime, with its controls on nuptiality and fertility, to avert a major Malthusian crisis. But while both of these factors – demographic and economic – are of obvious importance in the long-term, what needs to be emphasised here is that they were by themselves insufficient to solve the problem of the harvest-sensitive. Indeed, whatever their longer-term importance, they had consequences that exacerbated the problems harvest failure posed for this group in the period when population growth was most rapid and increasing output insufficient to eradicate periodic dearth.

An emphasis on economic factors – the provision of a grain surplus through the mechanism of the market – assumes an ability to gain access to grain through purchase on the market. In so doing, it ignores the important criticisms raised by Amartya Sen's work on famine.[20] Sen has argued that explanations that put an emphasis on food availability miss the impact of harvest deficiency on what he terms 'exchange-entitlements'. In an exchange economy, Sen observes, the ability to obtain food depends on the rate at which labour or commodities can be exchanged for food. Explanations that put the emphasis on the growing availability of grain therefore ignore the all-important problem of command over access to grain. A consequence of harvest failure for the upland pastoral economies was a collapse in the price of their product and an inability to afford grain from other regions: in Sen's terms, a trade-entitlement failure. A direct failure of entitlements also threatened at least some sections of the communities of lowland arable England. Fragile surpluses and a market insufficiently developed to wipe out local shortages meant that for the land-poor and labour-dependent, in towns as well as villages, the sharp rise in

[19] Clay, *Economic Expansion*, chapter 4 provides a good recent summary of agricultural developments in the period; Overton, 'Estimating crop yields', pp. 375–8; Wrigley, 'Corn yields and prices', below, pp. 257–9; Wrigley and Schofield, *Population History*, chapter 10 and pp. 677–8; Appleby, *Famine*, chapter 10–11.
[20] Sen, *Poverty and Famines*.

grain prices in years of shortage posed acutely the problem of access to grain.

The problems of these groups were compounded by the attenuated nature of the kinship system that was the corollary of the demographic regime. While the low-pressure demographic system offered a check on fertility through the norm of the nuclear family and a later-marrying population, it also created, in Peter Laslett's striking phrase, 'nuclear hardship'. The need to secure economic independence before marriage led to later age at marriage, migration, and the formation of neo-local marriages for many couples. These combined with patterns of lower life expectancy to produce low kinship densities in many communities.[21] While kin might represent 'a store of wealth . . . to be drawn upon as need arose',[22] an attenuated kinship system meant that protection against economic crises for the generally more mobile harvest-sensitive households had to be sought from within the collectivity, rather than from an extended family or kin.

While, therefore, economic growth and the relatively favourable nature of the demographic regime are of obvious importance in explaining the longer-term disappearance of famine, they cannot by themselves explain why famine was not a more general scourge in the period of greatest population growth. The argument here will be that, while the threat of famine has been exaggerated, the possible defences against that threat have been largely unexplored and, consequently, underestimated. In particular, there has been an uncritical use of the ambiguous evidence for famine that literary sources offer. The evidence thus derived has been married with what we might term a Malthusian model of social and economic change which exaggerates the depth of poverty in early modern England and, therefore, the extent of vulnerability to famine. This model, in its turn, has found support in a reading of price and wage series whose construction (probably) and applicability (certainly) need more critical scrutiny. Finally, an exaggerated emphasis on the economically-determined and market-dominated nature of relationships in early modern society has obscured the protection against harvest failure still to be found in such relationships. Together with the better-known crisis relief, this social economy insulated many of the poor from the full impact of harvest

---

[21] Laslett, 'Family, kinship and the collectivity' (I am grateful to Peter Laslett for letting me see a typescript of this paper); Wrightson and Levine, *Poverty and Piety*, pp. 82–94; Wrightson, 'Household and kinship', pp. 151–8.

[22] Cressy, 'Kinship and kin interaction', p. 69. Evidence of aid between kin in dearth years would provide an interesting test of Cressy's claims that dense and extended kin links were more common than has been allowed and that they provided 'a store of wealth'.

failure. It did so, however, in ways that constrained the poor's ability to articulate popular grievances in collective protest.

Literary evidence has not always been approached with the caution its use demands. Famine and starvation are words with an ambiguity of meaning. In contemporary usage this ambiguity was sometimes intentional or the product of alarmed apprehension.[23] For example, while reports from provincial authorities to the centre give an accurate sense of the alarm contemporaries felt when faced with the failure of the harvest, that same alarm sometimes clouded the accuracy of their judgement. When provincial magistrates were suitors to the central government for aid, this distortion was sometimes deliberate. There is the further danger with literary evidence that such reports, emanating from regions where there was famine, can be taken out of their regional context and married with other evidence taken to be indicators of crisis (sedition, riot) to (mis-)represent the 'national' experience of crisis in years of harvest failure.

Allied to this use of literary evidence has been the use of a particular model of social structure and social change which, if accepted, lends credence to contemporary reports of famine. At its most extreme, this model of social change emphasises the growth in the harvest-sensitive section of the population to the point that makes famine almost an inevitability. Thus, the Malthusian model, holds that there was already at the beginning of the sixteenth century a large proportion of the population dependent on wages. Population growth and inflation brought a polarisation of rural landholding under the stimulus of commercial agriculture and demographic attrition. Larger farms were built up at the expense of smallholdings as subsistence farming gave ground to commercialised agriculture. There was therefore a sharp increase both relatively and absolutely in those dependent on an uncertain market for employment (which was scarce) and food (which was expensive and subject to savage short-term increases). The logic of this model was that social and economic change resulted in a population that was living so close to the level of subsistence that a deficient harvest could have lethal consequences on a grand scale. As Professor Hoskins wrote in his pioneering study of harvest failure, 'In a country in which between one-half and two-thirds of the population were wage-earners, and a considerable proportion of the remainder subsistence farmers; in which about one-third of the population lived below the poverty-line and another third lived on or barely above it; in

---

[23] Rotberg and Rabb, *Hunger and History*, p. 1; Oddy, 'Urban famine', pp. 69–71.

which the working class spent fully 80 to 90 per cent of their incomes upon food and drink; in such a country the harvest was the fundamental fact of economic life.'[24]

The 'harvest-sensitive model' depends heavily on the analysis of fiscal records, buttressed by the estimates of contemporary social taxonomies. Analysis of early sixteenth-century taxation records has suggested that between a quarter to a third of the population was already dependent upon wage labour at the beginning of the sixteenth century, though even higher figures have been claimed for some regions. Similar analysis of hearth tax records for the later seventeenth century has yielded even higher figures, again with pronounced regional peaks reflecting the weaknesses of local economies. These have been taken to lend support to Gregory King's estimate that just under half of the population in the later seventeenth century were labourers, outservants, cottagers, or paupers.[25] It is this evidence of a growth in the number of the labouring poor derived from fiscal records which suggests the existence of a large harvest-sensitive group vulnerable to the vicious increases in grain prices that marked years of dearth. Nowhere in this analysis was the problem more acute than in the towns. Thus, according to Professor Hoskins' much-repeated estimate, 'fully two-thirds of the urban population in the 1520s lived below or very near the poverty line', a figure translated into national proportions in his work on harvest failure.[26]

Hoskins' reference to the poverty line has been widely followed, but the notion of the 'poverty line', a tricky concept even in current social scientific usage,[27] has scarcely been defined. If, as seems likely, Hoskins was proposing tax assessments as an approximation for the 'poverty line', then recent research might offer some grounds for challenging this usage. *Faute de mieux*, in the absence of anything approaching a national census historians are forced to make use of the snapshots provided by census-like fiscal records or contemporary social estimates to recover the profile of early modern society. To deny that these provide evidence of a growth in the size of the labouring population would be foolish. But there is now perhaps in the prompting of the demographic record a need to re-assess the meaning and validity of the commonly accepted and widely quoted figures derived from these sources. Taxation records register income inequali-

---

[24] Hoskins, 'Harvest fluctuations, 1480–1619', pp. 28–9.
[25] Everitt, 'Farm labourers', 397–9; Spufford, *Constrasting Communities*, pp. 31–3; Thirsk and Cooper, eds., *Economic Documents*, pp. 780–1.
[26] Hoskins, *Provincial England*, p. 84; 'Harvest Fluctuations, 1480–1619', p. 29.
[27] See, for example, the comments of Sen, *Poverty and Famines*, p. 11.

ties. Without further evidence, these should not be confused with levels of destitution.

Both types of source have their problems. Contemporary estimates are simply that and therefore subject to a margin of error. Thus, as has already been suggested, Gregory King in his widely quoted estimates of poverty for the later seventeenth century may have over-estimated the size of the labouring poor.[28] Fiscal records, despite their attractiveness, require for their use the resolution of technical and methodological difficulties, which hitherto have received inadequate attention from historians drawing on them. Equally important, they also demand a greater attentiveness to the social meaning of the figures derived from their exploitation.

Hoskins' estimates were based on the evidence of the early Tudor subsidies. Where detailed local sources have permitted a comparison to be made with other listings of wealth, it is clear that nil or minimum assessments should not automatically be equated with destitution. For example, Dr Phythian-Adams' study of Coventry, a town cited by Hoskins, led him to revise downwards for the early sixteenth century Hoskins' original estimate that between a third and a half of the population were vulnerable to harvest failure; perhaps something like a fifth were affected by bad harvests he suggests, a figure for which there is support from other urban studies.[29] Similar studies suggest the need for a downward revision of levels of rural poverty derived from early subsidy records.[30] Revision of the evidence furnished by analysis of the hearth-tax listings suggests a similar need for caution and a greater sensitivity to the way differing methods of assessment and collection determine the resulting record of levels of exemption. As the work of Dr Husbands has recently detailed, there are many serious problems involved in translating levels of exemption into levels of poverty.[31] Ignoring these has led historians to exaggerate levels of poverty in the later seventeenth century.

There is a further problem. Decontextualising fiscal records from their socio-economic, as well as their administrative, context,

---

[28] Lindert and Williamson, 'Revising England's social tables', pp. 387–91.

[29] Phythian-Adams, *Coventry*, pp. 13, 132–4, 240; Youings, *Sixteenth-Century England*, pp. 75, 279; cf. Dyer, *Worcester*, pp. 166–7; Slack, 'Poverty and politics in Salisbury', pp. 173–7; Beier, 'Warwick', pp. 53–61.

[30] Campbell, 'Re-evaluation of the 1522 muster rolls and 1524/5 lay subsidies'; Fieldhouse, 'Social structure from Tudor lay subsidies and probate inventories', p. 18.

[31] Husbands, 'Methodological pitfalls of the Hearth Tax returns' (I am grateful to Dr. Husbands for letting me see this important paper); Husbands, 'Hearth Tax and structure of English economy', especially chapter 6.

smoothes out significant contrasts in regional social and economic structures. These could give very different meanings to the significance of exemption or minimum assessments. The 'poverty' of the urban exempt was probably different from that of their rural counterparts. Within rural society differences in local ecologies drew further distinctions; the possession of common rights in an area of extensive commons and dual economy doubtless gave a very different social meaning to exemption from that implied by exemption from taxation of cottagers in an enclosed economy.[32] It is clear that we need more detailed local studies, to provide a context in which to assess the social meaning of exemption and, by exploiting record linkage, to provide a more accurate sense of the relationship between taxation assessments and levels of wealth, before we can feel confident in translating the categories imposed by state taxation into sensitive indicators of the vulnerability of the population to harvest failure.

If our sense of the proportion of the population that was impoverished needs scaling down, then so does the other side of the equation, represented here by Hoskins, by which vulnerability to harvest failure has been calculated. Although our knowledge of both diet and family budgets is woefully inadequate, Carole Shammas' research on household expenditure would revise significantly downwards Hoskins' figure for expenditure on food.[33] She suggests that food expenditure probably accounted for just over a half of poorer households' expenditure, a figure that, if correct, would have given greater flexibility in the face of harvest failure. Clearly, the evidence on income and expenditure needs more critical examination.

Using the standard source of the Phelps Brown and Hopkins' basket of consumables would seem to lend powerful support to the Malthusian model of a society with a large population of wage-dependent and harvest-sensitive poor. Their index shows real wages to have fallen drastically.[34] Demographic pressures and the inability of

[32] Husbands, pp. 18–19. The most careful assessment of ecological differences in levels and meaning of poverty is to be found in Wales, 'Poverty and parish relief in seventeenth century Norfolk' (I am grateful to Tim Wales for letting me see this important paper.) See also the comments of Appleby on the southern bias of measures used to measure the rural labouring poor, *Famine*, p. 45.

[33] Shammas, 'Food expenditure and well-being', pp. 89–100. Interestingly, the evidence of contemporary budgets of poorer households for the difficult years of the later seventeenth and eighteenth centuries give levels of expenditure on food in the range of 70 to just under 75 per cent of income.

[34] Phelps Brown and Hopkins, 'Seven centuries of building wages', 'Seven centuries of the price of consumables compared with builders' wage-rates; 'Wage-rates and prices: evidence for population pressures in the sixteenth century'. All these are conveniently reprinted in Phelps Brown and Hopkins, *Perspective of Wages and Prices*.

a pre-industrial economy to absorb and employ the surplus population meant that wages failed to keep pace with the rise in the price of essential foodstuffs. Those who became dependent on the market for both employment and food were therefore in a precarious situation. According to the Phelps Brown and Hopkins' index, wage-earners by the late sixteenth century were only able to purchase some 40 per cent of the basket of consumables that their wages would have brought them in the period 1451-75. Other estimates offer confirmation of this trend. However, the repeated flourishing of these figures, which have acquired the status of textbook orthodoxies, has meant that such 'statistics' have been accorded a status which seriously distorts either their utility or applicability. As a recent review of the republished articles of Phelps Brown and Hopkins noted, 'The conjectures, conclusions, and influences arrived at by applying the economist's traditional engine of thought to an incomplete historical record still call loudly for confirmation or refutation.'[35]

This is not the place to embark on that task, but there are serious technical and what we might call 'real' problems that question the use made of the wage and price data to underpin the Malthusian model. In both prices and composition the construction of the basket of consumables shows a strong southern bias. They find no place for oats which, even at the end of the eighteenth century, were an important component in northern and Celtic diets, nor do they reflect the fact that wage rates were lower in the pastoral north-west. Ironically, therefore, the index gives a poor guide to the experience of those areas where the threat of famine was a reality. (As Shammas suggests, food expenditure in her 'northern' region may have represented a higher proportion of family income and thus left less flexibility against harvest failure.)[36] The prices used are those paid by institutional buyers making bulk purchases of largely unprocessed products. The relationship between these wholesale prices, which were likely to have been sticky, and those paid by smaller consumers is largely unexplored. There are similar problems on the side of wages. The raw materials for the wage series is represented by payments to building craftsmen and labourers. These again reflect a southern bias and are payments made by institutional employers. The base years for the wage series – 1451-75 – represent a period of exceptional prosperity for wage-labour. The fall indicated in real wages is, therefore, from a high point in what Thorold Rogers called the 'golden age of labour'. Recent work has suggested

---

[35] Deane, *Economic History Review.*, 36 (1983), pp. 140–1.
[36] Brinsley Thomas, 'Feeding England', p. 332; Shammas, 'Food expenditure', pp. 96–7.

that for some building craftsmen the Phelps Brown index may have exaggerated the extent of the decline in their wages. Work on wages and prices in early modern London has suggested that real wages fell by 25, rather than some 40, per cent over the sixteenth century.[37]

But technical problems apart, some of them pointed out by Phelps Brown and Hopkins but ignored by consumers of their statistics, there are more fundamental problems with the index of real wages. The construction of the basket of consumables assigns an unchanging proportion of composite commodities over a period stretching from the mid fifteenth to the early twentieth century. In the inflationary conditions of the long sixteenth century, the proportion allowed for farinaceous products – 20 per cent – (a figure mirroring expenditure in a mid fifteenth century priest's household, the first of four budgets used in the construction of the basket) seems a poor reflection of the likely composition of the diet of wage labourers in the period. In turn, the proportion assigned to wheat within this farinaceous component of 37 per cent in 1500 rising to 48 per cent in the 1725 budget fails to take into account the ability of poorer consumers to trade down to inferior and less expensive grains, a practice particularly marked in conditions of dearth and, as Appleby argued, of growing importance in the seventeenth century.[38]

Wages are calculated on the basis of *per diem* payments made to individual workers. To translate *per diem* payments into annual wage rates it is necessary to confront contradictory assumptions. While the abolition of holy days after the Reformation would have increased the available days for employment, perhaps by as much as a fifth, this theoretical gain needs to be set against the growing problems of under- and un-employment. Moreover, a basic daily wage fails to reflect the importance of higher payments for seasonal or special tasks. Even given the successful resolution of these problems, the resulting annual wage would still provide an inadequate guide to income. Since in the conditions of the early modern economy the family, and not the individual, was most frequently the unit of production, it is the *family* income that the historian needs to recover, an even more challenging task. And even then, it needs to be remembered that the wage was for many (but how many remains unknown) only a contribution to that income. How many were solely dependent on wage labour for a living is unknown – as we have seen, the attempt to read off levels of wage

---

[37] Airs, *Making of English Country House*, pp. 182–9; Rappaport, *Social Structure and Mobility in Sixteenth Century London*, chapter 7, especially pp. 383–95; Bowden, 'Agricultural prices', p. 600.

[38] Phelps Brown and Hopkins, *Perspective of Wages*, pp. 13–20; Appleby, 'Diet', p. 108; Appleby, 'Grain prices', pp. 865–87.

earners from tax records is fraught with difficulty – but for many, not least building craftsmen, a smallholding or common rights continued to provide other sources of income which, depending on the nature of the local economy, might be extensive. Moreover, efforts to measure changes in wage rates depend upon an anachronistic simplification of what constituted the wage in a pre-industrial economy.[39] Monetary payment was often only one aspect of the wage. Depending on the form it took, the wage could offer the possibility of protection from the inflationary pressures of the market place through payment in kind or some other form of privileged access to food.

One final assumption in the use of the price indices to support the Malthusian model needs challenging. This is the belief that the impact of harvest failure on poorer consumers can be read off from the sharp upward movement of prices in the market. Again, this is a question of our ignorance. We do not know the proportion of the poor that purchased their essential foodstuffs, nor the proportion that bought in the market, from middlemen or at the farm gate. Nor do we know in what form they purchased their food. As Phelps Brown and Hopkins pointed out the decline in real wages would have been less marked for those who purchased processed food. Although the proportion of the population forced to purchase their grain in the market was undoubtedly increasing throughout the period, there is reason to believe that their numbers may have been exaggerated. If this were the case then this may be a further factor of some importance in making sense of the resistance of the population to harvest failure.

As Mark Overton has noted, the marketing process must be interposed between harvest quality and the subsequent price of grain.[40] Consequently, studies of dearth are more properly studies of prices. It is therefore possible to envisage situations in which, as indeed some contemporaries recognised, market prices either exaggerate or under-represent the extent of grain deficiency.[41] Higher prices in markets without access to good and cheap waterborne routes and

[39] Airs, *English Country House*, pp. 148–9; Durant and Rider, eds., *Building of Hardwick Hall*, 2 vols., part one, p. xxi; part two, p. lxxi; Woodward, 'Wage rates and living standards', pp. 28–45; Sonnescher, 'Work and wages', pp. 147–72.

[40] Appleby, 'Diet', pp. 109–10; Overton, 'Estimating crop yields', p. 366.

[41] See, for example, the comments of Sir Ralph Maddison reprinted in Thirsk and Cooper, eds, *Economic Documents*, p. 25. For price series in this period, see Hoskins, 'Harvest fluctuations, 1480–1619', pp. 28–46; 'Harvest Fluctuations, 1620–1759', pp. 15–31; Bowden, 'Agricultural prices', pp. 693–695, 814–70. These prices may not reflect the impact on poorer consumers. As has been pointed out Hoskins' series is based on wheat and therefore fails to reflect the ability of poorer consumers to switch to other grains: Harrison, 'Grain price analysis', pp. 135–55. For a fuller consideration of this and other issues, see Appleby, 'Diet', pp. 112–13; Wrigley, 'Corn yields and prices', below, p. 248.

which therefore experienced high transport costs reflected the reduced variety of weather zones from which grain could be drawn. The smaller the amounts of grain coming onto the market and the fewer the number of purchasers then the larger the amplitude of fluctuations in prices. It may be because the total quantity of marketable grain was small in relation to demand, and the number of regular purchasers small relative to the much larger numbers forced to depend on the market when their own small surpluses failed, that dearth could have such a seismic impact on prices.[42] If, however, the number of those who obtained their grain from the market was smaller than has been assumed, then the critical question becomes how did they obtain their grain and did they do so in ways that afforded them some cushioning from the full impact of dearth on market prices?

It could be argued, therefore, that the scale of poverty was less great and its growth less rapid than the Malthusian model assumes. Scaling down levels of poverty is not sufficient however to explain the absence of famine. Over time an increase in agricultural output may have raised the threshold of harvest failure, but for much of the early modern period harvest failure continued to threaten many with potential destitution. Poor law records perhaps provide better evidence of the contours of poverty. The levels of poverty they record can offer an important corrective to estimates of poverty derived from the records of taxation. They need, however, to be used with caution. Lists of those in receipt of poor relief undoubtedly underestimate the extent of poverty since their compilation betrays notions of eligibility and not necessarily need, and the restricted numbers of recipients reflect the limits of funds rather than the limits of the problem. Censuses of the poor, a relatively under-exploited source, avoid much of these problems. These exist for both rural and urban communities. Since they were taken most often in response to the failure of the harvest they offer the most detailed evidence of levels of harvest sensitivity. If the evidence of the poor law scales down estimates of levels of destitution, the evidence of the censuses underscores the problem of 'conjunctural poverty', that growth of the penumbral poor whose shakey independence and vulnerability to harvest failure are well brought out in the excellent series of records available for the Norfolk village of Cawston in the difficult years of the 1590s.[43] Poverty may

---

[42] Blanchard, 'Early Tudor Economy', p. 429; Postan, *Medieval Economy and Society*, pp. 256–7.

[43] Staffordshire RO, D 593 S/4/10/30, of which there is a brief analysis in Clark, *Provincial Society*, pp. 239–40; Slack, ed., *Poverty in Early-Stuart Salisbury*; Pound, ed., *Norwich Census of the Poor*; Beier, 'Warwick', pp. 46–85; Phythian-Adams, *Coventry*, pp. 59,

have been less than the Malthusian model assumed, but the existence of the 'conjunctural poor', vulnerable to exactly the problems of declining 'exchange-entitlements' that Sen emphasises, underlines the need for an explanation of why this potentially large group did not starve which goes beyond an emphasis on longer-term agrarian changes.[44]

A partial solution to this demographic conundrum might be found in a re-examination of the impact of change on the social and economic structures of early modern England. Demographic growth and the stimulus this gave to the intensification of agrarian capitalism was the dominant motif of change for much of this period; the increasing polarisation of society its chief consequence. But the end result of this process – an increase in the harvest-sensitive sector of society – was less rapid or complete than the enforced brevity of textbook accounts might suggest. Nor was it uniform. A fruitful place to begin an examination of why these changes were not also accompanied by a growing vulnerability to famine is with the reminder that society and economy in early modern England were local and regional. Clearly, at the level of individual strategies of survival to cope with harvest failure (historically the most difficult to recover)[45] the nature of the local economy played an important role. While these strategies might exhibit a common pattern, their success or failure was heavily dependent upon the nature of the local economy. Gleaning, which could provide the poor with a valuable and by no means insignificant source of grain, was likely to have played a larger role in the strategies of the poor in arable

---

134, 194; Goose, 'Comparative study of Cambridge, Colchester and Reading', p. 344; Hunt, *Puritan Moment*, pp. 68–9; Amussen, 'Class and gender relations', pp. 55–74; Wales, 'Poverty, poor relief and life-cycle', pp. 369–80.

[44] Thus, although the argument up to here has something in common with the revisionist reading offered by David Palliser ('Tawney's century; brave new world or Malthusian trap'), I differ from him in seeing the problem of poverty being greater than perhaps he allows.

[45] While there was a common thread to many of these responses for which evidence can be recovered (for example, eating seed-corn or more desperately eating unripe corn: Bowden, 'Agricultural prices', p. 634: Penry, *Three Treatises*, Williams, ed. pp. 41–2), evidence of other responses survives by chance; see; for example, the case of an Essex woman who gained grain after the harvest failures of the 1590s through prostitution: Emmison, *Morals and the Church Courts*, p. 17. Vagrancy examinations can occasionally give a vivid glimpse of the dynamic of individual adaptive strategies to cope with dearth; see the case of Humfrey Gibbons recounted in Clark, 'Migrant in Kentish towns', p. 143. For a detailed story of how one family in the north-west survived the famines of the 1590s, marrying aid from their friends and, when this was temporarily no longer available, mortgaging a future crop for the loan of meal, see Newcome, *Autobiography*, 1, pp. 82–4. For a general discussion of the range of food strategies, see Dirks, 'Social responses'; Colson, 'In good years and bad'.

areas.[46] By contrast, common rights in pastoral areas of wood and fen with extensive waste and common offered greater scope for obtaining alternative sources of food. Similarly, differences in local ecologies doubtless dictated the scope for food substitution – trading down in grains, making use of grain substitutes such as lentils usually reserved for animal feed and eating animals otherwise proscribed by (informal) dietary restrictions.[47] Together with differences in common rights they also determined the availability of other 'need foods'. In contrast to their known role in the Celtic fringe, not enough is known about the rôle of such alternative food sources in early modern England (our ignorance is perhaps a further subtle indication of the early lifting of fears of famine),[48] but when the harvest failed bread was baked out of meal ground from acorns and fern roots, and roots and young foliage provided a desperate diet.[49]

It was in communities practising monoculture that harvest failure was most damaging. The more mixed the economy the greater were the defences against harvest failure. That much of English agriculture, despite regional emphases, was mixed and regional specialization occurred within that context meant that continuing diversification

[46] John Cook acknowledged the value of gleaning in helping the poor through the hard winter of 1647/8: *Unum Necessarium*, p. 28. We lack as yet an adequate study of gleaning, but it is clear that in the then state of harvest technology it could provide the poor with a significant amount of grain to last them through the difficult winter months or in some places, as Francis Eden claimed in the 1790s, enough to feed themselves and a pig through the year; Bushaway, *By Rite*, pp. 141–3; King, 'Crime, law and society in Essex', p. 288. The value of gleanings may have been increased by a deliberate policy on the part of harvesters; one Lancashire gentleman who criticised his harvesters for unclean reaping was told, 'What shall we leave for the poor ones?': Gibson, ed. *Crosby Records*, p. 136. The loss of the protection gleaning afforded was one of the criticisms made by opponents of enclosure: Powell, *Depopulation Arraigned*, pp. 66–7.

[47] Everitt, 'Farm labourers', pp. 403–6; Thirsk, *Peasant Farming*, pp. 27–8, 119; Appleby, 'Diet', p. 105; Harrison, *Description of England*, p. 133; Anderson, 'Ethnography of yeoman foodways', p. 168; Salter, *Tudor England Through Venetian Eyes*, p. 73; Meeke, *Extracts from the Diary* p. 75; Thomas, *Man And Natural World*, pp. 53–5, 116.

[48] The success of, and need for, Richard Mabey's *Food for Free* perhaps provides a further indication of this.

[49] Sayce, 'Need years and need foods', pp. 55–80; Lucas, 'Nettles and charlock as famine food', pp. 137–46; Cullen, 'Population growth and diet', pp. 89–112. Platt, *Artificiall remedies against Famine* listed a large number of famine foods. For some examples of their use, see PRO, SP 12/188/47 (Gloucestershire 1586: cats, dogs and nettle roots); Pilkington, *Works*, pp. 611–12; Hartley, *Food in England*, p. 231; Dymond, 'Famine of 1527 in Essex', p. 31n.; Jones, *Tudor Commonwealth*, p. 116; Palliser, *Age of Elizabeth*, p. 192. It may be significant that many of the references to 'need foods' in the English record come in the context of polemical comment which draws on their use to heighten the exceptional nature of the events to which they refer disapprovingly. I hope to deal more fully with diet and the use of 'need foods' in early modern England elsewhere.

brought greater insulation against crop failure. For example, in the fen-edge village of Willingham in Cambridgeshire, the combination of mixed agriculture with dairying helped to avoid sharp increases in mortality in all but successive years of harvest failure. Similarly, a greater diversity within the arable sector offered further insulation. Where, as in the open fields of the Midlands, there was considerable acreage given to the cultivation of peas and beans as animal feed these could be used to offset failure of the cereal crops. As the Elizabethan proverb observed, 'hunger setteth his first foot into the horse manger'.[50]

One particular aspect of crop diversifiction may have been of special importance in mitigating the impact of harvest failure. As Professor Appleby argued, a growing emphasis on spring-sown crops – oats and barley – broke the symmetrical price structure in which harvest failure saw sharp increases in the prices of all grains. A better balance between winter and spring cereals lessened the impact of the failure of any one of the grains. Appleby argued that this had been achieved by the later 1650s. Regional evidence suggests that this important shift had happened earlier in some areas: for example, in Cornwall by the end of the sixteenth, in the Forest of Arden by the early seventeenth century, and in East Anglia by the 1630s. Richard Carew, doubtless making reference to his county's experience in the successive harvest failures of the 1590s, paid tribute to the value of spring-sown grain in his *Survey of Cornwall*

Barley is now grown into great use of late years, so as now they till a larger quantity in one hundred than was in the whole shire before and, of this, in the dear seasons past, the poor found happy benefit, for they were principally relieved and the labourers also fed by the bread made thereof, whereas otherwise the scarcity of wheat fell out so great that these must have made many hungry meals and those outright have starved.[51]

Like other peasant societies, medieval England had exhibited in its basic structures mechanisms for defence against the frequent failure of the harvest.[52] Recent work on the open fields, for example, has suggested that their logic can best be seen in terms of a subsistence–

---

[50] Spufford, *Constrasting Communities*, pp. 129, 152–4; Hoskins, *Midland Peasant*, pp. 154–6; 'Leicestershire farmer in sixteenth century', p. 161; *APC, 1596–97*, p.7; Leicester RO, Hall Papers BR II/18/14, no. 108; Harrison, *Description of England*, p. 133.

[51] Appleby, 'Grain prices', pp. 865–87; Skipp, *Crisis and Development*, p. 48; Overton, 'English probate inventories', p. 214; Carew, *Survey of Cornwall*, pp. 101–3; Whetter, *Cornwall*, pp. 37, 48; cf. Large, 'Urban growth and agrarian change'.

[52] For a stimulating discussion of the possible range of 'life insurances' against harvest failure, see Outhwaite, 'Dearth', pp. 37–9; see also Clark, *Provincial Society*, pp. 233–4.

sufficiency orientation. Thus, the persistence of practices whose demonstrable loss to output angered later would-be reformers represented a foregoing of potential profit for protection against probable risks. The scattering of strips and differing crops among the open fields were ways of mitigating risk.[53] If the winter crop failed, then fields could be resown with spring cereals, showing the value of a diversified portfolio of plots. To this we might add that where there remained commons, these provided a reserve from which additional land could be taken and put temporarily under the plough, a practice for which we have evidence from a number of communities in years of harvest failure.[54]

In some regions these defences were undermined by demographic growth and economic change that encouraged specialisation that ran ahead of the ability of a poorly integrated market to iron out regional shortages in grain. In others, their continuing vitality may help to explain the absence of crises of subsistence there. From the earliest date for which demographic evidence becomes readily available (though it should be noted that the earliest evidence is thin), some areas seem resistant to crises of subsistence. While more work needs to be done in the mapping of subsistence crises, it is clear that the broad explanatory divisions – between highland and lowland, north and south, pastoral and arable (but more properly mixed) – advanced to explain differing responses to harvest failure need further refinement.[55] These broad regional divisions themselves need opening up to explore the more local contrasts in economy and ecology that they contained and which may hold the key to anomalies in the existing maps.

Pastoral specialisation has been seen as an important factor in explaining the geography of famine. But it is probably the case that while some forms of pastoral specialisation rendered communities especially vulnerable, other forms may have afforded some protection against harvest failure. Specialisation in cattle-rearing, where capital investment was greater and tied up for several years, may have

---

[53] Hoffman, 'Medieval origins common fields'; McCloskey, 'Persistence of common fields'; McCloskey, 'Open fields as behaviour towards risk'. For an interesting discussion of the logic of peasant agriculture as a search for long-term stability and minimum subsistence, see Watts, *Food, Famine and Peasantry*; see also Colson, 'In good years and bad'; Scott, *Moral Economy*, p. 5.

[54] See, for example, Yonge, *Dairy Walter Yonge*, pp. 18–19; Hey, *English Rural Community*, p. 49. Taking land into cultivation, especially to sow extra spring crops, seems to have been common: Skipp, *Crisis and Development*, p. 37; Gough, *Human Nature Displayed*, p. 33; Griffiths, 'Kirtlington', pp.211–12; Coventry RO, A 14(a), fo. 131; Chester, 'Poor relief in Coventry', p. 36 and note. In Worcestershire, dredge (a mixture of grains) was sown as a form of insurance against excessively wet summers: Seavoy, *Famine*, p. 56.

[55] Wrigley and Schofield, *Population History*, pp. 670–2.

produced an inflexibility which led to destocking in unfavourable market conditions as a response to harvest failure. Hence, it was reported from the uplands of North Wales in the crisis of 1622/3 that the 'country [was] exceeding poor, past belief, because their cattle, whereon they lived for the past four years, bore no price' and that 'bread corn is at such a rate . . . that many die of hunger, and the rest bear the impression of hunger in their faces'.[56] By contrast, dairying gave a greater degree of flexibility which helped areas like the Somerset levels to escape famine.[57]

Rural industrialisation has also been seen as a form of specialisation which exposed communites to the threat of famine. But much may have depended on the exact nature of the inter-relationship between agriculture and industry. Where rural industry supplanted agricultural employment, promoting the growth of a workforce dependent on industrial employment alone for subsistence, then it may have weakened defences against harvest failure. The textile communities of Westmorland and the West Riding of Yorkshire were rendered doubly vulnerable as rural industrialisation encouraged population growth in grain-deficient, upland pastoral and harvest-sensitive economies. But where rural industry supplemented household economies that retained an agrarian base it contributed to a dual economy that offered greater protection against dearth. In the sheep-corn region of north-east Norfolk by-employments for women and children in the worsted cloth industry made an important contribution to the family economies of smallholders and agricultural labourers. In the Forest of Arden in Warwickshire the development of metal-working in an economy moving to a better balance between pasture and plough eased the previous ecological disequilibrium, a process similar to that observed in the metal-working districts of Staffordshire.[58] Much may have depended on the date at which specialisation took place. The

---

[56] Wynn, *Calendar of Wynn (of Gwydir) Papers*, p. 173 (I am grateful to Anthony Fletcher for bringing this source to my attention); for evidence of the limited arable land on these estates, see Jones, 'Wynn Estates of Gwydir', pp. 141–69. In the dearth of 1622/3, Henry Best in the East Riding of Yorkshire was taking in cattle in exchange for grain: Best, *Farming and Memorandum Books*, p. 168.

[57] P. Croot, The commercial attitudes and activities of small farmers in Somerset in the seventeenth century, paper read to the Early Modern English Economic and Social History Seminar, Cambridge, 10 November 1983.

[58] Thirsk, 'Industries in countryside', pp 82–3; Hudson, 'From manor to mill', pp. 124–44; (It would be interesting to know whether the socio-economic differences between areas of worsted – pastoral, upland, grain-deficient – and woollen production – lower land, mixed agriculture, larger farms, and tighter manorial controls – were reflected in differential patterns of harvest mortality); Wales, 'Poverty and parish relief', p. 67; Skipp, *Crisis and Development*, p. 62 and graph, p. 19; Rowlands, *Masters and Men*, p. 13; Hey, *Rural Metal Workers*; Large, 'Urban growth', pp. 173, 176.

earlier the specialisation, the less likely it was that market integration was sufficiently developed to iron out regional shortages or that the gains in overall output were sufficient to provide transferable surpluses. By contrast, later pastoral specialisation in a period of more favourable markets for livestock production, larger surpluses and better integration meant that communities – like those in the Northamptonshire forests where the equilibrium between grass and corn had by the seventeenth century been pushed too far in favour of the former – escaped any demographic penalty.[59] Poverty, then, needs to be understood in its regional and local context. Vulnerability to harvest failure was dictated by a complex of conditions which, while they coincided in some areas with disastrous results, were only partly present in others.

The resistance of some areas and some sections of those whose economic status was thought to render them sensitive to harvest failure should encourage us to challenge another aspect of the 'harvest-vulnerable' model. In a reading of social change which emphasises the increasing dominance of market forces and the economically determined nature of relationships, the impact of harvest failure is seen as being all the more disastrous on the landless since they were now no longer cushioned by the defences of community and neighbourliness. But the triumph of English individualism was perhaps less absolute than this interpretation might suggest. Relationships in which the nature of the exchange was not strictly conditioned by the market had a continuing vitality well into the eighteenth century. To see early modern England as a market society would do serious damage to the realities of social relationships in this period. In particular, it obscures the protection still to be found in those relationships for the land-poor or wage-dependent against the problem of declining exchange entitlements. For, as Sen himself acknowledged, 'even in capitalist market economies entitlements may not be well defined in the absence of a market-clearing equilibrium and in pre-capitalist formations there can be a good deal of vagueness on property rights and related matters'.[60]

Even clearly economic relationships offered some degree of protection against harvest failure by giving the possibility of privileged access to grain. Sharecropping, as in other societies, may have offered a form of 'subsistence crisis insurance'. Although nowhere near enough is known about the role of sharecropping in English agriculture, sowing

[59] Pettit, *Royal Forests of Northamptonshire*, pp. 152, 169.
[60] Sen, *Poverty and Famines*, p. 49.

to halves and thirds was, it has been argued, common. Robert Loder in Berkshire and Nicholas Toke in Kent, where the practice seems well established, both let to halves. If common, sharecropping may constitute an additional reason, along with the prevalence of sub-letting, for questioning estimates of landlessness based on the snapshots of manorial studies.[61] Though sharecropping on the continent in this period was predominantly associated with rural poverty, it may well be that this form of tenure represented a preference for minimal returns but maximum security against harvest failure. As Sen has pointed out, sharecroppers may have lower entitlements, but they can eat the returns to their labour directly without having to secure their subsistence through the vagaries of the market. Even if harvest failure left them with insufficient grain to meet the claims of the landowner and their own needs, then the reciprocities of their relationship with their landlord could give them, as in other societies, first claim on what grain there was and, if even this was not sufficient, the expectation of a grain subsidy.[62]

The nature of the labour market in early modern England could also provide direct access to food. Many were protected at least at one stage in their life-cycle from high food prices by residence as a servant in the household of their employer. A recent estimate suggests that as many as two-fifths of the rural labour force lived in the households of their employers, and in towns the proportion may have been even higher. On the basis of social structural listings, Ann Kussmaul estimates that some 60 per cent of the population aged between fifteen and twenty-four were employed as servants. Service, that 'refuge of the children of the poor' as one contemporary termed it, offered protection against harvest failure in two ways. It relieved harvest-sensitive families of the burden of feeding young adults and transferred this responsibility to the household of the employer.[63] If employment as a servant withstood harvest failure (and there is some evidence to suggest that the response of at least smaller employers might have been to put off servants when the harvest failed), then servants would continue to be fed in conditions of dearth at their employer's expense. As such, they might fare better than they otherwise would have done in their family of origin. In the early seventeenth century the Berkshire yeoman, Robert Loder, calculated the annual cost of his servants' diet at ten pounds each. At the end of the century, Richard Baxter thought

[61] Scott, *Moral Economy*, p. 56; Kerridge, 'Movement of rent', p. 18; Chalkin, *Seventeenth Century Kent*, p. 63; Harrison, 'Village surveys', pp. 82–9.
[62] Sen, *Poverty and Famines*, p. 5; Scott, *Moral Economy*, pp. 50–1.
[63] Kussmaul, *Servants*, pp. 11–42, 76; Beier, *Masterless Men*, p. 23.

the case of servants far easier than that of the poor tenants who were their masters for, 'they know their work and wages, and are troubled with no cares for paying rent, or making good markets, or for the loss of corn or cattle . . . or the unfavourable weather'.[64]

Annual hiring as a servant or non-resident farmworker, even hiring to task, could give privileged access to food through payment in kind and through the valuable perquisites, licit and illicit,[65] this brought. Both Henry Best and Robert Loder paid their farm servants partly in cash and partly in kind, and in this they were representative of others. Where Loder's servants did not live in as members of his household, he paid them 'board wages' with quantities of grain. In 1617, for example, Robert Loder's carter was hired to board wages for eleven pounds in cash, four bushels of wheat valued at sixteen shillings, four weeks' board in the harvest, also valued at sixteen shillings, and a hog's keeping all year, valued at 13s. 4d., which, as Loder noted, 'was exceeding great wages'.[66]

Payments in kind seem to have been made especially to those with particular skills. It was common for shepherds to receive additions to their cash wage. Two shepherds who petitioned the Wiltshire justices for the payment of their wages put their wages at three pounds and two bushels of wheat. A Norfolk shepherd received three pounds a year in cash, a tenement with an acre of land, the right to run eighty sheep with the lord's flock, furze and breaks for fuel, the 'tath' (pasturing) of two acres a year, the right to put three neats and one nag on the 'heath' for a rent of 6½d. and a hen, as well as other minor perquisites. The value of these perquisites as insulation against the threat of harvest failure can be seen clearly in the payments made by Henry Best to his farmworkers in the East Riding of Yorkshire. In June

---

[64] Robert Loder in his accounts showed a recurrent concern with the cost of servants; in the dearth of 1614 he noted, 'I judge it were good (in such deare yeares) to keep as few servants as possible': Fussell, ed., *Loder's Farm Accounts*, p. 90; Thirsk and Cooper, eds., *Economic Documents*, p. 182.

[65] Employment may have given opportunities for appropriating grain as a perquisite. Robert Loder, for whom 'pilfering' by servants and taskers was a continuing problem, noted on one occasion, 'Item that corne which my men doe steale (more then I allow of in a yeare); although it be a thing uncertaine, yet I think it may well be valued at xls.': Fussell, ed., *Loder's Farm Accounts*, p. 56; cf. pp. 24, 96, 127, 139, 163. Dearth may have made owners of grain more willing to treat such appropriation as theft; for examples of prosecutions of taskers and carters for taking grain, see Sharpe, *Crime: A County Study*, p. 99; King, 'Crime, law and society', p. 132.

[66] Fussell, ed., *Loder's Farm Accounts*, pp. 28, 47–9, 113, 136–7, 141; Best, *Farming and Memorandum Books*, pp. xxxix, 169 ff.; Everitt, 'Farm labourers', pp. 436–8; Rule, *Labouring Classes*, pp. 109–10. For a similar argument about the privileged access to grain enjoyed by certain categories of workers, see Vaughan, 'Famine analysis', pp. 183–4.

1622, John Bonwick, a farm servant who had worked for Best for a number of years, was hired for '£6 in money, 8 bushels of barley, 2 bushels of oats and a peak of oatmeal and a *frise* coat and a *stooke* of straw every week from Christmas to Lady Day'. The access this gave to grain must have been particularly valuable in the ensuing dearth that caused serious crises of subsistence in the north.[67]

Being hired as a servant or to task could also offer more direct protection against the problems of landlessness. For the fortunate, hiring might be rewarded by the grant of a piece of land which could be sown with grain. Robert Bulkeley paid a man to plough sixteen shillings and the ground to sow three-quarters of hemp seed or a *kip* of barley. One of Best's servants was hired for three pounds a year and 'the sowings of a mette [two bushels] of barley in the claye'. As we have seen the Norfolk shepherd also received an acre of land as well as grain. In Kent, sowing to halves represented a type of tenancy in which the rent was partly in the form of labour and partly in kind. Others, for example building craftsmen, may also have been given access to land as part of their employment.[68]

Even those without land or the protection offered by annual hiring might yet be protected from the problems of a decline in 'exchange-entitlements' by less formal relationships in the employment of labour. Those hired by the task might, like servants, receive part of their payment in kind, gaining access to grain in this way. Threshers, whose work gave them obvious opportunities for pilfering grain, regularly received part of the grain they threshed. On the Isle of Wight, Sir John Oglander, who cautioned his son, 'above all things, be sure your threshers are honest men', allowed his threshers one bushel for every twenty they threshed. The diary of Robert Bulkeley of Anglesey for the 1630s regularly records payments in cash and corn to those who did work on his house and lands. Henry Best in Yorkshire and Nicholas Toke in Kent made similar payments. In December 1623 Best paid two carpenters for sawing up a walnut tree and making furniture of it 10s. and one bushel of barley and a peck of oatmeal, and to two others for building a barn 13s.4d. and two pecks of barley. In July 1629, Nicholas Toke paid one Longe a load of wood and a bushel of wheat as well as 40s. in money.[69] That both these years were years of dearth underlines

---

[67] Wiltshire RO, Q/S Great Roll, Easter 1609/114; Simpson, *Wealth Gentry*, p. 186; Best, *Farming and Memorandum Books*, pp. lv–vii, 169; Kussmaul, *Servants*, p. 39.

[68] Bulkeley 'Diary of Bulkeley', p. 106; Best, *Farming and Memorandum Books*, p. 164; Chalkin, *Seventeenth Century Kent*, p. 63; Airs, *Making English Country House*, p. lxxii.

[69] Oglander, *Commonplace Book Sir John Oglander*, p. 207; Bulkeley, 'Diary of Bulkeley', pp. 81, 59–60, 71; Best, *Farming and Memorandum Books*, p. 179; Lodge, ed., *Account Book of a Kentish Estate*, p. 112.

the value of these relationships. Even employment by the day if it included meat and drink offered some insulation against dearth prices. Henry Best records payments to a man and wife for some seventeen days of work of both money, cheese, and grain. Those employed to plough for Sir Robert Spencer in the difficult autumn of 1596 received in addition to 6d. per day, cheese, breadcorn, malt, beef, and five sheep. Even some rural industrial workers could find some protection against the direct impact of harvest failure in the provision of food by their employers.[70]

Even those without access to land or food through these relationships may still not have been exposed to the full impact of famine-level prices as some discussions of the period assume. There were, in effect, two markets operating in early modern England. There was the sale of grain through the market place upon which attention has been concentrated and through local exchanges. To see the landless as dependent on the market place for grain is to mistake the experience of certain sections of the poor – notably the urban and rural industrial poor (and then probably not even all of these) – for that of the labouring poor as a whole.

Rural labourers, especially those in areas specialising in grain production, could obtain their grain through purchase from their employers or other farmers in the local community at farm-gate prices. Being able to buy farm produce at a concessionary rate from their employer was one of the perquisites most valued by farm labourers. Accounts and diaries frequently record the sale of small amounts of grain. Robert Loder sold grain both in the market and at home, as did Adam Eyre in Yorkshire. The diary of Adam Winthrop in Suffolk records the sale of small amounts of grain – to those who had threshed for him, those renting a cottage from him and to widows among others – in the dearth years of the 1590s. Henry Best's account book shows that it was a common practice for Best in the East Riding of Yorkshire to make sales at home of small amounts of grain, ranging in quantity from a single peck to several bushels, as well as to send grain to market.[71]

---

[70] Best, *Farming and Memorandum Books*, p. 175; Simpkinson, *The Washingtons*, appendix. Credit and the provision of cheaper food were one of the few benefits to the workers of the truck system, whose growth in the later eighteenth century, it has been suggested, owed something to the dearths of the period: Wells, *Dearth and Distress*, pp. 16–17.

[71] Kerridge, *Farmers of Old England*, p. 153; Fussell, ed., *Loder's Farm Accounts*, pp. 28, 47; Eyre, 'Dyurnall', pp. 50–2, 56–7; Robinson, *Winthrop Papers*, I, pp. 52, 113, 122–3, 130; *Farming and Memorandum Books*, pp. 163–207; see also Brooks, ed., 'Supplementary Stiffkey Papers', pp. 40–2; Hull, 'Agriculture and rural society', pp. 136–7. For evidence of the persistence of local sales into the eighteenth century, see Pounds, 'Food production pre-industrial Cornwall', p. 120.

Since sales in this alternative local market were often below market prices they offered otherwise harvest-sensitive groups valuable insulation against the full pressures of the market place. A report on the marketing of corn in Norfolk, drawn up in 1631 in response to the previous year's dearth, referred to 'labourers that buy it at an under price of them with whom they work'. From Sussex in the same year it was reported that 'those who have any corne to spare sell it better cheape at home to their poore neighbors then in the markets'.[72] Local sales had other advantages. They allowed the labouring poor to buy in small amounts without having to pay the higher prices that market sellers were complained of demanding on the sales of small quantities; nor did they involve the loss of work which trudging to the market entailed. Perhaps most importantly, purchasing grain directly in this way not only allowed the poor to buy at under-prices but also on credit. A memorandum of 1597 summarised these advantages

in those Countries where Corne is plentyfull most men of hability haue of their owne groweth both for their owne store and to spare for their Neighbors and the poorer sort do only buy in the market unles yt be for Seede Corne, and yt were more easy for the poore to fetch yt at the ffarmors house nere to him, where sometymes he is trusted by pecke and half pecke then to go to the markett, w[hi]ch does lose him a dayes labor, and the ffarmer will afforde a better pennyworthe at his house in Charity to a Neighbor then in open markett, where he doth bring Corne to make his best price.[73]

A final advantage was that the existence of this local market enabled labourers without money to pay for their grain with the promise of future work. In North Wales, Robert Bulkely when recording sales of small amounts of grain, usually a bushel, notes frequently, 'he shall pay me in work'. The 1631 Norfolk report pointed to the practice whereby the labourer in the sheep-corn region, 'hath now corn at home upon trust, or by agreement for work'. Again, the value of this to those otherwise vulnerable to the effects of harvest failure is graphically brought out in the large number of sales of grain in exchange for future work that Henry Best records in the severe harvest failure of 1622/3.[74]

---

[72] Thirsk and Cooper, eds., *Economic Documents*, p. 344; Fletcher, *Sussex*, p. 151. Local sales to labourers were specifically exempted from orders to sell all grain in the market in years of dearth: Brit. Lib. (hereafer BL), Lansdowne MS.51, fo. 89.

[73] BL, Lansdowne MS.84/13, fos. 30–31v; but cf. a speech in the 1601 Parliament; 'for the rich have two measures, with one he buyes and ingrosseth Corn in the Country, that is the greater, with the other he retails it at home to his poor Neighbours, that's by the lesser', D'Ewes, *Journals*, pp. 662–3.

[74] 'Diary of Bulkeley', passim; Thirsk and Cooper, eds., *Economic Documents*, p. 344; Best, *Farming and Memorandum Books*, pp. 163–207; cf. Robinson, *Winthrop Papers*, 1, p. 52.

Clearly the provision of grain through these various relationships offered a potentially powerful shield against harvest failure. But for this protection to be effective against the problem of declining 'exchange-entitlements', it has to be shown that these relationships were not undermined by the failure of the harvest and that prices within these local circuits of exchange remained below the dearth prices of the market place. That there was a market price and that the recovery of this is unproblematic is itself open to question. Again, we know far too little about transactions in the early modern market. Then, as now, prices might vary according to quality and quantity. But most relevant to the discussion here is the fact that prices might be expected also to reflect both the underlying economic and *social* relationships between the parties to the transaction. As the difficulties encountered by the Quakers in their refusal to bargain make clear, prices in the market were expected to be negotiable (though presumably within limits). Something of the force of these considerations is captured in the example of the sale of grain between two Oxfordshire women, where the seller gave the buyer 'advantageous terms' because she was her niece and 'a very poor widow . . . [with] many small children unprovided for'.[75]

Did the divergence in prices between market transactions and local exchanges persist even under the impact of harvest failure? Local transactions were clearly not uninfluenced by economic considerations. There were, as farmers like Best and Loder were well aware, costs in taking grain to market which could lessen profits. By contrast, as has been argued for eighteenth-century Massachussets, selling locally could tap a sizeable market. But there is also evidence to suggest that selling locally and at under-price was part of an expected relationship between master and labourers. The special nature of transactions in food between members of the same community may have made them, as in other societies, especially subject to social pressures.[76]

Without considerably more research (for which the recovery of local price series is crucial), it is impossible to generalise confidently, but on

---

[75] Mintz, 'Internal market systems', pp. 20–30; Marshall, ed., *Autobiography of Stout*, p. 90; Everitt, 'Marketing agricultural produce', p. 558. Richard Baxter urged his readers to take into account the quality of the party with whom they dealt and, if they were poor, to mix charity with justice: *Christian Directory*, part 4, 'Christian politics'. For a glimpse of the pressures around sales of grain to poorer consumers whose custom was to ask for a 'blessing' of grain over and above that for which they had paid, see Slack, ed., *Poverty Early Stuart Salisbury*, pp. 123–5.

[76] Thirsk and Cooper, eds., *Economic Documents*, p. 344; Fussell, ed., *Loder's Farm Accounts*, p. 138; Hobbs Pruitt, 'Self-sufficiency', p. 338; Ortiz, 'Concept of "peasant culture"', p. 328; Clark, *Provincial Society*, p. 121.

the basis of existing evidence it seems to have been the case that prices of local exchanges did rise in years of dearth, but they continued to lag behind market places and did not register the seismic leaps that took place in the market.[77] But whatever the exact relationship with market prices, it was of equal importance that as long as grain was available in this way, it could be paid for in ways that offered further protection against declining 'exchange-entitlements'. Grain could be exchanged on credit for later repayment or future work. Where repayment was in kind, changes in market price were irrelevant to the transaction; where grain was provided as part of the contract of employment or for future labour, then if valuations were customary (something about which we know next to nothing, but for which there is some evidence in the eighteenth century) or sticky (for which there is some evidence) this also afforded some protection.[78]

While harvest failure may have challenged these relationships, it is clear that they could and did survive the challenge. Indeed, as responses to inquiries from the central government under the Book of Orders issued in years of dearth make clear, selling locally at under price may have been more fully implemented in exactly those years. The practice reported from Hertfordshire in 1630 of allowing farmers and cornmasters a free market on condition that they relieved the poor at home at prices under those in the market seems to have been widespread. The obvious value of this in offsetting the threatened decline in 'exchange-entitlements' is brought out in a report of the Nottinghamshire magistrates in the same year. They reported their corn growers, 'to have been likewise willing to help their poor neighbours at home upon reasonable prices and upon trust, who otherwise would have tasted of want in greater measure than they have done'. There is evidence to suggest that even those 'greedy cormorants', the middlemen traditionally blamed for high food prices, were sensitive to these expectations and sought to moderate their prices accordingly. One Norfolk corn merchant in 1597 claimed to have, 'theis three dere yeares last paste . . . uttered great quantities to the poor w[hi]ch have fetched the same at his house or Barne by the

---

[77] There appears to have been a relationship similar to that found in work on probate inventories, although as Roger Schofield has suggested to me, the discrepancy between market and probate valuations may also reflect some allowance for wastage and discount to heirs; Overton, 'Estimating crop yields', p. 373; Marshall, 'Domestic economy lakeland yeoman', p. 219. Although difficult to interpret, Robert Loder's accounts show a lower valuation of grain given to his workers than the market prices he records: Fussell, ed., *Loder's Farm Account*, pp. 28–9, 125, 136–7.

[78] Schofield, 'Through a glass darkly', pp. 586–7; Rule, *Labouring Classes*, chapter 4. For examples of wage assessments (which, it has been argued, acted as wage norms) tending to stick after being increased, see Roberts, 'Wages and wage-earners', p. 218.

bushell, halfe bushell & Peck, and hath allwayes or for the most part
uttered the same . . . after the Rate of Twelve pence in the pound
cheaper then the price of the markett'. In the same year, another
Norfolk man claimed that, 'he hath Continewally this last and
other late deere yeers sold unto the poorer sorte of the towne where he
dwelleth and of the neiboure townes aboute him Corne for three
shillings the bushill when as it was at fyue shillings in the bushill in the
markett'.[79]

Recent research has emphasised the pervasiveness of credit in early
modern society.[80] Credit may also have offered a further source of
insulation against the full impact of harvest failure. If the proposal by
John Cooke in the dearths of the later 1640s to establish banks of piety
to lend to the poor without interest came to nothing, there were other
institutions and relationships through which credit was available to the
poor. Many of the large-scale market transactions were conducted on
credit. Although one of the disadvantages of the market for poorer
consumers was held to be the need to purchase with ready money,
there is some evidence to suggest that they might also purchase on
credit. Farmers, shopkeepers, and traders advanced credit to their
customers. As we have seen accounts and diaries record the loan or
sale of small amounts of grain on credit. In towns, small retailers may
have offered a parallel source of credit. Alehouses sold bread as well as
beer, and might serve as pawnbrokers. Bakers sold bread on account.
A small Oxfordshire village like Kirtlington had several bread sellers
visiting it while its manorial court records cases concerning the attempt
to secure repayment of small quantities of grain. Badgers could also
offer credit to their customers. John Veppen, a licensed badger in
Cambridge, claimed in 1597 to have sold barley to his poor neighbours
'better Cheape then they could buye anye in the markett' and 'for
relieffe of theire necessitie did gyve Credytt for the same'.[81]

The protection offered by these sources of credit differed according
to the nature of the relationship. Credit may have been given relatively
freely in some relationship, for example, those between neighbours or
kin. In others, credit may have been only reluctantly provided, but still
have been vital, for example, in the carrying of rent arrears by
landlords or in sales on credit by petty retailers anxious not to allow

---

[79] HMC, *Buccleuch MSS*. i, p. 272; PRO, SP 16/185/93; 16/177/50; STAC 5/A55/36.
[80] Holderness, 'Credit', pp. 97–109; Holderness, 'Widows', pp. 435–42.
[81] Cook, *Unum Necessarium*, pp. 49–50; Somerset RO, Q/SR 38/66 (husbandman
   bargained in market for two bushels of wheat and gave 6d. 'in earnest'); Clarkson,
   Pre-Industrial Economy, p. 148; Clark, *English Alehouse*, pp. 137–8; Clark, *Provincial
   Society*, pp. 233–4; Pendlebury, *Bolton*, p. 4; Griffiths, 'Kirtlington', p. 310; PRO,
   STAC 5/A55/36.

temporary crisis to disrupt longer-term relationships with their customers.[82] We do not yet know whether the poor of early modern England attempted, as did their counterparts elsewhere, to compensate for their vulnerability as consumers by concentrating their purchases on a particular seller, thus threatening the seller with the loss of all their custom,[83] but some such restraint may have faced middlemen bringing grain to sell in rural communities. Debts entered into within a community and within horizontal relationships may neither have carried interest nor have had a fixed term for repayment. Nor, as in eighteenth-century Massachussets, may they have been expected to be repaid in full.[84] By contrast, other debts may have carried rates of interests whose burden contributed to the increased pauperisation of those forced to enter into them. Distress sales of land, mortgaging land or sales of futures in next year's crops may have staved off starvation,[85] but at some cost to the ability to secure subsistence in the future. Much depended on the precise nature of the debtor–creditor relationship. But whatever the longer-term consequences of indebtedness, the availability of credit offered vital protection against the short-term threat of starvation. Thus, a further cause for the vulnerability of smallholders in the north-west to famine may have been the tendency Appleby noted for landlords there to favour rent exploitation rather than tenant cooperation.[86]

There were both strong positive and negative reasons why those with grain or money to spare should be prepared to advance aid to those rendered vulnerable by harvest failure. Apart from the promptings of church and conscience, neither of which should be underestimated in this period, it was often in the self-interest of the 'better sort'

---

[82] For evidence of the sharp increase in rental arrears following harvest failure, see Stone, *Family and Fortune*, p. 140; Phillips, ed., *Lowther Family Estate Books*, pp. 16–19. The economic conditions of the earlier part of the period when there was competition for land may have made landlords less ready to allow rental arrears than were their successors in the later agricultural depressions (Holderness, 'Credit', p. 102; Mingay, 'Agricultural depression 1730–1750', pp. 324–9), but it is clear that Sir Ralph Assheton, who ordered his steward to abate his tenants' rents after the harvest failure of 1648, was not alone in recognising this obligation of the landlord to his tenants: Wrightson, *English Society*, pp. 57–8; Holderness, *Pre-Industrial England*, p. 79; cf. Watts, *Northumberland*, p. 169; Marshall, 'Lakeland yeoman', p. 217. That landlords were expected to remit a portion of their rents when the harvest failed might be suggested by the polemical comments of Francis Trigge that, 'The incloser . . . will not abate one penie what weather soever come', *Humble Petition*, E2v.

[83] Stirling, *Turkish Village*, pp. 62, 64; Arensberg, *Irish Countryman*, pp. 143, 158.

[84] Wrightson and Levine, *Poverty and Piety*, p. 124; Hobbs Pruitt, 'Self-sufficiency', p. 353; Clark, 'Household economy Connecticut Valley', p. 173.

[85] Bowden, 'Agricultural prices', p. 632; Newcome, *Autobiography*, I, p. 83.

[86] Appleby, 'Agrarian capitalism', pp. 574–94.

to lend to the poor in conditions of dearth which highlighted inequalities and bred resentment. As the author of *Sundry new and artificial remedies against Famine* hinted, if Christian charity was not sufficient reason to remember the poor, 'yet reason, and civill policy might prevaile so much with us for our selves and those which are deare unto us, that we should not stay so long untill our neighbours flames take holde of our owne houses, nor try the extremities that hunger, and famine may work amongst us'. Relief against harvest failure was but one of the reciprocities expected of richer members of the community.[87] Meeting these expectations could not only displace hostility but also bring positive gains in terms of enhanced status and reputation. 'Lending to neighbour, in time of his need/Wins love of thy neighbour, and credit doth breed', counselled Thomas Tusser. As Thomas Fuller wrote of the yeoman in a work published in the difficult years of the later 1640s

> In time of famine he is the Joseph of the countrey, and keeps the poore from sterving. Then he tameth the stocks of corn, which not his covetousnesse but providence hath reserv'd for time of need, and to his poore neighbours abateth somewhat of the high price of the market.[88]

That this was more than wishful thinking can be seen in the need felt by one Kentish yeoman to employ a middleman to sell his grain, because he was 'loath himself to be seen to sell it'.[89] It was the strength of such expectations that prompted aid that ran from the loan of grain without interest to free distribution of grain.

The provision of grain in times of dearth was part of an expected relationship between wealthy and poor which might be extended, and expected, more generally. A moral prohibition on seeking to profit from dearth by selling grain into the highest markets might have been felt more strongly (though by no means always observed) by members of the landed classes. In Warwickshire, for example, members of the gentry were criticised on several occasions for their failure to fulfil this obligation. One of the grievances levelled against the encloser Sir John Newdegate in the aftermath of the Midlands Rising was his practice of selling his grain out of the locality, 'which if it had been brought to the Market would have been a great help to the poor commin[ali]te'; while at Warwick in 1626, Sir Thomas Puckering, the unsuccessful candidate in parliamentary elections for the borough, was compared unfavourably with his opponent, as 'but a stranger in the county and not so commodious by sending corn to market for the overall good of the

---

[87] Platt, *Artificiall remedies against Famine*, A3v; cf., Scott, *Moral Economy*, p. 5.
[88] Tusser, *Good Husbandry*, p. 19; Fuller, *Holy State*, pp. 106–7.
[89]·Clark, *Provincial Society*, p. 232.

people nor a man of such noble hospitality as that worthy family of the Lucys'.[90] If the obligation to provide grain was less formal than in France where, when famine threatened, the *seigneur* was expected to feed his *censitaires*, it was widely expected and frequently observed. (Indeed there were those in England who wished to make lords of the manor formally responsible for the relief of their tenants in harvest failure.)[91]

Successive dearths saw members of the landed classes respond to these expectations. In that of 1586 the Duke of Rutland was reported to have caused his grain in Nottinghamshire upon the first rumour of dearth, 'to be soulde to the porest by stryks and pecks & smale measurs in Nottingham, Newarke and Mansfelde, under the marketts iis. viiid. in every quarter, and so continueth the same wherby the gredines of a number was frustrated, the poore releued, and the expectancy of excessiue dearthe stayed'. Several years later the gentry in Lincolnshire were praised for sending their grain to market to be sold only to the poor and at prices below those prevailing in the market. In the aftermath of the dearths of the 1590s, the Norfolk cousin of Sir Robert Sidney met allegations that he had offended the law by not buying and selling in the market with the counter-claim that he had sold his corn in the market at below market prices and had relieved weekly four-hundred poor men at his door. In the dearth of 1608, Robert Cecil bought grain which he sold to his tenants at a considerable loss to himself of four hundred and sixty-one pounds.[92]

The distribution of grain at under-prices by members of the gentry shaded into more obvious examples of outright benevolence and charity. While many contemporaries believed hospitality and charity to be on the decline, moralists and government continued to urge its importance in combatting dearth. In years of dearth the repeated commands to the gentry to remain on, or to return to, their estates

[90] Warwickshire RO, CR 136/c 2614; Hughes, 'Warwickshire 1620–50', p. 72; cf. the complaints against an Oxfordshire landowner that 'he hath alsoe given nothing to his poore neighboures and Tennants theis twentie yeres to the value of one groate when wheate was sould for tenn shillinges the bushell'; PRO, STAC 8/142/16.

[91] Tilly, 'Food supply and public order in modern Europe', p. 412; Teall, 'Seigneur renaissance France', p. 140; Post, 'Famine, mortality', p. 24; HMC, *Buccleuch MSS.*, iii, p. 355: Lord Montagu to Lord Manchester, 6 Dec. 1630, 'Your first rule, for lords of manors to take order for their tenants is an excellent good one'. *Cf.* the complaints of the failure of their lord to maintain hospitality and relieve the poor made by one group of Kentish tenants after the dearths of the 1590s, Thirsk, ed., *Agrarian History*, 4, p. 63.

[92] PRO, SP 12/190/14; HMC, *De L'Isle MSS.*, ii, pp. 299, 302, 319, 324; Stone, *Crisis*, appendix; xxiii; *cf.* the actions of Cecil's mother in buying and distributing grain in the earlier crisis of 1586/7: BL Lansdowne MS. 103/51, fo. 118v.

reflected the government's belief in the important role they had to play in relieving (and, of course, if necessary, repressing) the poor. As a royal proclamation in the crisis of 1622 noted, 'by this way of reviving the laudable and ancient housekeeping of this Realme, the poore, & such as are most pinched in times of scarcity & want, will be much relieved & comforted'.[93] Despite the perennial lamentations of what we might term the literature of complaint, there are enough examples to suggest that for many the gentle household remained an important centre of relief until at least well into the eighteenth century. According to the historian of the aristocracy in this period, 'there was a steady flow of food and alms to the needy, a matter on which the nobility and gentry continued to set great store, to judge by what they liked to have said about themselves after they were dead'. Indeed the link between the two was sometimes made explicit in the bread doles left to the poor by gentlemen (as well as more humble testators). In Sussex in the 1650s both Sir Thomas Pelham and William Fettiplace gave money to be used to buy grain for the poor when the harvest failed; by the mid eighteenth century some seven- or eight-hundred men and women received at the annual distribution of the Pelham Dole bread, beer, and a few pence each.[94]

Though we need to know more about the practice, as opposed to the prescription, of noble charity, it was apparently more common in dearth, and in conditions of scarcity its role could be considerable. In just under three months in the dearth of 1597, Lord Buckhurst spent one hundred and fifty-four pounds on purchasing imported rye to give away to 'the hungry villagers' in six Sussex villages. In what was presumably also a reference to the harvest failures of the 1590s, Sir George Shirley was said to merit 'the glorious title of father and nourisher of the poor' for 'relieving during the great dearth 500 a day at his gate'. Of the Cheshire gentleman, John Bruen, it was said at his death in 1641, that 'he did usually to his great expence and cost, fill the bellies of great multitudes, which out of his owne and other Parishes, did twice a week resort unto his house . . . And in the deare years he made provision for them, almost every day in the week'. In particular,

---

[93] Greaves, *Society and Religion*, pp. 568–91; Heal, 'Hospitality', pp. 66–93; PRO, SP 14/187/109.

[94] Stone, *Aristocracy*, p. 47; Fletcher, *Sussex*, pp. 155–6; Bushaway, *By Rite*, p. 43. It may well be that further research will reveal that as important a source of relief was offered by the role of the gentle household as a considerable employer of labour. For example, it was reported of one Norfolk gentleman, Sir Francis Lovell, that 'he keepeth a great house at Harlinge, where the poor hath good releife'; Wales, 'Poverty, poor relief, life-cycle', p. 382; Wales, 'Poverty and parish relief', p. 21.

In the time of the great dearth, fearing that divers of his poore neighbours were in great want, as having neither money nor meate: He tooke an opportunity, when the most of his family were gone abroad . . . to call for the keyes of the Store-house, where the corn lay, and presently hee sent into the towne to such persons as were the greatest needers, willing them to bring their baggs with them . . . and so to supply their wants, hee gave them freely and with a cheerful heart, some fourteene measures of corne amongst them at that time.[95]

Although the encomiums of ministers for their dead patrons or of pious descendants for the memory of their ancestors should not be allowed to conceal the fact that noble charity represented only a fraction of noble incomes (nor that this 'generosity' was sometimes triggered by the threats of the poor), its value to the 'harvest-sensitive' was considerably greater. It is not possible to quantify the value of the food and money thus distributed nor number its recipients, but for those able to benefit from the more generous schemes, it could represent a not inconsiderable contribution to that 'makeshift economy' by which the poor survived. In Warwickshire, the charity of Henry, Lord Berkeley meant that the poor were given pottage, beef, mutton, bread, and beer three days a week, as well as receiving alms daily and at various festivals. On the estate of Lady Mildmay, there was a carefully planned system of loans and small bonuses and the provision of work to assist poor families in distress. Noble charity may have been especially important in areas which lagged behind in the introduction of parochial or crisis relief. After a succession of bad harvests, it was reported from Northumberland in 1625 that 'the multitude of poor people . . . would starve if they were not relieved out of the bounties and charges of the gentlemen and others here'.[96]

Charity was not solely the preserve or prerogative of the nobility. Reports of the death of charity are exaggerated, and the dating of its replacement by a more formalised system of poor relief in the late sixteenth century, premature. There is every reason to believe that the harvest crises of the late sixteenth and early seventeenth centuries that gave a powerful impetus to legislative change in poor relief also continued to witness increases in charitable giving. Those below the level of the gentry were also subjected to the same strong pressures – from above, from Church and State; from below, from the poor – to offer relief. In years of dearth the government called on the clergy to

[95] Phillips, *Sackville Family*, 1, p. 231; Shirley, *Stemmata Shirleiana*, p. 87; Hinde, *Holy Life and Happy Death John Bruen*, pp. 187–8; cf. Cliffe, *Yorkshire Gentry*, pp. 114ff.; Cliffe, *Puritan Gentry*, pp. 102–24; Foley, ed., *Records Society Jesus*, II, p. 427; Eden, *State of the Poor*, III, appendix. vi, p. cxxv; Jenkins, *Glamorgan Gentry*, p. 207.
[96] Stone and Fawtier Stone, *Open Elite*, p. 317; Smyth, *Berkeley Manuscripts*, Maclean, ed., II, pp. 368–9; Greaves, *Society and Religion*, p. 565; Watts, *Northumberland*, p. 203.

urge their parishioners, 'to relieve the poor and needy by good house-keeping, by setting them on work, and by other deeds of alms and brotherly compassion'. And, as is becoming increasingly recognised, far from providing a simple prescription for 'a new medicine for poverty', puritan preaching with its notion of stewardship continued to offer a powerful endorsement of the obligatory (if discriminatory) role of charity.[97] The response to such appeals offered the poor another layer of insulation against harvest failure.

Beneficed clergy were not only required to preach up the need for charity in years of harvest failure, but by residing on their benefices, 'to give good example to others in usinge hospitality, almes and releyving their poor neighbors', an injunction reminding them of the requirement in canon law to use part of their income for the poor. Whether the remission of tithe grain offered the land-poor another source of relief against dearth remains to be researched, but not surprisingly, it was often the clergy who took the lead in relieving the poor in years of harvest failure. Examples abound of the initiatives they took. William Shepherd, minister of the Essex parish of Heydon where harvest failure left two-thirds of the village in need of relief in 1579, noted in his register: 'This yer beyng very der yer of corne for whe[a]t was worth xxxs. a quarter, barley xxs. and all other grayn derer, not withstanding I sold my croppe to my power neyghbers so long as yt lasted After the rate as I had sold the yeares before.' At Dry Drayton in Cambridgeshire around about the same period, the minister Richard Greenham similarly provided out of his own corn and persuaded the farmers of the parish to provide a common granary from which the poor were supplied at less than half the market price.[98]

Recent work on the relief of the poor in early modern England confirms that many communities continued to see traditional forms of neighbourly reciprocities as an important source of aid for their own poor. If historians of poverty are right, as seems likely, in their emphasis on the continuing importance of charity, then its role in

---

[97] Slack, 'Poverty and social regulation', pp. 236–7; Sampson, 'Property and poverty' (I am grateful to Margaret Sampson for letting me see this valuable unpublished paper); APC, 1586–7, pp. 277–8; Strype, Life and Acts of Whitgift, III, pp. 348–50. For a good example of the obligations of the propertied towards the poor derived from the concept of stewardship see Perkins, Golden Chaine, pp. 91–100.

[98] APC, 1596–7, pp. 94–6; Youings, Sixteenth-Century England, pp. 255, 273; Hull, 'Agriculture and society', p. 476; Spufford, Contrasting Communities, pp. 51–2. Individual acts of clerical charity abound, but whether these amounted to the third of their income canon law required them to spend on the poor and hospitality seems doubtful; the Essex clergyman, Ralph Josselin, partly to compensate for his earlier failings, attempted to devote a tenth of his income to the poor, a level he did not always reach: Macfarlane, Family Life Ralph Josselin, pp. 51–2.

periods of dearth may have been the greater. If, and where, informal relief was on the decline, there were nonetheless compelling reasons why in conditions of dearth the wealthier sort should revert to earlier practice. Reciprocity and mutual aid were at the heart of the important notion of neighbourliness. In the past, harvest failure must have played a vital role in underwriting the value of this norm, one of whose most important springs was the need for mutual aid to combat the threat posed to all by an uncertain environment. In the early modern period, increasing social polarisation may have meant that wealthier villagers were less dependent on this form of social insurance against harvest failure. But while neighbourly reciprocity might have been on the decline in relationships between those being driven apart by very different levels of wealth, it is clear that charitable giving remained an important consideration in the evaluation of wealthier members of the community. The inner tensions between 'possessive individualism' and continuing membership of the 'moral community' advanced to explain the increase in witchcraft prosecutions point to the continuing force of the sanctions for neighbourly giving. It was reported from Northumberland in the 1660s that the local gentry wanted to prohibit begging, but they were afraid of the curses and clamours of the beggars who continued to be given alms 'for fear of their curses'.[99] Mental beliefs, moral pressures, magisterial directives and the menace of popular discontent all conspired to encourage the 'better sort' to assist their poorer neighbours. Moreover, what might be seen by these new elites of wealthier farmers as the distribution of charity may have had for them the more positive advantage of marking out their status and aligning themselves with the gentry as patrons of the poor.

Informal relief has not attracted the attention it deserves. A teleological obsession with the development of administrative schemes has blunted an awareness of its continuing importance. Despite legislative proscription of begging (in itself, less complete than often assumed), it is clear that toleration of local begging made this a continuing source of support to which the poor had greater recourse when the harvest failed. The decision of the authorities in the West Riding of Yorkshire in 1598 not to enforce parochial rates since, 'many are able to give relief which are not able to give money' is but one of many pointers to the continuing practise of informal relief. As late as the dearths of the later 1640s the poor in one Norfolk community were being relieved by informal means, 'itt being held fitter by our Minister

---

[99] Fletcher, *Reform Provinces*, pp. 184–7; Wales, 'Poverty, poor relief, life-cycle', p. 359; Hey, *English Rural Community*, p. 217; Macfarlane, *Witchcraft*, pp. 174–6; Gibson, ed., *Crosby Records*, p. 136.

to provide for the Pore rather by voluntary contributions then by rates and collections'.[100]

By its very nature, evidence of informal relief is elusive. For example, we only learn of the charity of William Blundell's aunt, who used 'sometimes to give a peck or bushel of corn to several particular persons of the poorest sort', because of the impudence of one recipient who is reported to have said, 'I hope, good Mrs., you will give me now some charity or overmeasure, according as others do after a measure of corn sold.' Not surprisingly, much informal relief took the form of giving small amounts of corn or other food. In Wiltshire in the dearth of 1630, a woman came to beg leave to gather a lapful of peas at a house where she had previously worked as a servant. In some areas the giving of food could assume the form of a right – at least in the eyes of the poor. In early seventeenth-century Anglesea, it was the custom for married couples to be allowed to beg for such gifts in the year after their marriage, the man for grain and seed, the woman for haulms and thrives. From Northumberland in the 1660s it was reported that, 'the beggars wherever corn is stirring (as in winnowing, sowing, etc.) do beg, *or as it were get by custom* a part of the same: and to that end many go about to beg in the time of seeding.'[101] The pressures such popular expectations could produce are graphically brought out in the series of orders recorded in the manorial courts of two Lancashire manors in response to the harvest crisis of 1623 which produced widespread famine there. Millers were to be fined if they allowed those without grain to linger in their mills, and the courts found it necessary to threaten with fines anybody bringing grain to be ground who 'shall give anie almes to anie poore folkes'.[102]

Something of these tensions were eased by forms of relief which, while still voluntary, exhibited more organisation. Of these, the most frequent was the fast. Fasting by the better sort was called for by the government and preached up by the clergy. An obvious attempt to lessen the scarcity, it served several other purposes. It purged society

---

[100] Beier, *Masterless Men*, p. 71; Slack, 'Poverty and social regulation', p. 234; Wales, 'Poverty, poor relief, life-cycle', p. 359. It would be interesting to know whether the spate of 'ales' (a gathering of neighbours to raise money for one of their number) recorded by Adam Eyre in Yorkshire during the harvest failures of the later 1640s represents another form of 'informal' relief against harvest failure: Eyre, 'A Dyurnall', pp. 40–1, 43, 63, 72–3.

[101] Gibson, ed., *Crosby Records*, pp. 136, 283 (my italics); Wiltshire RO, Q/S Great Roll M. 1630/132; Halliwell, *People of Anglesea*, p. 17; *cf.* Wiltshire RO, Q/S Great Roll E. 1634 (the examination of a labourer hired to thresh grain and approached by some poor to let them have a little grain).

[102] Winchester, 'Responses to the 1623 famine', pp. 47–8; *cf.* Newcome, *Autobiography*, I, p. 83.

of the sins that had prompted God to send the scourge of dearth and propitiated the poor. By fasting, the better sort were to taste of the dearth (albeit temporarily) and to relieve the poor out of the savings they made. Something of the symbolic importance of the fast can be seen in its highly publicised recurrence into the eighteenth century.[103] It is difficult now to judge how far fasting made a significant contribution to protecting the 'harvest-sensitive'. Despite intentions, its symbolic rôle may have been greater. But apart from providing a further example of those pressures encouraging the persistence of other forms of relief, it could lead directly to relief of the poor. The example of the Essex minister Ralph Josselin, fasting for one to two meals a week and giving what he saved to the poor in the form of money or meat broth, is one reminder of this. And fasting could make a more significant contribution. The minister Ezekiel Culverwell by his example encouraged his parishioners to fast once a week and out of the savings corn was provided for the poor at half the market price.[104]

The insulation offered by the mechanisms so far discussed was likely to have been greater in rural rather than urban communities. Years of harvest failure could produce peaks in patterns of urban mortality whose concentration in the poorer parishes reflected the social geography of the early modern town.[105] But though the 'harvest-sensitive' in at least the larger urban centres lacked the defences potentially available to the rural poor by virtue of their residence in the countryside, it seems likely that even these groups were not totally exposed to the dearth prices of the market place. As well as producing something of their own food, they also could employ food substitution to offset higher prices.[106] There were urban equivalents for many of the mechanisms so far discussed, and the greater wealth and organisation of urban society were available to offset the greater problem of urban poverty.

---

[103] APC, 1596–7, pp. 94–6; Gardiner, *Fasting and giving of Almes: verie needfall for these difficult times;* Vaughan, *Golde-groue,* R2v–R3r; Thomas, *Religion and Decline of Magic,* pp. 97, 133–6. In 1796 the Dorset justices met at Quarter Sessions and agreed to reduce their families' wheat consumption by a third: Holmes, 'Sources for history of food supplies', p. 97.

[104] Macfarlane, *Family Life Ralph Josselin,* pp. 51–2; Culverwell, *Treatise Of Faith,* preface.

[105] Slack, *Impact of Plague,* pp. 111–43. Since harvest failure did not see the wealthier citizens fleeing to the country, as was common when plague struck, towns were in theory better able to cope with dearth.

[106] We should be careful not to exaggerate the separation of the town from the countryside in this period; that pigs were being kept in almshouses in Canterbury in the 1590s provides an unusual reminder of the ability of the urban poor to meet some of their own food needs: Palliser, *Age of Elizabeth,* p. 208. For examples of substituting cheaper grains or mixing grains with beans in London, see City of London RO, Repertory 23, fo. 413v; *ibid.* Remembrancia, ii, no. 162.

As in the countryside, the nature of the labour market offered those, whose employment withstood the depressed trading conditions dearth brought, some protection against higher food prices. In Coventry in the early 1520s about a quarter of the population were living-in servants and most journeymen would also have been fed by their employers on working days. In towns, trade guilds offered an additional source of relief not available in rural villages.[107] Networks of credit must have offered a shield for some against harvest failure. The decision of the corporation at Winchester to remit poorer tenants their rent arrears provides one example of sources of urban credit to ease difficulties in dearth, about which we need to know more. Neighbourliness was also important in an urban context. While these ties may have been strongest amongst artisans and their neighbours, both the Norwich and Ipswich censuses of the poor record examples of those said 'to live upon their friends'.[108]

Even in the urban market, transactions in grain reflected the pressures that surrounded its sale, especially in conditions of dearth, and both sellers and purchasers might attempt to deflect popular hostility by reserving part of the grain for distribution or sale to the poor at under-price. Dealers set aside grain to be sold to the poor at under-prices. At Reading in 1631 the corn masters were reported to be setting aside a sack in every load to be sold in small quanties at the rate of twelve pence a bushel under the market price. In 1648 in the grain markets of Wiltshire the cornsellers agreed to set aside a bushel in every quarter to be stored and sold to the poor at a lower price. Purchasers of corn might also make allowances for the poor. At Woodchurch in Kent, Sir Walter Roberts purchased ten quarters of wheat in the dearth of 1631 and left half to be sold to the poor. While his example may reflect the strength of the pressures on the gentry to be charitable, this was a practice commonly followed in that county and elsewhere. Farmers and dealers supplying larger urban centres left grain to be sold at below market prices. From Faversham in Kent it was reported in 1597 that, 'the Countrye people . . . Gratefye the poore in selling twoe q[uar]ters of wheate in the markett after iiijs. the bushell for eu[er]ye skore they passed through the Towne to London, wheate [being] then worth viis. the bushell'.[109]

Informal relief, which again remains for the most part invisible or under-researched, also played a rôle in towns. Begging by the local poor

---

[107] Phythian-Adams, *Coventry*, pp. 134, 204; Pearl, 'Social policy', p. 130.
[108] Rose, 'Winchester', p. 157; Clark and Slack, *English Towns*, p. 122.
[109] PRO, SP 16/182/81; 16/191/4; Wiltshire RO, Q/S Great Roll H. 1648/not no.; Kent AO, Fa. AC3, fo. 44v.

was tolerated in cities as well as villages. In the capital itself, the Lord Mayor's response to the enforcement of the late Elizabethan statute on poor relief was to recommend to the aldermen that they should prescribe some fit time of day for the parish poor to seek relief from the houses of the richer sort. There may have been many like the Nantwich mercer who after the harvest failures of the 1590s calculated that he had spent all but five pounds of his reduced profits, 'by reason of the dearth and great charge I lived at and giving away to the poor, for corn was at such a very fearful price'.[110] The church was used also in towns, large and small, to exhort the wealthy to be charitable. At Southampton in the dearth of 1608, the Corporation ordered that the ministers after their sermons should 'give the people admonition to remember the poore' and church wardens were to stand at the door to take the collection. In the later dearth of 1631 at Dorchester voluntary contributions were gathered in the church for the provision of corn (and the rector's contribution compared very unfavourably with the bounty of others).[111] Fasting was not only recommended by the church, but also prescribed by city councils. In London in 1596, the abandonment of the livery companies' feasts helped to finance the distribution of four-thousand loaves weekly.[112]

If the gentry abandoned the country for the city, they could not escape the obligation to relieve the poor. For example, in the dearth of 1596, Sir Thomas Egerton was distributing weekly alms to sixty-two inhabitants of the London parish of St. Dunstan's. In the later dearth of 1608, the Lord Chancellor gave forty pounds to be distributed in bread to the poor of Coventry.[113] Neither was such giving confined to the capital nor to wealthy gentlemen or clerics. At Bristol in 1597, all the men of ability in the city were enjoined to give a meal of meat to upwards of eight poor people each. In the same year, the wealthiest citizens at Worcester 'took into their homes "above two hundred poor and aged persons" and supported them'. At Winchester in the earlier dearth of 1587 this obligation was made more formal with the maintenance of poor children being specified as a term in some of the city's leases.[114] Individual acts of philanthropy by wealthy urban patricians and others less wealthy, orchestrated on occasion by public fasts, could produce levels of giving that rivalled formal relief.

[110] City of London RO, Journal 24, fo. 289; Clark and Slack, *English Towns*, p. 108.
[111] Southampton City RO, SC2/1/6, fo. 71; Mayo, ed., *Municipal Records Dorchester*, pp. 616–17; *cf.* Colchester RO, D/Y 2/7/226.
[112] City of London RO, Journal 24, fos. 143v, 149v, 152.
[113] Clay, *Economic Expansion*, I, pp. 226–7; Coventry RO, A14(a), fo. 165v.
[114] Toulmin Smith, ed., *Maire of Bristowe Is Kalendar*, p. 63; Dyer, *Worcester*, p. 166; Rose, 'Winchester', p. 157. For the emphasis on the role of charity in combating the dearths

Collectively, their contribution to protecting the poor from harvest failure could be significant, as has been argued was the case in London in the 1590s.[115] Philanthropy that took the form of doles or bequests to endow regular distributions of bread had an obvious value in conditions of dearth. Some were intended specifically to afford the urban 'harvest-sensitive' insulation against high food prices. Coventry, Chester and the capital were all cities whose citizens benefitted from bequests to finance the purchase and distribution at subsidised prices of grain.[116]

What did distinguish urban relief was the greater degree of organisation. This was most apparent in the purchase and distribution of food in the form of grain or bread to the needy. Nevertheless, despite superior financial and administrative bases, towns found the call on their resources considerable. While urban elites sought to finance grain purchases through town revenues – an increase in rates or the re-allocation of other sources of incomes like market tolls, less commonly by desperate measures like the sale of town's ordnance as at Faversham in Kent–they too were forced to rely on less formal funding. The provision of grain in many towns depended on the 'charitable' inclination of members of the ruling group to advance loans or on persuading dealers to set aside grain to be sold more cheaply to poorer consumers.[117] While the manner by which urban grain purchases were financed illustrates the blurring of informal and formal attempts to relieve dearth, this policy is best discussed under the general heading of official policies to cope with harvest failure.

Official measures to combat the consequences of harvest failure provide a more familiar reason for early modern England's resistance to famine. The government's policies were codified in the first Book of Orders issued in 1586, but they clearly predated this and had been long anticipated by local, especially urban, government.[118] When prices

of the 1590s in London, see City of London RO, Journal 24, fo. 141.
[115] Archer, 'Social policy in Elizabethan London' (I am grateful to Ian Archer for allowing me to see this unpublished paper which contains the most complete analysis of the relative roles of formal and informal relief in an urban context); Pearl, 'Social policy', pp. 122–31; Herlan, 'Poor relief in London', p. 44; Herlan, 'Poor relief in parish of Dunstan', pp. 31–2.
[116] Greaves, Society and Religion, p. 584; Phythian-Adams, Coventry, p. 55; Chester, 'Poor relief in Coventry', pp. 192–3; Gras, Evolution English Corn Market, pp. 80–1.
[117] Ibid; Chartres, Inland Trade, p. 60; Leonard, Early History English Poor Relief, chapters 5, 7; Dyer, Worcester, pp. 166–7; MacCaffrey, Exeter, pp. 37, 85, 116, 157–8; Coventry RO, A14(a), fo. 132; Everitt, 'Marketing agricultural produce', p. 487; Kent AO, Fa AC3, fo. 44; PRO, SP 16/182/81; Essex RO, D/B3/479, no. 1.
[118] Leonard, Poor Relief; Slack, 'Books of Orders'.

rose, exports of grain were to be banned, censuses taken of grain stocks, the market regularly supplied and the storage and sale of grain closely regulated. All this was intended explicitly to ensure a supply of grain at prices which the poor could afford. These policies to police the marketing of grain were reinforced by the developing system of poor relief. Together they are held to have played a critical role in mitigating the impact of harvest failure. Much of what they intended is too familiar to need much discussion. But in the early modern state intentions were not achievements. There is still considerable scope for exploring how effective policies intended to ensure a supply of grain were in actually providing the 'harvest-sensitive' with grain. The history and geography of their local enforcement and the definitions of eligibility on which they were implemented await detailed research.

Parochial poor relief was not by itself adequate to offset the impact of harvest failure. Given full expression in the late Elizabethan legislation of the 1590s which provided for a public rate, this form of poor relief was slow to be fully implemented and in its funding, as much as in its expenditure, was highly vulnerable to the impact of harvest failure. As recent studies have shown, parochial poor relief normally offered support at moments of dependency within the cycle of family formation and dissolution to a relatively small percentage of the population. Harvest failure dramatically reversed the proportion of ratepayers (usually a minority) to those in need of relief. Indeed, it could create a vicious spiral in which the additional burden of poor relief pushed further families from independence into dependency. Some idea of this increased burden can be seen in the example of the Norfolk village of Cawston, where the harvest failures of the later 1590s resulted in assessments of ½d. to 20d. weekly instead of 'normal' rate of ½d. to 3s. 1d. per month.[119]

To cope with the crisis of harvest failure, relief was needed in much larger amounts and for the much greater numbers of the conjunctural poor. Consequently, dearth years saw sharp increases in poor relief expenditure. At Norwich in the dearth of 1631, the city's authorities were forced to rate 'the better rank of citizens' three times what they had previously paid and the rest of the citizens double. In some London parishes, the dearth of the later 1640s brought a doubling in the poor rate. Similar increases were recorded in both towns and villages.[120] While some increase would have been necessary to meet

[119] Wales, 'Poverty, poor relief, life-cycle'; Newman Brown, 'Receipt of poor relief', pp. 405–22; Amussen, 'Class and gender relations', pp. 73–4.
[120] PRO, SP 16/177/55; /178/26; Pearl, 'Social policy', p. 124; Wrightson, 'Puritan reformation of manners', p. 184; Emmison, 'Poor relief accounts', p. 114.

the higher costs of relieving regular pensioners, the scale of these increases reflected the greater burden placed on the parish as the precarious independence of the 'harvest sensitive' was undermined by rising prices. Relief for the conjunctural poor could take a variety of forms – the provision of work, the binding out of their children, monetary payments, or the provision of grain – but it was the last of these that was the most common. In many communities, the poor rate (even when doubled or trebled) was not sufficient to fund such a policy.

Policies for making grain available in dearth years were first implemented and were at their most developed in towns. From at least the early sixteenth century, many towns including London, had their own granaries. Urban granaries were not without their problems however, and a more common policy was to buy in grain when the harvest looked uncertain.[121] This was a risky policy and one which could provoke opposition from both magistrates and people in the areas of supply. But against the temporal risk-spreading offered by urban granaries, towns were able use their resources and patterns of trade to take advantage of the possibilities of geographical risk-spreading by importing grain from the Baltic. Although, significantly, this policy may have become less pronounced as early as 1608, imports of Baltic rye played an important role in the relief of both urban centres and their hinterlands in the crises of the sixteenth century. London, Norwich, Bristol, Shrewsbury, Worcester, Exeter, as well as smaller towns like Barnstaple or Maldon, were among those towns importing grain in the dearths of the 1590s.[122]

Urban grain stocks could be used in several ways to offer relief. They could be used as 'equalisation funds' to moderate the rise in prices in the retail market. More commonly, they were used to provide the poor with grain at subsidised prices. This was a policy widely implemented from cities like London, Norwich, Exeter, Winchester, Leicester, and Chester down to small towns like Lyme Regis in Dorset.[123] At Norwich in 1596 where rye had been selling at 6s 4d. or more, 4,600 quarters of rye were imported and sold at 4s. a bushel; at Shrewsbury, where rye

---

[121] Leonard, *English Poor Relief*, chapters 3, 7; McGrath, 'Marketing of food London area', pp. 140–2; Clark, '"Ramoth-Gilead of the Good"', p. 175.

[122] Zins, *England and the Baltic*, pp. 248–63; Federowicz, *England's Baltic Trade*, pp. 110–15; Dyer, *Worcester*, pp. 166–7; Leonard, *English Poor Relief*, pp. 122–4; MacCaffrey, *Exeter*, p. 85; Pound, *Poverty and Vagrancy*, p. 51; Wyot, 'Diary Philip Wyot', p. 105.

[123] Gras, *English Corn Market*, chapter 3; Sachse, ed., *Minutes Norwich Court of Mayoralty*; Leicester RO, Hall Papers BR II/18/14, no. 98; Stocks, ed., *Leicester Borough Records 1603–1688*, p. 204; MacCaffrey, *Exeter*, pp. 37, 85; Woodward, *Trade of Elizabethan Chester*, pp. 49–50; Whiteway, 'Diary of William Whiteway', p. 73.

had been selling for 12s. a bushel, 3,200 bushels were brought in and sold at 8s. the bushel. At Worcester in the following year £1,800 was spent on Baltic grain which was then sold in the market at some 10 to 20 per cent below current prices. Grain might also be baked and then sold to the poor in small loaves, as at Shrewbury or Maidstone. Less regularly it would appear, grain might be distributed free to those in most need. At Bristol in 1596 the authorites bought 3,000 quarters of Baltic rye (having spent £1,200 importing grain in the previous harvest) which they sold much under the market rate 'and many pecks were given among the poor of the city'.[124] If the volume of subsidised sales was sufficiently large, then the use of grain stocks in this way too could reduce prices in the market. The value of these schemes in shielding the urban 'harvest-sensitive' is shown in the example of Coventry. There, subsidized sales of oats from a store specially provided were made from tubs taken through the streets of the city. The scheme, which ran for just over a year from March 1597 to March 1598, supplied regularly some 500 to 700 households, perhaps as much as a third and, at its peak, a half of the city's population.[125]

A similar policy of selling grain at subsidised prices was also adopted by rural communities in dearth years. In 1595, the Privy Council had called on magistrates 'by charitable persuasions [and personal example] to every man . . . being of wealth and ability' to contribute to a stock with which to buy grain to sell to the poor in the market place at under-prices.[126] Norfolk provides a good example of the successful implementation of this policy. The 1631 report on the marketing of grain in that county noted, 'in Norfolk where corn abounds the inhabitants of the better and abler sort provide in a dearth for the poor in the market of their own town'. Their practice was 'to provide corn for the poor at home in their own town . . . at a very easy and under-rate'. As the report makes clear, this had been the policy from at least the 1580s. One of those called before Star Chamber in 1597 to answer charges of marketing abuses in fact turned out to have bought with others of the 'better sort' of Kenninghall in Norfolk twenty-five combs of rye to sell in small portions and at reasonable prices to their poor. In 1631 the justices of south-west Norfolk reported that parishes had at their command laid in a store of corn for the poor, 'which is daylie uttered amongst them att a farr lower price then the market doth

---

[124] Pound, 'Elizabethan census', p. 136; Leighton, 'Chronicles Shrewsbury', pp. 335–6; Dyer, *Worcester*, pp. 166–7; Everitt, 'Marketing agricultural produce', p. 481n.; Seyer, *Memoirs Historical and Topographical of Bristol*, II, pp. 254–5.
[125] Chester, 'Poor relief Coventry', pp. 168–70; *cf.* Sachse, ed., *Minutes Norwich Court of Mayoralty*, pp. 92–3, 119.
[126] HMC, *Buccleuch MSS.*, iii, p. 35.

yealde.' In the dearths of the later 1640s communities in Norfolk again bought in grain to sell to the poor at under-price or to distribute free.[127]

Both the geography and chronology of the rural implementation of this policy need further research.[128] It may well predate the introduction of the first Book of Orders. But it is the provincial reports this called for that first provide extensive evidence of this practice in rural areas. It became more frequent in subsequent crises, being perhaps most extensive after the issue of the Book of Orders of 1631. For example, in Hertfordshire in 1623 the justices and gentlemen had, 'by there good and charitable exsamples and perswasiones', provided grain at nearly half the market price in 'euery parish where need requireth'. In 1631 the 'princepall Inhabitants' of most of Essex's parishes had laid in corn for their poor, 'abateinge in some p[ar]ishes Two shillings, in some xviiid., others viid, ye bz. [i.e. bushel] of ye price of ye Market accordinge to ye necessitie of theire poore'; while from east Sussex in the same year the magistrates reported that, 'the most substantiall inhabitants of those parishes where the poore did most abounde . . . partly by the perswasions of us and of their ministers and of their owne charytable disposition have laid down in some one parish about thirty pounds, in another twenty pounds, some lesse, according to the extent and abilitie of theire parishes, above their assessments' to finance the purchase of grain. At its most organised, grain was distributed to the poor in their own homes under this policy, as in Cambridgeshire in 1631 where the poor had their grain at least twelve pence under market price. While the later crises of the 1640s saw further examples of this policy, it may well be that the period of the 1630s represented a peak in its implementation. Significantly, the later harvest failure of 1661/2, one of the most serious in the period, provides markedly less evidence of the formal implementation of this policy.[129]

Traditionally, the system of transfer payments operated under the poor law has been held to be an important part of the explanation for England's resistance to famine. Certainly, a comparison with explanations offered for the continuing presence of famine in other parts of the British Isles or the Continent would lend weight to this analysis.[130]

---

[127] Thirsk and Cooper, eds., *Economic Documents*, pp. 346–7; PRO, STAC 5/A55/36; Wales, 'Poverty and parish relief', chapter 5.

[128] Leonard, *English Poor Relief*, provides an introduction to the subject. The preliminary outline of the geography and chronology that follows is based on research in central and local papers, which I intend to report on more fully at a later date.

[129] PRO, SP 14/140/41; 16/177/43; /182/20; Fletcher, *Sussex*, p. 150; PRO, SP 16/189/75; Outhwaite, 'Dearth and government intervention'.

[130] Mitchinson, 'Control of famine in pre-industrial Scotland'; Smout, 'Famine and

Gains in agriculture raised the output of food to the point at which harvest failure produced spatial and social shortages which the organised transfer of reduced surpluses could overcome. Increases in the levels of regular relief offered to the parish poor (for which increases the renewed dearths of the period may be partly responsible) were likely to have been especially important in offering protection to exactly those groups (the elderly and the very young) that modern work has identified as being most at risk of starvation when the harvest fails.[131] Formal crisis relief with its policy of providing subsidised or free distribution of grain offered the much larger group of 'harvest-sensitive' poor the possibility of protection from the problem of declining 'exchange-entitlements' that Sen has identified as a major cause of starvation amongst this group.

In part, however, the prominence attributed to formal relief reflects the nature of the surviving evidence. By its very nature, poor relief has left a more visible impress in the historical record. But before we can be certain of the exact value of crisis relief, we need far more detailed studies of its local implementation – were the quantities of grain sufficiently large, the prices sufficiently low and the period of subsidy sufficiently long to offer effective relief against the problem of declining 'exchange-entitlements'? By contrast, the lack of an official (and hence record-keeping) framework has meant that other means of protection against harvest failure have not received sufficient attention.

The continuing importance of these forms of relief has been neglected because of the teleological distortions that disfigure the study of the history of social welfare. Studies of poor relief have tended to emphasise change at the expense of an attentiveness to continuity; discussions have been organised around a too-sharp transition from charity (itself a questionable label to describe earlier forms of relief) to legal provision. An anachronistic reading of early modern society as a market society marked by the triumph of economic individualism has helped to underwrite this interpretation. Although more work remains to be done, the evidence here collected cautions against a premature tendency to see early modern England as a fully-fledged market society in which the social impact of harvest failure can be read off from the evidence of wage rates and price series. In a world in which the content of relationships is perhaps better captured by considerations of

famine-relief in Scotland'; Post, 'Famine, mortality', p. 22; Sogner, 'Demographic crisis', pp. 127–8.
[131] Watkins and Menken, 'Famine in historical perspective', pp. 654–6. Both the level of wages and relief payments seem to have risen after the mid seventeenth century: Wales, 'Poverty and parish relief', Roberts, 'Wages and wage-earners', p. 196.

oeconomy, rather than economy, protection against harvest failure was also to be found in a much wider set of relationships: amongst others the relationship between landlord and tenant, farmer and labourer, master and servant, rich and poor.

Rather than seeking to evaluate the respective contribution of 'formal' or 'informal' relief in offering protection against dearth, it would be better to emphasise the degree of overlap between them. There was a similarity of language between church sermon and government decree in dearth years. Both employed the vocabulary of compassion and obligation. The government called for contributions to the purchase of grain for sale to the poor to be given 'according to their devotions, and as charity requireth in this time of dearth'; the church was to 'exhort the rich sort to be liberall to help the more with mony or victuall nedfull'.[132] This confusion of language was made necessary as much by the inadequacies of parochial assessment to fund the large purchases of grain necessary as well as by the apparent legal uncertainty over the government's ability to dictate to holders of grain the prices at which they should sell to the poor. Formal relief succeeded to the extent that it reflected not simply the degree of political centralisation, but also drew on the attitudes (of both fear and charity) that underpinned the protection afforded by informal practices and exchanges. Similarly, while emphasis has been given here to the continuing importance of patterns of reciprocity, it would be a mistake in turn to exaggerate their importance. Because evidence of the protection offered by these forms of informal relief is necessarily diffuse, it is difficult to gauge or to quantify the protection they afforded. Taken singly their value might have been slight. What was important was the opportunity they offered to the poor to piece them together with more formal relief to secure access to food. The 'harvest-sensitive' in early modern England survived by being able to marry together the protection offered by formal and informal relief.

But, while it was the inter-relationship between formal and informal crisis relief that offered protection against harvest failure, it is clear that the relationship between the two was far from uniform. The balance varied from community to community and from region to region. Nor was acccess to either of these forms of relief uniform. Neither was freely available to all. The protection they offered against famine was socially as well as geographically selective. A fuller exploration of the

---

[132] HMC, *Buccleuch MSS.*, iii, p. 35; Goring and Wake, eds., *Northampton Lieutenancy Papers*, pp. 30–2. Compare the situation in eighteenth-century Norway where poor relief was provided for those not looked after on 'good farms', Sogner, 'Demographic crisis', pp. 124–5.

selective nature of crisis relief will provide a final and finer-grained explanation for the patterning of famine-free and and famine-prone areas and point up its consequences for the maintenance of order in the face of harvest failure.

Both forms of relief presupposed membership of a community. To take advantage of the full panoply of protection required membership of a community which not only had a surplus to transfer, but also local social and administrative structures to secure that transfer. Grain-deficient upland communities in the highland zone, with limited arable and low yields and a pattern of dispersed settlement, may have lacked both the surpluses and structures to cope with the impact of harvest failure. While further research might be expected to reveal that they had their own mechanisms to minimise the impact of harvest failure (prominent among them migration),[133] it is probable that the economic specialisation which pulled them out of a subsistence–sufficiency orientation weakened these. To the greater natural risk faced by these poor soil uplands with less favourable climate was added economic risk. Where self-sufficiency in arable production had predominated, the under-development of market networks in grain meant that when the harvest failed it was harder to transfer surpluses into these regions. Where, as has been argued was common, communities in these areas were marked by a greater degree of social homogeneity, groups with surpluses to transfer informally to their neighbours were likely to have been fewer. The general absence of a resident magistracy and weak parochial administration, as well as the lower density of gentlemen in such regions, meant that there were not the administrative structures to compensate for these weaknesses by organising formally the import and distribution of food.[134] Evidence of crisis relief is, significantly, noticeably absent for famine-prone areas like Northumberland, while the implementation of parochial relief lagged behind progress in the south-east.[135] The vulnerability of smallholders and labourers in communities with these characteristics is reflected in the patterns of migration in early modern England. The dominant pattern was one of movement out of the marginal uplands of the north and west and into the lowlands of the south and east, a

---

[133] There is considerable evidence to suggest that migration was a common response in these regions (*e.g.* Beier, *Masterless Men*, pp. 118–19) but, as in other societies and periods, its frequency may be a telling indication of the absence of available alternative strategies to combat harvest failure.

[134] Appleby, *Famine*; Thirsk, 'Seventeenth century agriculture', p. 167; Thirsk, *Peasant Farming*, pp. 45–7; Everitt, *Change in the Provinces*, p. 22–3; Everitt, 'Farm labourers', pp. 409–11; Malcomson, 'Kingswood colliers', pp. 85–127.

[135] Watts, *Northumberland*, pp. 202–3; Fletcher, *Reform Provinces*, pp. 183–228.

pattern of movement from upland to lowland reflected in microcosm in individual counties. When the harvest failed there may have been many like Lancelot Brown of the village of Greystoke in Cumberland who, when famine struck in 1623, 'went forth of the country for want of means'.[136] A disproportionate number of those poor wandering men and women whose anonymous burials are recorded in parish registers thoughout England probably wandered from such communities or their equivalents in Wales and Scotland.

By the later seventeenth century the shadow of famine had been lifted from these previously vulnerable communities. They, like the rest of the country, were the beneficiaries of a slowing down in the rate of population growth, an increase in agricultural output and in real wages that brought better market integration for pastoral economies in particular. But if this convergence of factors brought an end to crises of subsistence in even previously vulnerable areas, this did not mean an end to the insecurities that dearth brought. Dearth retained its prominence in popular culture and consciousness. Almanacs and oral weather omens, for example, reveal a continuing popular anxiety about the quality of future harvests, while diaries continued to record the consequences for the poor of sudden, sharp increases in prices.[137] At the very end of the seventeenth century Charles Davenant drew attention to the limited carry over of grain even in good years, and well into the eighteenth century harvest fluctuations remained the dominant cause of economic instability.[138] Indeed, the underlying increase in the numbers of those dependent on the market for both food and employment made the problem of falling 'exchange-entitlements' potentially that much greater when the harvest failed. Harvest failure thus continued to exacerbate the problem of 'hidden hunger' among the labouring poor and, as the later mortality crises of the 1720s and 1740s vividly demonstrated, it could still give a vicious twist to the complex relationship between poor nutritional status and disease that made the impact of epidemics so devasting.[139] The disappearance of

---

[136] Beier, *Masterless Men*, p. 37; Laslett, *World We Have Lost Further Explored*, p. 131.

[137] Capp, *Astrology*, pp. 63–4, 114, 204; Jones, *Seasons and Prices*, pp. 54–5; Heywood, ed.; *Diary Rev. Henry Newcome*; Turner, ed., *Autobiography and Diaries Rev. Oliver Heywood*; Henry, *Diaries and Letters Philip Henry*; Meeke, *Diary Rev. Robert Meeke*.

[138] Thirsk and Cooper, eds., *Economic Documents*, pp. 814–15; Ashton, *Economic Fluctuations*.

[139] Carmichael, 'Infection, hidden hunger'; Taylor, 'Synergy'; Scrimshaw, 'Contemporary food and nutrition studies'; Foster, 'Demography in the North-West', pp. 5–6, 53; Gooder, 'Crisis of 1727–30 in Warwickshire'; Chambers, *Vale of Trent*; Johnston, 'Epidemics of 1727–30 in South-west Worcestershire', pp. 283–4, 286; Skinner, 'Crisis mortality in Buckinghamshire'. In the Cambridge Group's analysis, 'one-star crises' (in which mortality was between 10 and 20 per cent above trend) showed little diminution over time: Wrigley and Schofield, *Population History*, p. 335.

'crises of subsistence' precisely defined as a demographic measure should not be allowed to obscure the fact that for individuals the threat of starvation might remain very real. In 1683, for example, the overseers of the poor of a Worcestershire parish recorded the allocation of a bushel of wheat to one Henry Best, 'when he was almost starved'. Famine might have disappeared, but starvation as a 'class phenomenon' remained.[140]

The continuing threat harvest failure posed to the poor's subsistence thus made crisis relief, both formal and informal, of great importance to the 'harvest-sensitive' even in areas not subject to famine and in the period after famine's disappearance. But, if such relief was becoming geographically more widespread, access to such relief remained socially selective. It presupposed membership of a community. Without such membership there was claim to neither the protection offered by the social economy nor the formal defences of poor relief, a fact grimly attested to by the fate of those wandering poor who died in the streets of early modern England's villages and towns. Nor did residence automatically guarantee relief. To qualify for formal relief required a stated period of residence and, in conditions of rising expenditure on relief, authorities were probably quick to see this enforced: for example in the dearth of 1596/7 the constables of one Suffolk town were paid to remove almost 250 newcomers.[141] Similarly, crisis relief allowed those in charge of its distribution to define eligibility. In Wiltshire during the dearths of the later 1640s, the justices ordered that apart from the impotent poor only those who could show a certificate from their minister and four or five of the 'chief inhabitants', declaring that 'they are laborious & painefull & by reason of their hard charge of children they are not able to mainteyne their familie by their hard labour', were to receive subsidised grain. This same group were to decide how much grain they should receive.[142] If further research confirms that formal crisis relief was in decline in the later seventeenth century, this is a trend that can only have increased

---

[140] Barnard, 'Some Beoley parish accounts', p. 21. For evidence suggesting the cumulative impact of 'hidden hunger' on the harvest-sensitive, see Lee, 'Short-term variations in vital rates, prices, and weather', pp. 357, 372; Skipp, *Crisis and Development*, pp. 13–39. It is to be hoped that socially-specific reconstitution studies will be able to answer the problem of whether aggregative studies mask a continuing vulnerability of a part-population – the labouring poor – to harvest-related mortality.

[141] Styles, 'Evolution Law of Settlement', pp. 44–5; McIntosh, 'Responses to the poor in late medieval and Tudor England'; *cf.* Palliser, *Age of Elizabeth*, p. 121; Winchester, 'Responses to the 1623 famine', p. 48. The peaks in vagrancy in years of harvest failure therefore may, in part, reflect a greater sensitivity on the parts of the authorities to the problems of vagrants.

[142] Wiltshire RO, Q/S Order Book 1, H. 1647/8.

the poor's dependency on relief controlled by local elites who were thus able to define eligibility.

Protection, therefore, demanded membership of a community, whose rules and boundaries were defined increasingly by those chief inhabitants for whom growing wealth made redundant the reasons for observing customary patterns of mutual aid against dearth. Access to that membership was itself becoming more selective. The loss of land progressively restricted the circuits of exchange within the social economy in which the land-poor might be qualified to enter, and in the longer-term harvest failure gave a powerful push to a more conscious and restrictive definition of membership and 'rights', such as gleaning, by local elites.[143] In towns as well, there is evidence to suggest that harvest failure prompted a more restrictive definition of eligibility for relief.[144] While emphasis has been given here to the persistence of some forms of informal relief, it would be a mistake to ignore the evidence of the literature of complaint that these were under threat. While some relationships withstood change, it was undoubtedly the case that the abnormal situation of dearth prompted a temporary return to practices that had been, or were in the process of being, abandoned in the growing pursuit of possessive individualism. It was the fact that 'traditional' practices were being repudiated or their observance made discretionary, rather than obligatory, that gave elites scope for greater control. That the same relationship, for example the sale of grain locally, could be treated either as an exercise in 'neighbourliness' or as a commercial transaction in which a market price was exacted further emphasised the importance of the recipient's status.[145] That economic relationships, offering potential protection

---

[143] For an example of harvest failure leading to an intensification of local controls, see Ingram, 'Ecclesiastical justice', pp. 375–7. The uncertainty that surrounded the poor's right to glean (Ault, *Open-Field Farming*; Bushaway, *By Rite*, pp. 138–41) made it vulnerable to more restrictive definitions; for example, in one Norfolk village in the 1630s gleaning was annexed to the poor rates and access to it made contingent on a certificate from the churchwardens and overseers of the poor; Wales, 'Poverty and parish relief', p. 43. For evidence of discrimination in access to gleaning and the favouring of certain groups amongst the poor, see Best, *Farming and Memorandum Book*, pp. 25, 46.

[144] For an example of harvest failure leading to a discrimination between deserving and undeserving poor, see Phythian-Adams, *Coventry*, pp. 64–6.

[145] Payments in kind or assistance against harvest failure can also be seen as combining good economic, as well as political, sense to employers. It allowed them to make a *temporary* adjustment to the conditions of dearth over which they retained control. By contrast, an increase in wage assessments, called for by legislation, but only sporadically enforced, might have seen a permanent increase and would have denied them the leverage over their labourers that discretionary relief permitted them. On wage assessments see, Foot, *Effect Elizabethan Statute Artificers on Wages*; Roberts, 'Wages and wage-earners', p. 192.

against harvest failure, such as service or harvest employment, were both subject to cyclical trends eroding their use and vulnerable to harvest failure underlined the importance of reputation in the local labour market. That harvest failure itself encouraged a temporary, more restrictive access to areas of the social economy offering relief – for example, gleaning, harvest labour – had the same effect.[146] The young Somerset groom, before the courts for a theft of a peck of wheat in dust 'to releiue him in his necessities, for that he being without a Master, and unsettled, was like to famishe for want of food' exemplifies the problems of those without claim to relief.[147] In circumstances such as these the labouring poor's dependence could be used to demand a shift in the 'rate of exchange' in those relationships between superiors and inferiors central to the maintenance of order in early modern society.

Such a shift was not achieved without contest. (Nor was the change complete: in many ways this contest over the range and nature of the responsibilities of rural elites towards their neighbours remains at the centre of rural conflict well into the nineteenth century.) The continuing threat of harvest failure underlined the value of such relationships for both these groups since both, in contrasting ways, remained vulnerable. For the poor they offered protection from famine, for the propertied protection from the fear of disorder and the validation of their authority. Characteristically, Hobbes captured the nature of this exchange when he wrote that what men usually called charity was either a 'contract, whereby they seek to purchase friendship, or fear, which maketh them to purchase peace'.[148] In this sense years of dearth continued to provide an arena in which the nature of social responsibilities between the poor and their betters could be continually re-negotiated.[149] But over time this often bitter,

---

[146] Kussmaul, *Servants*, pp. 97–119; PRO, SP 14/137/16; Roberts, 'Wages and wage-earners', pp. 260–1; for examples of the restriction of those allowed to glean in years of dearth, see Ingram, 'Ecclesiastical justice', p. 75; Wales, 'Poverty and parish relief', p. 18; *Notes and Queries for Somerset and Dorset*, 1, pp. 211–12; King, 'Crime, law and society', p. 288.

[147] Somerset RO, Q/SR 64.1/121. Contemporaries believed dearth encouraged masters to put off their servants: Standish, *Commons Complaints*, p. 16; Cook, *Unum Necessarium*, p. 5. The vulnerability of servants and the independent young (a group that enjoyed a weak position in the social economy outside of their employment) is reflected in their predominance among arrested vagrants, as well as their appearances in criminal records and disorder in the period: Beier, *Masterless Men*, pp. 24–5, 44; Walter, 'Oxfordshire rising', p. 123 and note 113.

[148] Hobbes, *The Elements of Law*, p. 34, quoted in Hill, *Society and Puritanism*, p. 290.

[149] Thus, until the end of the eighteenth century, years of harvest failure saw a reversion to earlier practices under the threat of harvest failure; *e.g.* Stevenson, 'Food riots in England', p. 48.

but unequal contest over the obligatory nature of relief resulted increasingly (if never finally) in a redefinition of reciprocities as discriminatory and discretionary charity. Where this was achieved, it allowed the propertied to pass off as the gift what had prevously been perceived as a right. That the gift could take the form of food gave this exchange added significance in a society in which the giving and receiving of food was encrusted with meanings. We might see this as, in Raymond William's terms, a transition from a 'charity of production' to a 'charity of consumption'. By exercising what they now chose to call charity when the harvest failed, local elites contributed to a myth of community which helped to soften and disguise the nature of those expanding inequalities, whose existence dearth otherwise high-lighted.[150] The poor were encouraged to choose the solidarities of 'community' against those of class. As the shifting geography of the food riot suggests this was by no means a uniform process. Both the geography of the food riot (predominantly located in urban or rural industrial grain-deficient areas with more 'individualistic' economic relationships) and the increasing frequency of this form of popular political action provide a rough guide to differences in the availability of formal and informal relief. But the absence of the food riot from many purely agricultural areas and, until a very late date in its history, the general absence of the agricultural labourer from such disorder suggests that if the poor of early modern England escaped a 'crisis of subsistence', many fell victim to a crisis of dependence.[151]

[150] Heal, 'Hospitality'; Mennell, *All Manners of Food*; Mauss, *The Gift*, p. 72; Williams, *Country and City*, pp. 43–4. I intend developing at greater length elsewhere this reading of the shift in social relationships in the later seventeenth century as an attempted recreation of 'community' by local elites.

[151] Charlesworth, ed., *Atlas Rural Protest*; Charlesworth, 'English rural proletariat', pp. 101–11; Malcomson, 'Kingswood colliers'; Bohstedt, *Riots and Community Politics*; Stevenson, *Popular Disturbances in England*, chapter 5. By contrast, the abandonment by farmers of selling grain at under-prices has been seen as one factor in explaining riots by farm labourers in the nineteenth century: Dunbabin, *Rural Discontent*, p. 18.

3

Death in Whickham

KEITH WRIGHTSON and DAVID LEVINE

The emergence of historical demography in the decades since the Second World War has rendered English historians only too familiar with the demographic facts of mortality in the Tudor and Stuart period. The jagged peaks in burial statistics derived from the aggregative analysis of Anglican parish registers are in themselves sufficient to lacerate the complacency of a western culture in which death, though inevitable, has become postponed, confined, effaced from public view and muted in public consciousness. The patient piecing together of marriages, baptisms, and burials in family reconstruction studies demonstrates less dramatically, but in more compelling detail, the stark realities of an age in which high infant and child mortality and the premature deaths of spouses were perennial threats to the survival of the individual family. Graphs, tables and histograms, simulations and back-projections, the proliferating weaponry of the demographic arms race, combine to bring home to the modern student what every contemporary knew: that life was tenuous; that few could hope to live out the biblical span and die already retired from the immediacy of family responsibilities; that for most death came both unexpected and untimely, cutting them off quite literally in the midst of life.

The facts of a demographic regime in which high mortality was a central characteristic are clear enough. Far less apparent are the implications of such realities. Demographic statistics can be abstracted from the contexts of the local societies in which actual individuals were born, married, reproduced, and died. They can be manipulated with

Our research on Whickham is part of a project which has received support from the Social Sciences and Humanities Research Council of Canada, the Wolfson Foundation, and the University of St Andrews Research Fund. This chapter was drafted during Keith Wrightson's tenure of a Canadian Commonwealth Research Fellowship in 1983/4. We gratefully acknowledge the support of these various bodies.

an almost clinical precision to provide an analytical account of long-term trends in mortality. It remains true, however, that a neglect of the socio-economic context which helped to shape demographic realities entails a truncated understanding of the significance of those trends. Moreover, too narrow a preoccupation with statistical evidence leaves unexplored whole dimensions of the mortality regime of early modern England, the realities of which need to be weighed as well as counted.

No one was more aware of this than Andrew Appleby. In his *Famine in Tudor and Stuart England* he placed famine in Elizabethan and Jacobean Cumbria within a regional and national context which gave a deeper historical meaning to that experience. Characteristically, however, Appleby was not complacent with regard to his own achievement. In concluding his book he drew attention to further problems and argued that

Some of the questions that remain can only be answered by detailed local studies. If such a study combined the skills of the demographer – in a reconstitution – with all the literary evidence available in the records of manorial and church courts and wills and inventories, it might enable us to evaluate the true dimensions of the demographic crisis of the late-sixteenth and early seventeenth centuries and its effects on the family and on the village social structure.[1]

In this chapter we wish to pay tribute to the memory of Andrew Appleby by taking up that challenge and examining mortality and the experience of death in a particular locality in north-east England: the parish of Whickham, Co. Durham. In doing so we will not discuss every specific question raised by Appleby, for Whickham had its own history and it was one very different from that of Appleby's Cumbrian parishes. It is, however, in the spirit of his work that we have tried to reconstruct the demographic realities, the socio-economic impact, and the individual experience of death in Whickham.

I

The parish of Whickham lies on the south bank of the river Tyne, some four miles upstream from the city of Newcastle. It was a large parish, almost 6,000 acres in area, and it contained several distinct settlements. Whickham town was situated about one mile from the river on the brow of a steep hill rising sharply from the meadowlands along the riverside. To the north-east the township of Dunston in the 'Lowhand'

---

[1] Appleby, *Famine*, pp. 190–1.

quarter of the parish marked the point at which the river Team joined the Tyne at the eastern boundary of the parish. To the north-west, the confluence of the Derwent and the Tyne was similarly marked by the township of Swalwell. Behind Whickham town the land rose steadily from the common fields of the manor of Whickham to the 'Fellside' quarter of the parish, comprising Whickham Fell, the Hollinside estate of the Harding family, the Gibside estate of the Blakiston family and the extensive rough pasture of Marley Hill.[2]

For the student of mortality Whickham has the particular interest of being situated in an area of north-east England identified by Andrew Appleby as suffering severe mortality crises at the turn of the sixteenth and seventeenth centuries. Indeed, within that area Whickham may have been peculiarly vulnerable to such crises.[3] It was not this aspect of its history, however, which initially drew our attention to Whickham. The parish has a significance of an altogether different order in the economic and social history of early modern England. For between 1580 and 1630 Whickham emerged as the most significant centre of coal production in Britain. As the coal industry of Tyneside boomed in the last decades of the sixteenth and the first decades of the seventeenth centuries, primarily in response to the demand for domestic fuel exerted by London and the towns of south-east England, Whickham played a disproportionate role in the expansion of output. By the 1630s the parish produced possibly a quarter of the entire 'vend' shipped from Tyneside.[4] Whickham was at the very heart of the extraordinary early industrial experience of Tyneside, a focal point in a nascent industrial society within a largely 'pre-industrial' world.

This is not the place to present a detailed account of the industrialisation of Whickham which took place within the first half of the century covered by the chapter. The principal features of that process, however, must be briefly rehearsed. In the first half of the reign of Elizabeth I, Whickham was a relatively populous, predominantly agricultural, parish in which most households held land and almost all enjoyed pasture rights which were crucial to their well-being. The ecclesiastical returns of 1563 reveal that at that date the parish had a population of ninety-three households. A rental of the principal manor of Whickham, compiled only a few years later, lists fifty-nine copyhold tenants, of whom sixteen were virtually landless cottagers; nine had small holdings of up to six acres; twenty-eight held between ten and thirty-six acres and only six held more than forty acres (the largest

[2] Bourn, *Whickham Parish*, pp. 1–2, 41, 83, 117; Fordyce, *Durham*, 2, pp. 687–95.
[3] Appleby, *Famine*, pp. 134, 147; Hodgson, 'Demographic Trends', p. 31.
[4] Nef, *Coal Industry*, 1, pp. 19–21, 361 and appendix I.

single holding being of some sixty-two acres).[5] All enjoyed pasture rights on the extensive fells to the south of Whickham town. In addition, the parish included freehold lands which were not listed in the rental and the lands of the smaller manors of Farnacres, Axwell cum Swalwell, Hollinside, and Gibside, all of which had their tenants. It seems reasonable, therefore, to conclude that the majority of Whickham households held land, usually in small-to-medium-sized holdings. Moreover, they held their land securely, either by freehold or copyhold of inheritance, and copyhold rents and fines were both small and fixed.[6]

The husbandry which they practised on their land was overwhelmingly pastoral. A survey of Whickham farming inventories for the period 1557 to 1589 reveals a pattern of small, predominantly pastoral farms in which livestock generally accounted for over 70 per cent of the total farm value.[7] Cattle raising was the principal activity. Crops, mainly rye and oats, were grown in relatively small quantities. Whickham, like most of the north-east, was a 'corn-poor' parish, dependent on buying in grain to meet its bread needs in return for the profits made by the sale of locally raised cattle.

The special place of the parish in the history of the coal industry really begins in the last two decades of the sixteenth century. While it is true that Whickham had been involved in coal production since at least the fourteenth century, activity was on a small scale and was carefully restricted by the Bishops of Durham, lords of the manor of Whickham. In 1576 there were only four working pits in the parish.[8] In 1578, however, Queen Elizabeth obtained from the newly appointed Bishop of Durham a lease of all coal mines 'as well opened as unopened' within the manors of Whickham and Gateshead. This lease, which became known as the Grand Lease, was renewed in 1582 for a period of ninety-nine years, fortified with full powers of lordship over the two manors, and passed ultimately into the hands of the mayor and burgesses of Newcastle-upon-Tyne.[9]

---

[5] Brit. Lib., Harleian MS. 594, fo. 188v; Harrison, 'Census', p. 18; DPD, Church Commission MS., Box 20, No. 189721. This detailed rental is undated, but can be dated to the mid 1560s.

[6] Surtees, *County Palatine of Durham*, 2, pp. 237–56; James, *Family, Lineage and Civil Society*, p. 39; Horton, 'Durham Bishopric Estates', pp. 225–8.

[7] The Whickham wills and inventories used in this study are housed in the DPD. A modern index exists for the period 1534–1616 only. Hereafter individual wills and inventories will be cited as DPD Probate, followed by the name of the deceased and year.

[8] Blake, 'Medieval Coal Trade', p. 22; Nef, *Coal Industry*, 1, p. 137; Brit. Lib., Lansdowne MS. 66, nos. 84, 86, 87.

[9] Nef, *Coal Industry*, 1, pp. 150–5; Trevor-Roper, 'Bishopric of Durham'.

For the merchants of Newcastle, the securing of the Grand Lease was a dream come true: lordship over one of the richest and most accessible collieries in Britain. From the point of view of the inhabitants of Whickham its granting brought both advantages and disadvantages. During the first quarter century of increased mining activity, however, its seems probable that the benefits of industrial growth were most apparent. In the first place there was little interference with the husbandry of the parish. Mining operations were initially confined to the traditional sites allocated to mining on the abundant rough pasture to the south of Whickham town. Farming inventories for the period 1590 to 1610 reveal an agricultural pattern very similar to that of the preceding thirty years. No attempts were made to alter the tenure, rents or fines of the copyholders, and a reconstruction of the distribution of land in 1591 and 1600, based on surviving rentals, shows a remarkable stability in the landholding structure of the manor of Whickham, which in itself suggests the undisturbed well-being of the tenants.[10]

Again, industrial development brought some substantial benefits to the local inhabitants. The expansion of the coal industry provided work at the pits and staithes. Cottages could be erected and let to migrant mineworkers. Victuals could be supplied. Freeholders could lease the seams beneath, or rights of 'wayleave' across their land to the Grand Lessees, whose privileges did not extend to freehold property. Above all, the copyholders of Whickham were able to benefit from the preferential position accorded to them as 'wainmen' employed to transport coal from the pits down to the riverside staithes whenever coal fleets lay in the Tyne to be served. Given such welcome supplements to their incomes, it is hardly surprising that surviving inventories of household goods suggest that the living standards of Whickham's people were rising significantly during the first phase of industrial expansion. All in all, it would appear that the early developments of the Grand Lease colliery brought real gains to Whickham. A new economy and society was growing up in the parish, but as yet the old was able to coexist with innovation with relative ease and benefit besides.[11]

The balance of advantages and disadvantages from the point of view of Whickham's copyholders was to change, however, as industrial

---

[10] Full details of the development of mining operations in Whickham will be provided in our forthcoming book on the parish. For the rentals of 1591 and 1600, see DPD DDR Halmote Court III F 19, fos. 173–174v; DPD DDR Halmote Court Rentals, Box II, Bundle 5, No. 193323.

[11] These matters will be explored in detail in our forthcoming book.

expansion proceeded, and by 1620 the problems of industrialisation had become only too apparent. The 1610s in particular appear to have been a watershed on the pace of exploitation of the Grand Lease, as for a variety of reasons the Newcastle coal owners found it advantageous to intensify their operations in Whickham. The number of new sinkings increased dramatically in the copyhold lands of the manor of Whickham, while there was further intense activity elsewhere in the parish. Pits were sunk for the first time in the prime arable, meadow, and pasture lands of the manor. Land was buried beneath industrial refuse and polluted with coal dust. New 'coalways' for wain traffic were laid out with scant regard for the damage inflicted on field and pasture. Springs and wells were destroyed by mining operations or polluted by 'cankered' water from the drainage channels of the pits. By 1620 it could be plausibly claimed that 'more than a full third part of the said town is laid quite waste'. In 1647 and 1652 when the manor and colliery of Whickham were surveyed by parliamentary commissioners, it was reported that of the nineteen fields of the manor listed as arable, meadow and pasture, no fewer than sixteen had been worked by the Grand Lessees, many of them to exhaustion. East Field, for example, had had fifty-four pits sunk in it; Corn Moor had thirty. The common pasture of the manor was described as for the most part 'totally spoiled'.[12]

The consequences for the agrarian economy of Whickham can easily be imagined and are well-attested in the complaints of the aggrieved copyholders, who unsuccessfully challenged the Grand Lessees' proceedings. Throughout much of the parish agriculture had been disrupted. Industrial employment, formerly a seasonal and secondary occupation, had developed a far larger place in the domestic economies of the tenantry of Whickham. Moreover, the survey of 1647 reveals that the structure of landholding on the manor of Whickham, so stable between the 1560s and 1600, had undergone a process of polarisation. At the top of the landholding hierarchy there were now five copyholders with accumulations over sixty acres, as compared with only one in the 1560s. At the bottom, there were now sixty-six cottage holdings without land, as compared with sixteen. Small holdings of between one and seven acres had also increased in number from nine to eighteen, while the middle range of holdings of ten to thirty-nine acres had been reduced in number from twenty-eight to eleven. The customary 'oxgangs', which had retained their integrity to 1600, had

---

[12] DPD Church Commission MS., Box 205, Nos. 244227–244236, 244238; PRO DURH 4/1, pp. 205–6; *Parliamentary Surveys*, ed. Kirby, pp. 81–3, 105–6, 135–9.

frequently been split up piecemeal and redistributed, some as fragments, others as parcels of large accumulations.[13]

By the mid seventeenth century, then, the world of the copyholders of Whickham had undergone transformation. An older agrarian economy had been undermined – quite literally – and an industrial economy had come into being. At the same time, Whickham had experienced a social transformation, for already by the second quarter of the seventeenth century the greater part of the inhabitants of Whickham were not members of copyholder families and never had been. A new society had grown up in Whickham as the old declined.

The coal industry brought not only change to the established families of Whickham, but also an entirely new population of industrial workers. In 1563, as we have seen, Whickham was inhabited by ninety-three households (a total population of perhaps something over 400). By 1620 there were already said to be over a thousand men, women and children in the parish. In 1666 the hearth tax assessment listed 367 householders, suggesting a total population of just under 1,600.[14] Whickham had thus witnessed close to a fourfold increase in population in the course of a century, as compared with an estimated increase of 70 per cent in the population of County Durham as a whole between 1563 and 1674.[15] Indeed, the population expansion in Whickham may have been even more dramatic than these figures suggest. The Protestation return of 1642 lists 782 men over the age of eighteen in Whickham. If, as one might assume in a 'normal' parish, these adult men constituted perhaps 36 per cent of the population, and if the sex ratio of the over-eighteens can be assumed to have been 100, then the total population of 1642 might have been as high as 2,200. If

---

[13] *Ibid*, pp. 85–105. A number of the 1647 holdings are not described in detail. These have been identified by reference to two copies of a rental of 1638. DPD DDR Halmote Court Rentals, Box II, Bundle 5, No. 193324 and Gateshead Public Library, Cotesworth MS. CN/1/304.

[14] For the ecclesiastical returns of 1563, see note 5 above. The 1620 estimate was made by the Attorney of the Bishop of Durham. DPD Church Commission MS., Box 205, No. 244236, p. 7. The 1666 Hearth Tax assessment is to be found in PRO E 179 106/28. For conversion of hearth tax households into a total population estimate, we have adopted the multiplier 4.3 suggested by Arkell in 'Estimating population totals from the Hearth Tax'. In converting the 1563 return into a population of 'perhaps something over four hundred' we mean a total somewhere between that obtainable using Arkell's multiplier and that obtainable by using Peter Laslett's familiar muliplier of 4.75. As will be evident from the discussion below, Whickham presents special problems for any methods of estimating overall population.

[15] For the county as a whole, see Hodgson, 'Demographic trends', p. 15. Although the statistics given for Whickham's population growth might imply a linear trend, it is more likely that there was a series of spurts and periods of retrenchment in accordance with the pace of industrial development.

this was so, there must have been substantial population loss by 1666. Such dramatic fluctuation seems unlikely, however. A more plausible explanation may be that the population of Whickham included a substantial number of single men living in lodgings or in temporary 'hovels' thrown up around the coal workings.[16] Their numbers may have been at their greatest during the periodic bursts of frenetic activity which punctuated the history of the industry. The implications of the existence of such a population for the multipliers used to derive total population from the numbers of households listed in the hearth tax can only be guessed at. What we can say is that the population of Whickham underwent a remarkable expansion by the standards of the day, that the increase probably took place in a series of waves after 1580, and that it was intimately connected with the process of industrialisation.

Population growth of this order inevitably entailed both considerable growth in the housing stock and a major increase in the population density of the parish. In 1563 Whickham had not been outstanding among Durham parishes in its population density. By the mid-seventeenth century, however, it was the most densely populated parish in the county if we exclude the towns of Durham, Sunderland, Gateshead, and Hartlepool. The population density of the parish as a whole had risen from 15.5 to 61.0 households per 1,000 acres. Such global figures, however, give a misleading impression of the actual density of settlement. To judge by the Hearth Tax return of 1666, which divides the parish into 'quarters', the greater part of Whickham's population was heavily concentrated between Whickham town and the rivers Tyne, Team, and Derwent. In places its density may have been three or four times higher than the parish average.[17]

If Whickham's population was large and dense by contemporary standards, it was also quite remarkably volatile. Population growth had owed little to natural increase (between 1577 and 1659 there were only 5,350 recorded baptisms in Whickham to offset 5,244 recorded burials). The swollen population of the parish was the result of heavy

---

[16] *Durham Protestations*, ed. Wood, pp. 47–53. For the suggested figure of 36 per cent, see Wrigley and Schofield, *Population History*, appendix 3, data for 1641. These are, of course, national estimates of population structure and their applicability to Whickham's exceptional circumstances is very doubtful, as we have suggested.

[17] For contemporary statements concerning the proliferation of cottages and 'lodges' erected for coal workers, see DPD Church Commission MS. Box 20, No. 189721; DPD Halmote Court Rentals, Box II, Bundle 5, No. 193323; Kirby, *Parliamentary Surveys*, pp. 81, 84; DPD Church Commission MS., Box 205, No. 244238, p. 5. For Whickham's population density as compared with other Durham parishes, see Hodgson, 'Demographic Trends', p. 13 and Kirby, 'Population density', p. 89; PRO E 179 106/28.

and sustained immigration. The long-term effects in terms of population turnover can be indicated by the fact that of those surnames recorded in the parish registers in 1629–54, as many as 50.4 per cent were new to the parish, only 43 per cent having been recorded in the period 1603–28 and as few as 6.6 per cent in the period 1578–1602.[18] Surname analysis, however, provides only the roughest indication of population turnover. Far more striking evidence of the transience of the population can be provided. As a means of illustrating this phenomenon we have taken as our sample those families entering observation in the family reconstitution study whose surnames began with the letters A, B, and C. We have then distinguished those families which are regarded as 'wastage' for the purposes of the reconstitution study (by virtue of the fact that only one event was recorded for them), and those which can be regarded as 'persisting' in the sense that they retained representation in the parish into the next generation. In the period 1590–1619, of the 275 families entering observation, 50.9 per cent were categorised as 'wastage', only 12.9 per cent as 'persisting'. For the period 1620–49, 314 families entered observation, of which 39.7 per cent were 'wastage' and 13 per cent 'persisting'. The implication is that outside a core of relatively stable families the population of Whickham was in constant flux. At any given point in time it would seem that most of the people living in Whickham were birds of passage.[19]

The new population of Whickham, then, was large, dense, volatile, and probably unbalanced in its sex-ratio. It was also overwhelmingly wage-dependent. The farmers of the parish, large or small, were rapidly outnumbered by those who earned their livings as pitmen, or as transportation workers and who formed part of the emerging industrial workforce of Tyneside. If they could earn decent daily wages by the standards of the agricultural labouring poor of the period, they were also subject to the seasonality of employment which remained a feature of the coal industry. Moreover, they were chronically vulnerable to stoppages in the Tyne coal trade (which were all too frequent as the result of war, piracy, blockade or commercial boycott). Contemporaries had little doubt that the coal workers were poor and their judgement is confirmed by the hearth tax assessment of 1666. Of the Whickham households listed, approximately 78 per cent were ex-

---

[18] Lasker and Roberts, 'Study of a Tyneside parish', p. 301.
[19] Between those families regarded as 'wastage' and those 'persisting', there were, of course, very many families which recorded more than a single event, yet appear to have remained in the parish only a limited time (often only a few years) and were not represented in the next generation.

empted from the tax by reason of their poverty or smallness of estate, the exemption rate varying from some 65 per cent in Swalwell to approximately 85 per cent in both Lowhand and Fellside quarters, the principal areas of mining operations at this date. Those exempted were not so much destitute as *relatively* poor, of course. Even so, the rates of exemption in Whickham were extraordinarily high by the standards of rural England in general and very high even as compared with areas of domestic cloth industry. Rates of this kind would be more typical of the impoverished suburban parishes of England's larger cities. They were higher than the 75 per cent exemption rate of the poorest district of the city of Newcastle in 1665 – the Sandgate, home of the Keelman who ferried Whickham's coal to the London colliers.[20]

Whickham, then, was a parish undergoing transformation from a small farming, pastoral economy to one based upon the extraction and transportation of coal. That process brought new opportunities and the possibility of a new degree of material comfort for some. It also involved physical devastation, massive population growth, redistribution of the land and the emergence of a large, transient, wage-dependent, workforce housed in makeshift 'hovels' concentrated along the riverside and near the 'going pits' of the parish. It was an altogether extraordinary story of drastic change largely accomplished in only two generations. In what ways was that experience reflected in the history of mortality in Whickham?

II

The parish registers of Whickham begin in the later 1570s – baptisms and burials in 1577 and marriages in 1579. During their first century they are broken for various periods of time – most seriously for our present purposes by complete breaks in burial registration between July 1620 and the end of 1624, and from August 1661 through March 1667. In all the registration of burials is either missing or else defective for 15.5 per cent (186/1,200) of the months in the period 1577–1676.[21] If demographic analysis had been our only concern we would have rejected this parish as the focus of our efforts. As we have already shown, however, Whickham's history has claims upon our attention which far outweigh the technical deficiencies of its parish register.

---

[20] For stoppages, see Nef, *Coal Industry*, 2, pp. 181–96. For Hearth Tax exemption, PRO E179 106/28; Howell, *Newcastle-upon-Tyne*, pp. 10–12; Wrightson, *English Society*, p. 148.

[21] Whickham Parish Registers 1577–1676, DRO EP/Wh/1–2. An excellent transcript of registers is available in Newcastle-upon-Tyne Central Library.

Moreover, we hope to demonstrate that even the imperfect registration of mortality in Whickham can be supplemented with other sources so as to provide an enhanced understanding of the social consequences of industrialisation on Tyneside.

In figure 1 we have presented an annual series of burials in Whickham for the century after 1577, the onset of registration. Rather than smooth out the annual differences by means of a moving average, we have chosen to present the data in a 'raw' form which will highlight this variability. The outstanding characteristic of the resulting graph is the explosive annual variation of the mortality statistics.

Wrigley and Schofield's recent reconstruction of *The Population History of England* has made it clear that recurrent, crisis-level mortality was not the usual experience of rural English parishes, though to some extent all parishes so far studied have displayed dramatic year-to-year and even month-to-month swings in mortality.[22] What was remarkable about Whickham's experience was the profound impact of repetitive, annual crises at the end of the sixteenth and beginning of the seventeenth centuries. Our eyes are immediately drawn to this period in the graph. The jagged peaks of the mortality series are unmistakable to anyone who has studied the impact of epidemic and famine in the early modern era. In 1587 there were 112 burials recorded in the parish register; in 1588, just thirty-eight; but in the next year, 1589, there were 101. The situation more-or-less stabilised for the next six years and then the grim reaper returned to exact a terrible toll – 122 burials in 1596 and then 139 in 1597. Once again, from 1598 through 1603 there was a period of quiescence before the terrible mortality of 1604 killed 254 of the parishioners. In this eighteen-year period, 1587–1604, when there was no apparent break in the registration of burials, 1,243 men, women, and children were given Christian burial in Whickham. Of this total almost 60 per cent (728/1,243) died in the four bouts of catastrophic mortality to which we have alluded. Nor were the harrowing years at the turn of the sixteenth and seventeenth centuries the only period when crisis-level mortality touched the population of Whickham. In fact, if we define 'crisis' to mean years when annual burials were more than double the surrounding, 'background' level, then there were seventeen identifiable crises in Whickham during the first century of parochial registration.[23]

[22] Wrigley and Schofield, *Population History*, appendix 10.
[23] Wrigley and Schofield use rather different measurements and consider mortality crises on a monthly basis by means of a computer-assisted algorithm, *Population History*, appendix 10. Our measurement of annual mortality is much less sophisticated. We also face the problem, in dealing with Whickham, that some of the 'normal' years used to establish 'background' mortality, witnessed death rates which would be

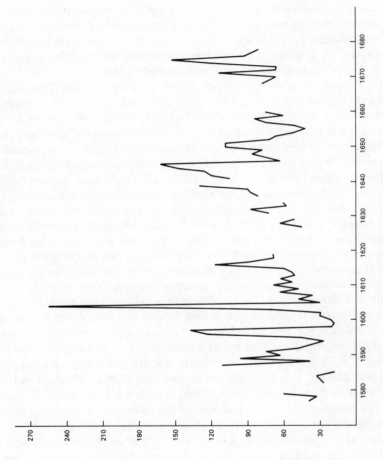

Figure 3.1 Burials in Whickham, 1577–1676

Determining the causes of these explosions of mortality involves the combination of quantitative and qualitative evidence. The seventeenth-century crises would seem to have been invariably the result of epidemic disease rather than famine. The parish register is quite definite in describing the cause of death as 'plague' in 1604, 1610, and during the recurrent crises of the 1640s. This evidence is substantiated in 1604 by several independent references in the local records. Thomas Pearson was buried on 28 July 1604. His inventory, drawn up a few months later, includes a payment 'for clensing the howse' to rid it of the pestilence. A Durham Chancery case of 1606 mentions the fact that Martin Wilson, his wife, and child all died 'of infection' after being 'visited with the plague'. They had been buried in August 1604. William Marshall was buried on 10 November. In a case in the Consistory Court of Durham it was recorded that he too had been 'visited with the infection of the plague'.[24] Later, in 1610 and 1645, the parish register mentions that the parishioners were living in 'lodges' on Whickham Fell to escape the pestilence. In several other years also there were occasional mentions of plague deaths in the parish register, though the mortality did not reach crisis proportions. Indeed still further references to plague in Whickham can be gleaned from county records, though the local impact does not seem to have been particularly severe. The Durham Quarter Sessions Order Book mentions plague in Gateshead, South Shields and Whickham in April and July 1626, while in July 1638 the justices ordered the payment of eighteen pounds for the relief of 'the towne of Whickham, lately infected with the plague'.[25]

Let us look a little more closely at the exceptional mortality of the principal plague years. That of 1604 towers over all the other years of catastrophe. Perhaps a fifth to a quarter of the inhabitants of Whickham were buried in the space of five months. Analysis of other seventeenth-century epidemics has made it clear that plague deaths tended to be bunched in family units.[26] In Whickham too some households were ravaged while their neighbours were completely

considered high by the English standards of the day, e.g. 1590–92. In the absence of really firm data on population size any estimates of mortality rates can be no more than educated guesses. What is clear is the severity of the mortality regime in Whickham, and the frequency of crisis years.

[24] DPD Probate, Inventory of Thomas Pearson (1604); PRO DURH 2/2/51; DPD DR V/8 fols. 31–32v.

[25] DRO Q/S OB 1, pp. 252, 261; Q/S OB 2, p. 276. In the case of the 1626 outbreak the parish register of burials seems patchy and we are unable to assess the dimensions of the mortality (which may have been severe) with real confidence.

[26] Schofield, 'Anatomy of an epidemic', pp. 95–126; Slack, *Impact of Plague*, p. 177 ff.

untouched. The young family of George Gilchrist and his wife
Margaret Blacklock, for example, was frightfully maimed. The couple
had been married on 1 June 1596. In the next two years they had a son,
Peter, and a daughter, Margaret. Thereafter, the family seems to be
unobserved by the registration process for six years. At the beginning
of July 1604, an unbaptised child, Will, was buried at the outset of the
epidemic. Ten days later Margaret Blacklock Gilchrist was buried.
Another ten days passed and six-year-old Margaret Gilchrist joined her
mother and brother in Whickham churchyard. Within the space of
three weeks, then, George Gilchrist saw his family disintegrate about
him. The Gilchrists' experience was representative in a number of
ways. In the first place, they were not 'in observation' continuously.
Perhaps they had moved in and out of the parish so that it was
fortuitous, in the most macabre sense, that they were located in the
records of the family reconstitution study. Indeed, only fifty-one of the
plague deaths could be linked with a family in the reconstituted
population. As we know, the parish had a very substantial floating
population of sojourners or short-term residents and it seems clear that
this section of the population suffered dreadfully. The second sense in
which the Gilchrists' experience was representative was that they died
together, within a short space of time. Among the fifty-one parishioners who could be traced, fully twenty-eight deaths (55 per cent)
occurred in such family clusters with mortality worst among infants
and young children.[27]

Analysis of the plague of 1645 presents a similar picture. Of the 161
burials in 1645, ninety-eight were of people stated to have died of the
plague. The seasonal distribution of burials was not as clear-cut as in
1604, but the register is quite explicit in attributing ninety-eight deaths
to the epidemic.[28] In contrast to the earlier period, when little over
one-fifth of the victims could be linked with a family in the
reconstitution study, by 1645 the figure was only a little under
three-fourths (72/98). On the other hand, the age- and family-
specificity of the later epidemic was quite similar to the figures

[27] Of the traceable burials, thirty-nine (80 per cent) were of infants and children. It can
also be remarked that of these very nearly half (seventeen) had not been baptised in
Whickham, even though the family had seemingly been 'in observation' as a result of
being in residence at some earlier date. This pattern of seemingly haphazard
registration characterised Whickham's parochial records in this period and testifies to
the extraordinary mobility of some of the parishioners. One final point needs to be
made about the quality of the parish register: the annual totals are not dramatically out
of line with what one might expect from a community of Whickham's approximate
size. Rather, it is the lack of continuity within families which presents problems for
the historical demographer.

[28] The seasonality of burials will be discussed below.

provided by the smaller samples of traceable victims of 1604: half the victims were children (48/98) and over half of the burials (58/98) occurred in family-multiples. Perhaps the disparity in the ratio of successful linkages between the reconstituted populations of 1604 and 1645 is further testimony to the extraordinary upheaval in Whickham's population at the turn of the sixteenth and seventeenth centuries.

The crises of the early seventeenth century can thus be attributed confidently to plague outbreaks. Plague may well have been endemic on Tyneside by this date.[29] The crises of the late sixteenth century, however, are more problematic. Of particular interest is the crisis of 1596/7. In attempting to distinguish plague from other forms of epidemic mortality, and disease from famine, Andrew Appleby ingeniously employed a method of specifying each factor's demographic 'footprint' in regard to its seasonality.[30] Following his method, for example, it is quite clear that the Whickham mortality of 1604 provides a classic instance of the correlation between warm weather and plague. In the first six months of that year there were thirty-one burials recorded. In July burials rose to seventy; in August eighty-three villagers were laid to rest; in September the impact began to diminish with thirty-two burials, followed by nineteen in October, fourteen in November and just five in December. The seasonal pattern of burials in 1596/7 was quite different. Heavy mortality was concentrated in five winter months. Between November 1596 and March 1597 there were 164 burials recorded in the parish register, which made up 62.8 per cent (164/261) of the total for the two-year period. This monthly pattern would seem to suggest a classical 'subsistence crisis' precipitated by food shortage.

There is other evidence to support such an interpretation. It is well-established that the mid 1590s witnessed a succession of disastrous harvests throughout northern Europe. Andrew Appleby found famine in north-west England in 1596–8 and similar evidence has been uncovered for other areas in these years.[31] In the north-east specifically, the coal owners of Newcastle complained late in 1595 of 'the darthe of . . . victuals' and the hardship which this entailed for their workers. By 1596, rye prices in Newcastle, which had stood at sixteen shillings a quarter in 1591 had reached twenty-four shillings a

---

[29] For the frequency of epidemics (usually plague) in the Tyneside area, see Howell, *Newcastle-upon-Tyne*, pp. 7, 319–20; James, *Family, Lineage and Civil Society*, pp. 8–10; Hodgson, 'Demographic trends', pp. 24–30; Slack, *Impact of Plague*, p. 62. Of course, it remains uncertain as to whether plague was constantly present in the area or whether it was very frequently reintroduced via trading contacts with London.

[30] Appleby, *Famine*, chapter 7.

[31] *Ibid*, pp. 109–21, 133–45. cf. Slack, *Impact of Plague*, pp. 73–4.

quarter and serious food shortages were reported in Northumberland and Durham.[32] By January 1597 some relief supplies had reached Newcastle by sea and were said to have saved thousands, but these shipments were certainly inadequate to meet the situation. Throughout the autumn and winter months of 1596/7 the commander of the garrison at Berwick, which was similarly dependent on imported supplies, wrote graphic accounts of shortage and it was stated in March 1597 that only a fifth of the usual supplies had reached the city. Some had been withheld from shipment by anxious local authorities in Yorkshire and Lincolnshire, while ships laden had been unable to reach the north-east because of many weeks of adverse weather. In July 1597 rye was being sold at ninety-six shillings a quarter and above in Newcastle, despite the arrival of three grain ships, while as late as September further shipments had brought prices down only to thirty-six shillings a quarter and the Corporation records spoke of 'poor folks who died for want in the streets'.[33]

In view of such well-documented conditions, it seems probable that the crisis of 1596/7 in Whickham was indeed the product of famine. Perhaps the swelling population of the parish had suffered the terrible consequences of a dependence upon regular food imports which had been dislocated by shortage elsewhere and adverse weather. Moreover, the industrial workers and cottagers of Whickham may have faced rocketing food prices at a time of year when their earnings were at their lowest, since the mortality coincided with the dead season of the coal trade. Against such an interpretation might be placed the facts that conceptions were not markedly inhibited during the months of highest mortality (there were three per month on average during the crises, as against an average of 4.5 for the other nineteen months of 1596 and 1597), and that plague was reported in Whickham in July 1597.[34] Nevertheless, it is entirely possible that conceptions in Whickham were little inhibited because the effects of malnutrition were largely concentrated among particular sections of the population, notably the poor and young, unmarried migrants. As for the flurry of burials which may be attributable to plague in the summer of 1597, these came after the main period of crisis. On balance, we must conclude that

---

[32] *Records of the Company of Hostmen*, ed. Dendy, pp. 5–7; Watts and Watts, *From Border to Middle Shire*. p. 49; James, *Family, Lineage and Civil Society*, p. 8.

[33] *Cal. S. P. Dom. 1595–7*, pp. 348, 501; *Calendar of Border Papers, 1595–1603*, pp. 128, 138–9, 185–6, 200, 231, 273, 281–2; *HMC Salisbury* VII, pp. 295–6. We are grateful to Dr R. B. Outhwaite for making available to us his file of references to the crisis of the 1590s. Cf. Appleby, *Famine*, p. 113.

[34] Richardson, *Local Historians Table Book*, 1, p. 231. There were also reports of plague in Newcastle in the late spring and summer of 1597, *Cal.S.P.Dom. 1595–7*, p. 420.

Whickham endured a crisis of subsistence in the winter of 1596/7.[35]

By way of contrast, the mortality of 1589 was clearly the result of a plague outbreak: fifty-three burials out of a total of 101 for the whole year were recorded in the eight weeks from late August to early October. Finally, the mortality pattern of 1587/8 seems remarkably similar to that found in Cumberland and Westmorland by Appleby. In most of the north-western parish registers he surveyed there were elevated burial totals in the latter part of 1587 and then a drop in the new year. He suggested that typhus was the likely villain of the piece. Appleby went on to argue that the 'footprint' of typhus is particularly evident in its age-incidence, but unfortunately the laconic nature of the Whickham parish register at this date makes it quite impossible to determine the age-specific impact of this crisis.[36]

In figure 2 we have attempted to illustrate the dissimilar patterns in the seasonality of the crises of 1587, 1589, 1596/7, and 1604. What is obvious is that despite their dissimilarities these mortality crises had in common the fact that they were long-lived and spread across several months. Their impact was of a different order of magnitude from many of the crises identified by Wrigley and Schofield, which only lasted a month or two and necessarily carried away fewer people. The long duration of the 1587 and 1604 crises in Whickham is particularly significant in view of Wrigley and Schofield's comments.

Crisis mortality of several months' duration cannot be sustained by airborne infections in populations of the size of most villages and market towns in pre-industrial England. These local crises were therefore likely to have been caused by diseases transmitted by insect vectors (*e.g.* typhus [by the body-louse and often associated with over-crowded conditions] or in certain circumstances bubonic plague) or to have encompassed a series of onslaughts

---

[35] It is of interest that Slack feels unable to attribute the heavy mortality of 1596/7 in Newcastle to plague alone: *Impact of Plague*, p. 62. See also his discussion on pp. 73–4 of the relative importance of famine and disease in the mortalities of the later 1590s.

[36] Appleby, *Famine*, pp. 102–8. A parish register can only be useful for age-specific analysis if it gives some supporting details of family relationship and/or covers a long time-frame and records a relatively stable community. In Whickham's case we are unable to deploy all the techniques applied by Appleby. It is important, however, to recognise that the reason why we cannot do so is, in fact, an essential element of Whickham's historical experience rather than a block to its recovery. One additional point can be made from the surviving Whickham records. 1586/7 was certainly a year of dearth, but it seems unlikely that famine lay behind the winter deaths of 1587 since the inventories of two of the victims of the crisis record well-stocked farms and supplies of grain: DPD Probate, inventories of Richard Arnold and Robert Donkin (1587). However, there remains the possibility that Whickham may have suffered what Slack has termed a 'mixed' crisis, involving both food shortage and deaths from typhus. See Slack, 'Mortality crises'. On the available evidence the problem cannot be resolved satisfactorily.

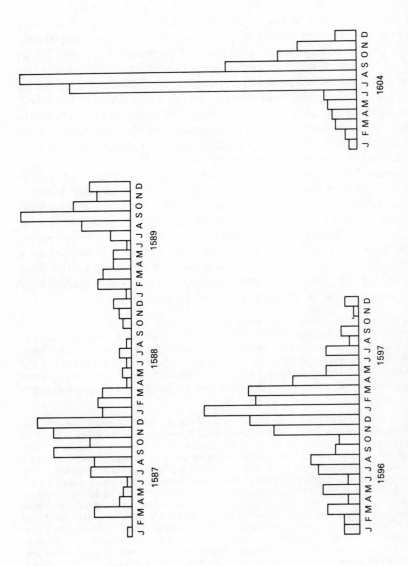

Figure 3.2 Seasonal distribution of burial in three mortality crises (a) January 1587 to December 1589 (b) January 1596 to December 1597 (c) January to December 1604

by a number of different micro-organisms, as the resistance of the human hosts was progressively weakened by successive infections.[37]

Considering the huddled state of the housing of Whickham's transient population, this description seems to fit the parish perfectly. The four swingeing mortality crises of the 1587–1604 period – caused successively by typhus, plague, famine or famine related diseases, and then plague again – all seem to have been intimately connected to the industrialisation of Tyneside in general and the social environment which it produced in Whickham in particular. The consequences of Tyneside's industrial expansion and closer incorporation into networks of national and international trade were double-edged. Whickham benefitted from trading ties which brought income and kept it well-supplied with food in most years. Yet it witnessed the growth of a wage-labouring population which was chronically vulnerable on the exceptional occasion on which these supplies were interrupted.[38] Moreover the parish was incorporated not only into a trading pattern, but into a unified system of disease transmission.[39] It developed a mortality regime more like that of a city than that of a rural parish.

The emergence of such a mortality regime in Whickham is confirmed by cohort statistics derived from family reconstitution which describe mortality in the parish in the first half of the seventeenth century. Despite the deficiencies of the parochial registration system in Whickham, these mortality figures are higher, not lower, than those derived from a survey of twelve widely dispersed English parishes over the same period. The fact that this difference is picked up in our calculations lends some confidence in the ability of computer-assisted

[37] Wrigley and Schofield, *Population History*, p. 663. cf. Paul Slack's comments on the rising population density and 'deterioration in the quality of the environment' which helped to create the distinct topography of the plague in London's suburbs: *Impact of Plague*, p. 159.

[38] We have no reason to believe that Whickham was vulnerable to outright famine after 1596/7 (though we would be more confident in making that judgement if burial registration survived for 1623, the last year of widespread famine in north-western England). By the mid seventeenth century Newcastle was known as a major receiving port for grain shipments from both southern England and the Baltic and in 1649 it was described as 'an Aegypt to all the shires of the north (in time of famine)': Gray, *Newcastle-upon-Tyne in 1649*, p. 33. There is, in fact, good reason to believe that this role was well-established for the area surrounding the city by the later sixteenth century. The crisis of 1596/7 resulted from exceptional circumstances, above all the nationwide shortages of that year and the adverse weather which prevented coastal shipping from reaching the city.

[39] cf. Slack, *Impact of Plague*, pp. 105–7 where the increasing severity and more widespread incidence of epidemics in seventeenth-century Essex is attributed in part to greater commercialisation, the growth of poverty and the increasing population density of the weaving townships of the county.

reconstitution analysis to discard families whose experience seems to suggest broken registration histories. The cost of the discrimination is that the Whickham statistics largely relate to settled and not transient families. This bias was likely to have been socially-specific to the extent that most settled families were located higher up the social scale than transients.[40] However, given that none of the seventeenth-century crises appear to have been famine-related, and because our data relate to the 1600–49 cohort in Whickham, it is probable that this bias is of only minor significance: epidemic disease did not respect social station.

Life expectancy at birth in Whickham was in the order of four years less than in Terling, which was broadly representative of the average of twelve villages cited by Wrigley and Schofield. Similarly, adult male life expectancy at 25–29 was some four years less than in Colyton. Whickham women's mortality, surprisingly, was somewhat better than that of their counterparts in the Devon village. The structure of adult men's mortality in Whickham is particularly interesting. The exceptional result of the Whickham family reconstitution study was the excess *male* mortality in the early years of marriage. This is precisely the period when, due to the risks associated with childbearing, one would have expected more female deaths and therefore higher, excess female mortality. If, as in Whickham, this period of high female risk was one of excess *male* mortality, then obviously men were involved in an activity several times more dangerous to their lives than 'pre-industrial' childbirth was to the life-chances of their womenfolk.[41]

The parish register confirms our suspicion as to the nature of that activity. Between November 1630 and April 1652 it was kept with unusual care and the burial register tells of fifty working miners killed in Whickham's pits. On 30 November 1632, for example, the register notes that Thomas Surrett and his son James were 'Slaine in a pitt at Jacks Leazes'. From the family reconstitution study we know that Thomas had entered the parish in or before 1617 and that his son James was a youth of fourteen whose baptism had been celebrated in Whickham. In addition, the register provides details of a further ten

---

[40] On the question of the selectivity of mortality measurements, see Schofield, 'Representativeness and family reconstitution', pp. 121–5.

[41] Female deaths could be related to birth events at the rate of ten per thousand (27 dying/2,738 births). It should be noted that this level of risk was for *each* birth and that a woman who gave birth to five children would have had a cumulative risk of roughly fifty per thousand. This would suggest that one woman in twenty who had lived long enough after marriage to give birth to five children might have died in childbirth or shortly thereafter as a result of complications. For a recent discussion of maternal mortality in other parishes, see Schofield, 'Did the mothers really die?', pp. 231–60.

Table 3.1 *Mortality in Whickham, Terling and Colyton*

A) Infant and child mortality (both sexes)

	At Risk	Dying	Rate/000	Expectation of life at birth	Corresponding Rate/000
Whickham (1600–24)					
0–	1917	325	169	42.78	168
1–4	1052	118	113		118
5–9	553	23	42		28
10–14	360	13	36		17
Terling (1550–1624)					
0–	1059	136	128	46.61	137
1–4	665	48	72		95
5–9	388	14	36		27
10–14	241	10	41		19

Note: The figures for expectation of life at birth are derived from Ledermann, *Nouvelles Tables-Types de Mortalité*, p. 134. The figures for Terling fit into the middle of the distribution of twelve villages discussed by Wrigley and Schofield in *Population History*, p. 249.

B) Adult mortality (Life expectancy at various ages)

	Whickham (1600–49)		Colyton (1600–49)	
	Male	Female	Male	Female
25–29	27.6	31.4	31.3	29.1
30–34	25.5	29.1	27.8	26.1
35–39	23.4	26.7	25.1	22.5
40–44	21.5	24.2	22.0	19.7
45–49	18.9	21.2	19.5	17.1
50–54	16.8	18.4	17.0	15.1
55–59	14.7	15.8	13.9	12.4

Note: The Whickham statistics are derived from combining 'optimistic' and 'pessimistic' assumptions about age-specific mortality. This procedure was required because so few of the adult villagers stayed in observation long enough to be traced through to their deaths. This method was devised to allocate death-dates to these birds of passage. Of course, the Whickham villagers whose burials were registered form the parameters within which these other deaths were allocated.

industrially-related deaths (nine of them before 1652), which did not involve underground workers. Men were slain by industrial machinery at the pit-heads, or in transportation accidents. Children were killed by coal wains or wagons, or by falls into disused and abandoned, sometimes flooded, pits.[42] In all, during the period of exceptionally detailed registration 1630–52, the fifty-nine burials which were either directly or indirectly attributable to coal mining represented 3.2 per cent of all burials registered. Those who died, where they can be traced, were overwhelmingly young men, a number of whom were married and had young families, so that the impact was in all likelihood significantly more focussed within the population than this global figure suggests. The reconstitution bears out this surmise in its description of excess male mortality.

If the development of the coal trade did much to enhance the general levels of mortality in Whickham, then, the activity of mining coal made its own quite specific impact on the life chances of the parishioners. In the foregoing discussion we have attempted to introduce both the socio-economic context and the demographic realities of death in Whickham. These structural parameters formed the essential framework within which the people of the parish lived and died. In the remaining sections of this chapter we wish to consider the social impact of the recurrent mortality crises of 1587–1610 upon the local community and the manner in which the inhabitants came to terms with the realities of death.

III

Between 1580 and 1620 the parish of Whickham was industrialised. In the same period it suffered four major mortality crises, followed by a minor outbreak of plague in 1610. We have already suggested how the pattern of mortality which emerged in Whickham may have been intimately connected with the process of industrial and commercial development which swept over the parish. It remains to explore the possibility that Whickham's dreadful mortality history may have exerted an independent influence on social change in the parish.

Social–structural change in Whickham involved two crucial develop-

---

[42] It is worth noting that after 1652 there were a further five scattered references to pitmen killed at work. Of the total of sixty-five deaths which related to industrial accidents, nineteen (29 per cent) could not be linked with the family reconstitution study. It will be remembered that twenty-six of the ninety-eight plague victims of 1645 (27 per cent) could not be traced in the reconstitution. In as much as these two attempts at linkage cover much the same time-period, the similarity of their results is striking.

ments: first, the dissolution of the agrarian economy of the copy-holders and the recasting of the landholding structure; secondly, the creation of a new industrial population which was remarkable for its volatility. To take the first of these processes of change, it seems reasonable to ask whether the heavy and chronologically concentrated mortality of the period 1587–1610 might have been a factor in the restructuring of agrarian society – perhaps by extinguishing tenant families; perhaps by facilitating the redistribution of land in a community in which tenure was very secure. We have tested this possibility in two ways. First, we have examined the influence of crisis mortality upon the transmission of property in the Halmote Court of the manor of Whickham between 1585 and 1614. Secondly, we have explored the survival of copyholder families across the period of industrialisation. The results are perhaps surprising.

The Halmote of Whickham did not meet in the years 1587, 1588, and 1589, perhaps as a result of the crisis conditions we have already described. When the court met again on 24 June 1590, it made up for lost time by recording twenty-six property transfers, as compared with nine in the court of 1585 and six in that of 1586. Some of these entries in the court book related to dated transactions of the period 1587–9 which had taken place outside the court and were only now formally registered. Five of these preceded the 1587 crisis. Following the June meeting, the Halmote met again in October 1590 and recorded a further three transactions.[43]

How far did this flurry of activity derive from the mortality of 1587? The answer would seem to be that the influence of crisis deaths was very small. Ninety Whickham people had been buried between July and December 1587. Yet of the twenty-four property transactions recorded in 1590 which post-dated the beginning of the crisis, only two can definitely be linked to crisis deaths, while a further two were probably so linked. Tracing on through the courts of 1592 and 1593, which recorded a further twenty-eight transactions, we find only one further case which appears linked to the crisis of 1587. Crisis-linked property transfers, then, were few in number. Nor does their nature suggest a dislocation of agrarian society in Whickham. In three of the five cases, the crisis deaths merely accelerated a succession which would probably have taken place in the fullness of time. John Dalton, for example, was admitted to his father's holding in 1588. Agnes Scott was admitted to the holding of her dead husband Robert in widowright, holding the tenement in trust for her young son

---

[43] DPD DDR Halmote Court III, F 18: Whickham Halmote Court Book, 1585–1632.

Christopher. William Shafto was admitted as son and heir of Roland Shafto. In the remaining two cases the effects of crisis deaths were to divert inheritance within a family, bringing to a fortunate individual property which he might not otherwise have gained. The Arnold family provide the clearest example. Christopher Arnold was buried on 24 July 1587 at the outset of the mortality crisis. In the normal course of events his holding would have passed to his son Richard, perhaps with a life interest to Christopher's widow Margaret. Richard, however, was buried on 27 July after making a deathbed will naming his brother Thomas and sister Margaret as principal heirs of his goods. His mother Margaret was buried on 3 August; his brother Thomas on 19 August. Ultimately the holding passed to a third brother, Nicholas, who had been left only a small token in Richard's will. In January 1588 Nicholas was appointed administrator of the goods of his deceased father and mother and in June 1590 he was admitted to the holding. The Arnolds had suffered a drastic culling, yet the family name continued in the person of Nicholas, who was, in fact, to emerge later as one of the leading figures among Whickham's tenants.[44]

The crisis of 1587 thus had a very limited impact on landholding in Whickham. The somewhat more severe crisis of July to October 1589 appears to have had even less effect. Of the sixty-nine transfers in the Halmote meetings of 1590–95 which postdated the crisis, only two can be linked to crisis deaths. Margaret Matfen inherited from her father Lawrence and James Leigh from his brother Ralph.[45] Turning to the transactions which followed the prolonged crisis of 1596/7, however, we find a situation which suggests, at first glance, a more profound impact.

No Halmote met in 1596. The court met in April 1597, in May 1598, and then twice in both 1599 and 1600. Of the ten property transfers recorded in the 1597 court which postdated the commencement of the crisis, only one can be linked to a crisis death. In the court of 1598, however, ten out of twenty transfers were linked to the crisis and the reverberations of crisis mortality continued to be felt in a muted form in 1599 (one out of fourteen transfers) and 1600 (two out of twelve transfers). All in all, a full quarter of the transfers recorded in the courts of 1597–1600 were connected to deaths during the 1596/7 crisis. To look at the impact of the crisis in another way, six of the sixty-one copyhold tenants of the manor of Whickham listed in the 1591 rental died in the crisis of 1596/7, while a further two tenants died who had not been

---

[44] *Ibid*, fols. 11, 15v, 18; DPD Probate, Will of Richard Arnold (1587), Administration Bonds of Agnes Scott (Bond 64, 1587) and Nicholas Arnold (Bond 463, 1587/8).
[45] DPD DDR Halmote Court III F 18, fols. 12, 17.

listed in 1591. The crisis had literally decimated the Whickham copyholders.[46]

Nevertheless, it would be mistaken to assume that this decimation involved an upheaval in landholding on the manor. Of the copyholders who died, only one held as much as six acres. Most held only houses and gardens or tiny cottage holdings carved from the waste of the manor. The copyholder victims of the crisis were almost exclusively drawn from the very lowest stratum of the manorial hierarchy – a fact which further reinforces our suggestion that the crisis of 1596/7 was primarily the result of famine conditions. Again, continuity of succession rather than dislocation is the dominant theme when we come to consider the nature of the transfers precipitated by crisis deaths. Seven of the eight copyholders who died were succeeded by a son and heir, the eighth by a daughter. The crisis thus served to accelerate, and on occasion to divert, succession within particular families. It did not obliterate family lines, though in the instance of inheritance by a daughter the family name ultimately passed from the land.

We can deal briefly with the epidemics of 1604 and 1610. The former was, as we have seen, a ghastly culling of the parish. Yet once again the crisis had only marginal effects on the land market. No Halmote met in 1604 or 1605. The courts of 1606 to 1608 recorded sixty-eight transfers postdating July 1604. Only two of these were related to the crisis. Elinor Blenkinsop took her dead husband's holding in widowright. Margaret Arnold was admitted as heir to her father's holding following his death and the deaths of her mother and elder brother. Finally, the relatively minor plague outbreak of 1610 seems to have had no impact whatever on landholding. Of fifty-three recorded transfers between the outbreak and July 1614, not one can be linked to a plague death.[47]

We began this analysis with the hypothesis that the terrible, repeated, crisis mortality in Whickham at the turn of the sixteenth and seventeenth centuries might have had a profound effect on the copyholder families of the manor of Whickham. Our findings suggest that although the effects of the crises were felt, their influence caused no dislocation of the landholding pattern. Certainly the copyholder families were not immune from these crises. Some of them suffered terribly. Yet their suffering did not extend to familial extinction. As we have seen, even where sudden death wreaked havoc in a household, carrying off both members of the parental generation and several children, there was usually a survivor to carry on the family line. This

[46] *Ibid*, fols. 25–49v; DPD DDR Halmote Court III F 19, fols. 173–174v.
[47] DPD DDR Halmote Court III F 18, fols. 64v–102, especially fo. 77.

was the more so when there existed married sons already established in households of their own, which escaped the crisis. Alternatively, where a wife and children died, remarriage and resultant birth could restore the demographic vitality of a family with remarkable swiftness.[48] The influence of crisis mortality would appear to have been above all an acceleration of inheritance, either by minors whose mothers held in widowright pending their majorities, or by adult children. The land market was affected only when a holding passed to an heiress as the result of the deaths of her brothers, or when an adult heir already established elsewhere chose to alienate the copyhold inherited in Whickham as the result of a crisis death. Both circumstances were known, but neither was more than occasional. For the rest, we have found not one instance of a copyhold falling vacant as a result of crisis mortality.

The general resilience of the copyholder families is further illustrated by the fact that of the copyhold families listed on the manorial rental of the mid to late 1560s, some 22 per cent were still represented in the male line among the Whickham copyholders of the 1647 survey. In a well-known calculation, E. A. Wrigley estimated that under the 'normal' conditions of fertility and mortality in pre-industrial England, a family would have approximately a 59 per cent chance of being succeeded by a male heir. In Whickham a generation can be taken to have been approximately thirty-three years (the period between the mean age of parenthood of the first and second generations, given an average age at first marriage of about 25–27 for both men and women and a cessation of childbearing at about 40). On these assumptions, we might expect some 29 per cent of Whickham copyholder families to have survived in the male line from 1567 to 1647. Actual survival, then, was rather less than might be estimated under 'normal' conditions. Of course, conditions in Whickham were not 'normal'. Given the context of Whickham's experience, it is perhaps surprising that the surival of copyholder families was so high.[49]

---

[48] To take an example from the plague of 1645, Henry Winshop lost his wife Barbara, one daughter and two sons between 20 July and 6 August 1645. Within months he had remarried. By the time of his own death in 1649 he had two new daughters and an infant son to add to the four children of his first marriage who had survived the epidemic: DPD Probate, Will of Henry Winshop (1649). We might add that the plague of 1645 does not appear to have affected landholding in Whickham in any significant way.

[49] Wrigley, 'Fertility strategy', pp. 135–54. Our calculation depends on the legitimacy of the assumption that Wrigley's extinction rate for a single generation can be converted into an annual rate. Provided that the copyholders listed in the starting document were evenly spaced by age of father (another assumption) we would argue that the conversion is defensible. Again, we have had to assume for the purpose of our

If individual families survived quite well, however, the structure of landholding on the manor of Whickham did not. As we have seen it underwent a process of polarisation between the rental of 1600 and the survey of 1647. Pursuing the full ramifications of that change is not our present purpose. What seems clear is that it owed little to the direct influence of the demographic crisis of the later sixteenth and early seventeenth centuries. It was related, rather, to economic factors prompting first the alienation and restructuring of holdings and second the proliferation of cottages. Both processes were, of course, part and parcel of the accelerating industrialisation of the parish after 1600.

One final point must be made concerning the mortality crises of late-Elizabethan and early-Stuart Whickham. While every crisis affected some of the copyholders of the parish and while most epidemics carried off individuals of considerable consequence in Whickham – plague being no respector of persons – it is abundantly clear that the vast majority of those who fell victim to the crises were drawn from the volatile mass of Whickham's new population of industrial workers. This much has already been suggested by the finding that only a fifth of the people buried in the crisis of 1604 could be linked to a family in the reconstitution study, and it is borne out by such evidence as we have of the identity of individuals. This was also, of course, the period when the degree of 'wastage' in the family reconstitution study was at its highest. By 1645 the population of Whickham was somewhat more stable and plague victims could be linked more readily to reconstituted families, though most remained socially obscure. The Elizabethan and Jacobean mortality crises, then, can be said to have had a direct influence on Whickham's social structure in that they contributed to the volatility of the population of the parish. There was a constant need for replacement among the immigrant industrial population of Whickham, comparable to that felt in the cities of the period, those 'devourers of mankind'. Again like the cities, Whickham experienced a surplus of burials over baptisms in the period 1577–1605 (1,622 as against 1,234). The phenomenal growth of the parish population clearly required immigration of a scale capable of replacing the deficit and permitting further growth.[50] Only after 1606

calculation that copyhold families wished to retain their holdings and did not alienate them from the male line voluntarily. We recognise that in practice some holdings were voluntarily alienated. Our calculation, then, involves several assumptions and we certainly do not wish to place too much weight upon it. We put it forward simply as an attempt to estimate the degree of survival in the male line which might be expected on the above assumptions.

[50] Cf. Paul Slack's assessment of the influence of plague on London's population: 'plague was both a symptom of urban instability and an independent variable which

did baptisms begin to outnumber burials and even then the surplus was fairly small. We might conclude that there was a marked dualism in the effects of the mortality structure of Whickham. Families possessed of real property (however modest), by a secure tenure and benefitting from the accompanying use-rights and a preferred place in industrial employment, had every reason to remain in Whickham. They proved themselves able to survive the vicissitudes of the mortality regime and to retain representation in the parish over at least two generations. The immigrant workers of the parish, in contrast, were more isolated, less likely to be 'settled', less liable to have several branches in the parish. They were attracted and held primarily by the prospect of wage work in and around the pits and staithes. Mortality crises obliterate such isolated individuals or less firmly rooted families. Acting alongside the fluctuations in employment opportunities which could stimulate renewed movement, the crises were a significant influence on the structuring of the social world of the early industrial workforce of Tyneside.

IV

High mortality was a fundamental feature of the social experience of Elizabethan and Jacobean Whickham, though its social structural significance varied between the different parts of Whickham's population. Mortality crises were a collective trauma. Their impact, however, was essentially individual and familial. This was, of course, equally true of mortality in general and serves to remind us that statistical description of the 'mortality regime', however sophisticated, inevitably fails to recapture the existential dimension of death in Whickham. Crucial to that experience was not the statistical average, but rather the unpredictability of individual mortality.

Some Whickham people died full of years, their children grown, their obligations discharged, already partly retired from the world. More, however, were cut off in their prime and the arbitrariness of death could have a drastic effect upon a family's fortunes. The history of the Scott family provides a particularly tragic example. Robert Scott held a tenement and garden in Swalwell. He died at the beginning of the crisis of 1587, leaving a widow Agnes, who took his copyhold in widowright, and three young children. One of the children, Isabel, died in January 1597. Of a second daughter we know nothing. By the

aggravated it, raising death rates which were already abnormally high and accelerating a turnover of population which was already rapid', *Impact of Plague*, p. 161.

time of Agnes' death in 1603, however, her son Christopher had reached adulthood. In September 1607 he was formally admitted as his father's heir in the Halmote, by which time he was married and had an infant son, Robert. By the end of the year, however, Christopher was dead: buried on 27 December. His widow Jane became the second successive Widow Scott to take the family copyhold in widowright. To make matters worse, Christopher had died at a time when he had substantial debts. Jane was sued by one of his creditors and in April 1612 she transferred the copyhold to that creditor, presumably as part of a settlement.[51]

Circumstances such as these make it clear enough why one strand in the quasi-magical popular beliefs of the period was a preoccupation with preservation against sudden death.[52] They also make it unsurprising that where we have evidence of the attitudes of Whickham people in the face of death, in the form of wills, it is a product of an anxiety to cope in advance with the social disturbance liable to be created by their imminent deaths (for most made their wills quite literally on their deathbeds).

Of course, not every parishioner made a will. In fact, only a small minority did so. The transference of family property between the generations was not solely dependent on death. Both land and goods or money were often enough transferred to adult children during the life of the parental generation.[53] Moreover, even transfers occasioned by death were not effected solely by wills.[54] Nevertheless last wills and

---

[51] DPD DDR Halmote Court III F 18, fols. 15v, 76v, 91v, 101v; PRO DURH 2/6/101. The child, Robert Scott, was buried within a month of this transfer. Jane Scott herself was buried within three months. For a further example of a family to whom sudden death brought disaster, see PRO DURH 2/6/21, 2/6/71: the case of Mathew Harrison, whose untimely death in 1607 not only left his widow 'utterly impoverished' but also brought down heavy financial penalties on two kinsmen who were his guarantors in a coal-mining sub-contract left unfulfilled as a result of his death.

[52] Thomas, *Religion and Decline of Magic*, pp. 37, 39, 134, 375.

[53] For some examples of property transfers during life, see DPD DDR Halmote Court III F 18, fols. 68, 83, 83v, 84v, 85; DPD Probate, Will of Robert Donkin (1587), Will of Beatrice Kirsop (1622). As might be expected, such transfers were often associated with marriage.

[54] Copyhold property was not devised by will. Heirs were recognised in the Halmote, according to the custom of the manor, and if there was no obvious heir, rival claimants were subject to the adjudication of the manorial jury. As for the goods and chattels of intestates, administrators (usually the widow or next of kin) could be appointed by the ecclesiastical courts, usually on condition that the children of the deceased received in due course the 'filiall and childes portions' guaranteed under the custom of the province of York (see Swinburne, *Treatise of Testaments*, pp. 183–98). Again, in some cases it would appear that the goods of a deceased person were simply taken over, without challenge and without formal process of any kind, by surviving spouses and heirs whose rights were tacitly acknowledged by kin and community alike. For an instance of this kind, see DPD DR V/12, unfoliated, Stobbs vs. Parmerley.

testaments were made by some Whickham people of all social levels
above the poor (though as might be expected testators were most
commonly drawn from the ranks of the relatively wealthy). In addition
to the general desire to specify the legacies due to each of their
dependents, they would appear to have been impelled by a variety of
specific motives. Some seem to have been anxious to leave a careful
record of the debts which they owed and which were owing to them.[55]
Some wished to use their wills to make explicit recognition of their
obligations to, or affection for, specific individuals.[56] A number wished
to appoint a specific 'tutor' to look to the interests of minor children, a
procedure permitted under the custom of the province of York.[57]
Others were anxious to influence the future behaviour of heirs by
placing conditions on their legacies.[58] A few may have feared the
falling of their estates into the hands of administrators whom they
could not trust – a possibility illustrated well enough by occasional
court cases arising from the maladministration of estates.[59] And
finally, some were moved by a desire to pre-empt possible conflict
among their heirs and survivors.[60]

[55] It is often clear that lists of debts and credits were dictated by the testator on the
deathbed. For some explicit examples, see DPD Probate, Wills and Inventories of
Thomas Wigham (1590), John Middleton (1603), Anthony Rodham (1614), John Nixon
(1644). John Nixon, indeed, resolved to make his will 'after he had begun to compute
and reckon up such debts as was due and owing unto him'. According to Prayer Book
rubrics the minister visiting sick parishioners should encourage them to declare their
debts and make a will: Gibson, *Codex Juris*, p. 460.

[56] This might be as simple as the statement of the smallholder and pit 'overman' Edward
Newby 'that what estate he had, he together with his wife Jane had got it by their
industry and therefore he gave and bequeathed all his whole estate to his loving wife,
to be at her disposall, and that if it were more, his said wife deserved it well'. It might
be as complex as that of the yeoman and 'wainman' Roger Colson who, in addition to
providing for his wife and three daughters, left legacies to his stepson, two
grandchildren, a brother, two sisters, a nephew and a godchild. D.P.D. Probate, Wills
of Edward Newby (1659), and Roger Colson (1608).

[57] Swinburne, *Treatise of Testaments*, pp. 168–80 outlines the law with regard to 'tutors' in
the province of York. For some Whickham examples, see DPD Probate, Wills of
Margaret Hirst (1576), Richard Harrison (1587), Henry Hall (1615).

[58] Ralph Hall left a legacy to his brother George 'if that he will keepe himself of good
conversion'. Anthony Barras said his son Ralph should have nothing if 'by sute or
otherwise' he tried to 'vex or molest' his brother Gregory: DPD Probate, Wills of Ralph
Hall (1581), Anthony Barras (1594). Other examples can be found in the wills of
Anthony Grundie (1600), Robert Fawdon (1603), Beatrice Kirsop (1622).

[59] For cases of alleged maladministration, see *e.g.* PRO DURH 2/6/81; DURH 4/3,
pp. 281–3.

[60] Anxiety over future conflict can be seen in Richard Hedworth's statement 'that
because he doubted his friends wold endeavor to wrong his said wife he desired to
have his said will all written up as it might stand by law': DPD DR V/9 unfol.,
17 October 1607. Again, John Blakiston drew up his will, 'considering . . . the
uncertainty of Mans Life, which in a moment may be taken away, after which many
tymes discords, variances and suites fall amongst their nearest kinsfolkes and deerist

Any or all of these motives might influence a testator and leave their traces in the formal record provided by the will itself. Taken together they bring out the extent to which the dying person was faced not only with the responsibilities of transmitting property, but also with the management of what could be a very complex web of personal relationships, with their attendant obligations and competing demands. Such detailed accounts of actual deathbed scenes as survive vividly illuminate these realities. They indicate that if the deathbed was certainly the scene of a formal settlement of material and emotional obligations contracted in life, it could also be the focus of a kind of familial diplomacy.

Thomas Harrison lay dying at the beginning of August 1603. He was an unmarried man and during his sickness he was kept in the house of his mother Jane and his stepfather the formidable village patriarch Nicholas Arnold. There he was attended and nursed by his sister Ann, a young married woman who had travelled from her home in Weardale to be by his side in his last days, and Elizabeth Pearson, a 'cosen' of the Harrisons. All these people were present, together with Agnes Harrison, another kinswoman, when he declared his wishes concerning his estate, early in the morning of the Saturday preceding his death. His 'nuncupative' will, however, was not committed to writing. On the following Thursday evening he was visited by George and Dorothy Dalton, two more 'cosens' and by Elizabeth Pearson's husband Thomas. Thomas Pearson later described how they 'found him lyinge sicke in Bedd' and 'after they had asked him howe he did and staied there a little', the conversation happened to turn to his will. George Dalton promptly attempted to persuade him to leave his nine acres of land to his brother Mathew rather than his brother Henry. Dorothy Dalton urged him to give a certain cow to Ann Watson, rather than to his mother. According to Pearson, Thomas resisted both suggestions, saying of the cow that 'he would not geve her from his mother who had disirved more of his goods'. George Dalton told a rather different story. According to him, the dying man took him by the hands and complained 'that he would faine have made his will and disposed of his goods but his mother and other his friends would not lett him'. Though his true desires were thwarted, he was prepared to acquiesce, saying 'they would not be contented and therefore lett them do with it what they will'. At this point Nicholas and Jane Arnold allegedly interrupted and prevented further discussion of the matter.

friends for want of perfect settling of their estates in their lifetimes': *Wills and Inventories from the Registry at Durham, Part 4*, Wood, ed., p. 307. In this context 'friends' means kinsfolk.

Exactly what transpired around Thomas Harrison's deathbed can never be known with certainty. The principal terms of the nuncupative will eventually accepted by the probate court, however, have an air of compromise. Brother Henry was named heir to nine acres of land. Brother Mathew was to have Thomas' stock, wains and gear and was to be given a lease of Henry's land for a term of twenty-one years. Nicholas Arnold got Thomas' best hat. Thomas' mother got her cow.[61]

Such deathbed diplomacy was not unique and could involve a variety of people who were far from backward in voicing their opinions as to how the testator should act. The Rector of Whickham, Henry Ewbank, urged a dying man in 1624 'to be good to his . . . wife' and to provide for her with greater care 'for that she had bene a carefull wife to him'.[62] William Marshall, a plague victim of 1604 was unwilling to make a will, declaring 'that he would not whilst he lived given and dispose his goods to anye'. He was won over by William Bainbridge, a neighbour, who urged him.

to consider of the great paines and charges that Adam Hogg his sonne in lawe had and was like to bestow upon him in the tyme of his visitacon and to consider of the same in giving to him his goods as he had proved a good sonne in lawe to him, so herein to show himself a kind father.[63]

Martin Wilson was also dying of the plague, which did not prevent several of his friends being present when he told his wife, 'Honye, I wolde thou would remember they sister . . . she hath taken pains for us, I wold thou would give her two kyne'. Back came the retort, 'I have rewarded her, we are not so far behind with her as you trow, if you gives her two kyne what shall I have to bring up my child'. Martin took the point. 'Nay, said he, take you all during your life to bring up my child and at your death consider of your sister'. No will was drawn up in this case 'for want of pen and inke'. We know of this discussion only because Martin's death from plague was rapidly followed by those of his wife and child, and settlement of various claims on his small estate involved the taking of depositions from witnesses of his deathbed wishes.[64]

The deathbed, then, was a public place, even a public forum of debate, and its principal concerns were those of settlement. The material and emotional obligations of a lifetime were recognised. Provision was made for the discharge of the family responsibilities which weighed heavily on the minds of the dying. Efforts were made to minimise the social disturbance which might be occasioned by

---

[61] DPD DR V/7, unfol., 22 Oct. 1603; DPD Probate, Will of Thomas Harrison (1603).
[62] DPD Probate, Will of Henry Harrison (1624).
[63] DPD DR V/8, fols. 31v–32.   [64] DPD DR V/8, fol. 32v; PRO DURH 2/2/51.

imminent death. That accomplished, if indeed it could be accomplished, the individual faced death with such comfort as could be provided by the presence of family and neighbours and such resolution as might be derived from religious beliefs.

Wills give an impression of dignified resignation in the face of death and of firm confidence in an afterlife to come. To judge by such evidence, it would appear that the testators of Whickham died calmly and devoutly, in accordance with the contemporary ideal of a 'good death'. This impression, of course, is inevitably coloured by the formal nature of these documents. Not all can have died well – there must have been pain too, and mental anguish, fear, and squalor. We know that William Marshall was not reconciled to the inevitability of death at the time he was persuaded to make his will: he was described walking restlessly before his door in a mood of bitter defiance. Nor is piety and repentance to be assumed. We know of testators enough whose attendance to their religious duties had been erratic or perfunctory in life. Nevertheless, the very public nature of death may have provided both support for the dying and social pressure to conform themselves to shared expectations of an appropriate comportment in the face of death. William Marshall was persuaded by a neighbour to calm himself and make his will. And there was a settlement to be made with God as well as with man. Every written will save one between 1547 and 1669 began with the bequest of the testator's soul to God. The terms in which these clauses were couched, of course, were devised by the scribes who wrote the wills. Yet even so, there were many scribes of wills in Whickham besides the clergy of the parish and all shared the same basic concept of the spiritual significance of death. It seems fair to assume that the testators did too and that they died for the most part 'in sure and certain hope' of the salvation promised them by their church. Indeed in the case of Thomas Harrison we know that after declaring his will he 'did for the most part of all the daie perfectly readd praiers in a Booke'.[65]

Moreover, conventional religious belief not only assured the dying of a life to come; it also helped to ease the smart of sudden death by insisting that death was neither random nor arbitrary. The language used by witnesses in depositions or by testators in the body of their wills indicates a view of death as purposeful, as a providential calling upon the individual soul by God. William Bainbridge persuaded William Marshall to settle his affairs in case 'it please God to call upon him'. John Whitfield in 1583 made provision for an alternative descent

---

[65] For the Marshall and Harrison cases, see notes 61 and 63 above.

of his property, 'if it happen that God call my child'. John Swan's will in 1633 included the phrase, 'after it shall please God to call me'.[66]

The providential call and the return of the soul 'to God that gave it' might be the fundamental significance of death to the individual. Yet Whickham testators were far from indifferent to the fate of their earthly remains or to the funeral rites which would mark their passage from the world.[67] Testators dying before 1640 almost invariably specified that they wished to be buried in Whickham church or Whickham churchyard, while before 1610 almost half the surviving wills contain even more specific instructions. Some wished to be buried 'at the east end of the church', 'at the queer end', 'in the queyre' or 'nere the quere door' – a preference quite common up to the 1580s and perhaps indicative of a desire to lie near the altar, at the 'holier' end of the church or churchyard. A few asked to be interred 'nighe unto my owne stall', 'near unto my stall', or 'under the pewe where I did sitt', a more personal expression of attachment to a specific place within the parish church and perhaps, by implication, within the social order of the parish. Rather more wished to lie not so much in particular places as by particular people – near a deceased wife, brother, husband, sister, mother, or father, or in two cases 'by those of my friends deceased' and 'neer unto the burials of my auncestoures'. Such requests, which are quite individual and unrelated to the identity of the scribes of wills, surely indicate both the continued power of family ties sundered by death and a sense of belonging to a community which embraced both the living and the dead within Whickham.[68]

If many Whickham testators had clear ideas about just where they wished to be laid to rest, they also had firm views about the appropriate manner of their burial. Sixteenth-century testators frequently specified that they should 'be honestly brought forth', a phrase repeated with small modifications in numerous wills. The actual costs of funerals, which are sometimes recoverable from inventories, varied considerably, both as absolute sums and as a proportion of the total value of a person's inventoried goods. It is clear enough, however, that each

---

[66] DPD DR V/8, fol. 31v; DPD Probate, Wills of John Whitfield (1583), John Swan (1633).
[67] The following discussion is based upon an analysis of all surviving Whickham wills and inventories for the period 1547–1669 (sixty-six wills; eighty-four inventories). Since the completion of this analysis and drafting of this chapter the whole question of funerals in early modern England has been greatly illuminated by Gittings, *Death*. As will be evident there are many similarities between Clare Gittings' findings for other parts of England and our study of Whickham. See also Laquer, 'Bodies, death and pauper funerals'.
[68] Cf. Gittings, *Death*, pp. 86–7 on the desire to be buried at a specific place or near a specified individual.

family had a good notion of what constituted an 'honest' funeral, and that an appropriate degree of pomp and circumstance mattered greatly both to the testator and to his or her survivors. One heir, William Thompson, actually went into debt to the tune of forty shillings in the midst of the crisis of 1596 to see his father, a modest yeoman, buried in the manner which he had requested.[69] Detailed funeral expenses in inventories indicate that certain items of expenditure were more or less fixed and that the overall costs of a funeral tended to depend upon the amount spent on the 'forthbringing' itself. This would appear to have been the carrying of the body from the house of the deceased to the church, a ceremony which was clearly preceded or accompanied by the dispensing of food and drink among the neighbours present. In the 1560s this might cost only five shillings for a modest cottager like Thomas Turner, thirteen shillings and four pence for yeoman like Lawrence Sotheron. Nevertheless, each received his 'outbringinge honestlie amonge [the] neighbours'.[70]

Taken together, the various aspects of the process of death which we have examined might be described as manifestations of a communal culture of death: a complex of attitudes, values and 'rituals of inclusion' which enabled the parishioners to cope on individual, familial, and community levels with both the emotional trauma and the social disturbance occasioned by death.[71] Yet if this was so, it must be emphasised that full participation in this culture of death became more socially circumscribed over time and that its more public features were subject to change. The way of handling death which we have described was most clearly that of the settled families of manorial Whickham. In reflecting on its significance it must be remembered that it was closely related to the ownership of property (albeit sometimes modest property), to personal connectedness within the existing community, and to a sense of identification with the community of the past. By 1600, the vast majority of the parishioners of Whickham were birds of passage, lacking extensive webs of kinship or deep roots in the parish and possessing little property beyond a few personal chattels. They made no wills. Few of them recorded transactions in the Halmote court. They took out no bonds of administration and appointed no

---

[69] DPD Probate, Will and Inventory of Cuthbert Thompson (1596).
[70] DPD Probate, Inventories of Thomas Turner (1569), Lawrence Sotheron (1562). See Gittings, *Death*, pp. 60ff., 89ff. and 151ff. For discussion of the intensity of the desire for proper burial, the mounting of funerals commensurate with the standing of the deceased, the large attendance at funerals and the hospitality provided.
[71] The phrase 'rituals of inclusion' is from Laquer, 'Bodies, death and pauper funerals', p. 112. These, he argues, 'expressed the deceased's place in the local community rather than in the social order generally'.

tutors for their children. They could not afford elaborate funerals. Of their methods of handling and celebrating death, we know almost nothing. Moreover, as the older community was inundated by the transient inhabitants of the new Whickham and as the copyholder families of the sixteenth century gradually died or moved away and were replaced by newcomers, the very context within which the propertied villagers conducted their affairs changed. This transformation of the social environment was reflected in the changing nature of the parishioners' culture of death.

Three processes of change can be identified. In the first place, a new element in funeral ritual emerged in the shape of the dole to the poor. Prior to 1580 bequests to the poor were rare and when they were made it was usually in the form of a small donation to the 'poor man's box'. Larger donations to the poor of twenty to forty shillings began to emerge in the later 1580s and by the early years of the seventeenth century wealthy testators usually specified that the sums bequeathed were to be distributed at their funerals by their executors. This was a new element in the 'forthbringing' and one of considerable significance. The commensality of eating and drinking among 'neighbours' was being paralleled, if not eclipsed, by the differentiation embodied in a public dole to 'the poor'.[72] Secondly, detailed funeral accounts of the early seventeenth century reveal a further innovation as compared with sixteenth-century accounts. This was the holding of a private dinner for relatives of the deceased which was quite separate from, and considerably more elaborate and expensive than, the public 'forthbringing'. Here was a second contribution to the devaluing of the 'forthbringing' among the wealthier parishioners, and it is surely significant that after the opening years of the seventeenth century the 'forthbringing' was no longer referred to by testators. A central pillar of the older corporate culture of death was crumbling. Thereafter, specific funeral instructions involved only the bequest of a sum for distribution to the poor or the placing of a limit on the money to be spent on the funeral. By the mid seventeenth century a new convention had emerged whereby a testator merely dismissed his funeral arrangements to 'the discretion of my executors'. Thirdly, after the first decade of the seventeenth century it became exceedingly rare for testators to request burial in a specific location or near a particular person in the manner which had been so common in the later sixteenth century. Between 1608 and 1669 there were only three such requests – in 1636,

---

[72] In this particular Whickham varied from the burial customs described by Gittings. She sees the dole to the poor as a medieval custom which was slowly declining in the later sixteenth and seventeenth centuries: *Death*, pp. 161–2.

1645, and 1667 – and it is perhaps significant that all three cases involved testators who were members of unusually long-established copyholder families. By the mid seventeenth century, in fact, some testators no longer even troubled to state that they wished to be buried in Whickham. The implication of these changes is that there was a diminishing sense of attachment to place among the testators of Whickham, a weakening sense of belonging to a community which embraced the living and the dead.[73]

In the gradual transformation of the ritual accompaniments of death in Whickham we find the cultural echo of the processes of socio-economic change which overwhelmed the parish in the first half-century of its industrialisation. Whickham's experience was unique, and yet it also represents a particular variant on patterns of change which have been observed at work elsewhere in England. At the turn of the sixteenth and seventeenth centuries provincial England witnesses what was perhaps the most intense phase of a process of socio-economic incorporation which was to produce both a more tightly integrated national society and a more highly differentiated local society. In Whickham such developments were felt with devastating force by virtue of the pell-mell exploitation of its subterranean wealth. The consequences were played out in the ways of life of the people of the parish and reverberated no less significantly in their ways of death.

---

[73] Gittings interprets change in funeral practices as an aspect of 'a changing conception of the self and a heightened sense of individuality' in early modern England, which expressed itself in 'an increasing anxiety over death', 'a growing desire to separate the living from the dead' and a 'gradual breaking down of the older communal solidarity which had previously assisted survivors': *Death*, pp. 13–14. This is certainly an arguable case. Our contribution to the emerging history of England's ways of death is to stress that changes in both attitudes and practice take on greater substance when they can be located in specific social contexts of the kind which we have attempted to provide in the case of Whickham.

4

The response to plague in early modern England: public policies and their consequences

PAUL SLACK

We may keep our Shipping to strict Quarantaine, we may form Lines, and cut off all Communication with the Infected, we may barricadoe up our Cities and our Towns, and shut ourselves up in our Houses, Death will come up into our Windows, and enter into our Palaces, and cut off our Children from without, and the young Men from the Streets.

William Hendley, *Loimologia Sacra*, 1721[1]

As it turned out, William Hendley was wrong. Death in the form of plague did not return to England during the 1720s, despite the scares aroused by its savage attack on Marseilles and other parts of southern France. Yet his profound scepticism about the policies adopted to control plague in England was widely shared; and it had been voiced by critical observers ever since those policies began in the sixteenth century. For quarantine had plainly not always protected England from the import of infection from the continent. Neither had strict watches against goods and travellers from London, when there were visitations there, prevented epidemics in provincial towns. The enforced isolation of infected families in their own houses, with their doors nailed up and guards outside them, had similarly failed to stop the movement of plague from household to household in stricken cities. Indeed, many critics had argued, such measures could not be expected to work. Plague was a divine punishment, and when God's hand struck, no human defences could ward off the blow. From the later sixteenth to the early eighteenth century the efficacy of precautions taken against plague was a matter of fierce controversy.[2]

It remains controversial. Although the theological element which was so prominent in earlier debates has faded away, historians

[1] Hendley, *Loimologia Sacra*, p. 59.
[2] These controversies are described in Slack, *Impact of Plague* and Mullett, *Bubonic Plague and England*.

167

continue to argue about the reasons for the disappearance of plague from single towns, countries, or the whole of Europe, and about the part played by human intervention. Some have attributed a decisive role to human action.[3] Others have argued that it was always partial and fallible, and that major changes in disease patterns must have been determined by broader developments: either biological – such as fluctuations in human or animal resistance to infection; or social – in the form of improvements in hygiene or diet or new patterns of intercontinental transport and trade.[4] These arguments have formed part of a more general discussion about the reasons for the stabilisation of European mortality since the eighteenth century; and they have raised the further, and equally important question of how far social policies have an effect, whether in the short or the long term.[5]

This chapter will seek to make a modest contribution to our understanding of these issues by describing the public policies which were adopted against plague in early modern England and by asking whether they might, on occasion, have worked. There will be no unqualified answer to this latter question; but a consideration of some relevant evidence should at least make it clear why the problem perplexed contemporaries and thus help us to comprehend some of the diverse responses to plague in the past.

I

England was late in adopting the policies invented and developed in other European countries in response to the Black Death and succeeding epidemics. Before the early sixteenth century there were no public orders controlling the infected or prohibiting contact with them, as there were in fourteenth-century Italy, in fifteenth-century France and even in Edinburgh by 1500.[6] The first steps were taken only in 1518, on Cardinal Wolsey's initiative. A proclamation ordered that infected houses in London should be marked with bundles of straw hung from their windows for forty days, and that their inmates should

---

[3] Especially Biraben, *Les hommes et la peste*. See also Flinn, 'Plague in Europe and the Mediterranean countries', pp. 139–46; Slack, 'Disappearance of plague', pp. 469–76.

[4] See, for example, Appleby, 'Disappearance of plague', pp. 161–73; McNeill, *Plagues and Peoples*, pp. 172–4; Shrewsbury, *Bubonic Plague*, pp. 485–6.

[5] Cf. Kunitz, 'Speculations on European mortality decline', pp. 349–64; Flinn, *European Demographic System*, pp. 95–101. Similar questions are raised by contemporary responses to dearth and the decline of 'subsistence' mortalities, a subject which also interested Andrew Appleby: see his 'Grain prices and subsistence crises', pp. 865–87.

[6] Biraben, *Les hommes et la peste*, 2, pp. 102–5; Mullett, 'Plague policy in Scotland', pp. 436–8.

carry white rods in their hands when they went into the streets.[7] Gradually, over the next fifty years, more elaborate and rigorous instructions were built on these foundations, first in London where the Privy Council was always pressing the Corporation for more forceful action, and then also in provincial cities such as York, where the Council in the North played a similar role.[8] Attempts were made to confine the sick and their families wholly to their own homes, to isolate some of them in specially built pesthouses, to set watches on infected households and pay for it all by local rates. By the early 1570s close control was being exercised over the sick in Cambridge and Shrewsbury, and there were new plague regulations in such towns as Chester and Hull at the same time.[9]

In 1578 these haphazard local endeavours were orchestrated by the central government and a uniform policy imposed on the whole kingdom. The Council published a Book of Orders to be enforced wherever outbreaks of plague occurred, and these printed regulations dictated English policy until almost the last breath of the disease in England. They were reissued with little alteration in 1592, 1593, 1603, 1609, 1625, 1630, 1636, and 1646, and radically revised only in 1666.[10] The main burden of administration was placed on justices of the peace, acting in their county divisions. They were to receive reports on the progress of infection from 'viewers' or searchers of the dead in each parish, to supervise the activities of constables and overseers of the poor, and to 'devise and make a general taxation' for the relief of the sick. The clothes and bedding of plague-victims should be burned, and funerals take place after sunset to reduce the number of participants. Above all, infected houses in towns should be completely shut up for at least six weeks, with all members of the family, whether sick or healthy, still inside them. Watchmen were to be appointed to enforce this order, and other officers should provide the inmates with food. Only in small villages where one house was distant from another could men be allowed out to tend their crops or cattle, and they must distinguish themselves by some mark on their clothes or by carrying a white stick in their hands.

These recommendations had foreign precedents. Certification of

---

[7] *Tudor Royal Proclamations*, Larkin and Hughes, eds., 3, pp. 269–70.

[8] E.g., *York Civic Records 5*, Raine, ed., pp. 23, 28, 49, 82. For London, see Wilson, *Plague in Shakespeare's London*, chapter 2.

[9] Cooper, *Annals of Cambridge*, 2, pp. 321, 335–6; HMC, *15th Report App. X*, pp. 18, 52 (Shrewsbury); Morris, *Chester*, p. 78; Hull Corporation Records, Bench Book 4, fos. 138–41.

[10] Slack, 'Books of Orders', pp. 3–4, 21. The 1592 edition is printed in *Present Remedies against the Plague*, intro. W. P. Barrett, Shakespeare Association Facsimile 7, 1933.

deaths, appointment of searchers, control of times of burial, and the fundamental policy of household segregation were all part of precautions widely adopted in Europe against epidemic disease. On one point the printed orders were silent. They did not dictate the sort of rigid restraints on movement of goods and people out of infected towns which brought the economy of some Italian cities in this period almost to a standstill. The English government did, however, regularly issue directions closing fairs in an effort to limit contact between towns during epidemics; and municipal councils themselves were quick to organise watches to prevent the introduction of infection from elsewhere, despite the damage this might do to an urban economy.[11]

Moreover, the English orders were uniquely strict in another respect. Other countries sometimes mitigated the rigours of household quarantine. In the Netherlands, for example, visits to the sick were not only permitted but to an extent encouraged, for purposes of religious consolation and medical help; and inmates of infected houses might be allowed out to 'refresh themselves' as long as they carried distinguishing marks.[12] There was no similar laxity in English towns. The incarceration of whole families in infected houses characterised English policy between 1578 and 1665, and it was this which stimulated most controversy. It was often attacked as inhuman and unchristian, and some critics thought it counter-productive: they argued that it virtually guaranteed contagion between members of a family and thus increased mortality rates rather than reducing them.[13]

Nevertheless, the practice was given the powerful sanction of parliamentary statute in 1604. Watchmen now had legal authority to use 'violence' to keep people shut up; anyone with a plague sore found wandering outside in the company of others was guilty of felony and might be hung; anyone else going out could be whipped as a vagrant.[14] The fiercest penalties envisaged by this Act were not enforced. No cases have been found of plague victims being prosecuted for felony. But the policy which it supported was being implemented in towns all

---

[11] E.g., York Corporation Records, House Book 32, fos. 279r, 316r, 321; Winchester Corporation Records, Proceedings of the Corporation 1593–1605, fos. 1–4, 57r. Cf. Cipolla, *Public Health and the Medical Profession*, pp. 28–9, 60–1.

[12] Van Andel, 'Plague regulations in the Netherlands', pp. 410–16; Chadwick, 'Plague in Yorkshire', pp. 467–75 (Hague regulations 1557). Household segregation was as strict in Italy as in England, and almost as strict in some parts of France (those shut up were allowed out only at night); but pesthouses were more common in both countries, giving more opportunity for isolation of the infected elsewhere: Cipolla, *Cristofano*, pp. 167–8; Biraben, *Les hommes et la peste*, 2, pp. 169–70; Deyon, *Amiens*, p. 18 and n. 5; Croix, *Nantes*, p. 146.

[13] See, for example, Brit. Lib., Lansdowne MS. 74, fos. 75–6; *Shutting Up Infected Houses*, London, 1665.   [14] 1 James I, c. 31.

over the country in the first decade of the seventeenth century. When plague arrived, councillors banned public assemblies, shut up houses, and set watchmen to guard their doors. Lists of infected households were kept in Reading, showing the sums paid to them every week while they were isolated. In Salisbury 411 different households, containing 1,300 people—one-fifth of the population of the town—were supported in the course of an epidemic in 1604. Not all of them can have been effectively guarded, day and night, of course, but weekly payments would not have continued if they had wandered completely free. Similar efforts were made in much smaller places. In Stone, Staffordshire, 115 families received aid during an epidemic in 1609; in a small Hampshire village six years earlier, eighteen infected households were attended to. In Nantwich, Cheshire, in 1604, fifty-five households were relieved by the parish, and there were significantly large payments to watchmen and constables, as well as to 'overseers' of the infected and buriers of the dead.[15] Household segregation and support had become the immediate reaction of local authorities when plague arrived.

Government policies to protect the whole country from the importation of plague developed much more slowly. England had no regular mechanism for controlling communication with infected ports abroad before the middle of the seventeenth century. The central government simply acted *ad hoc* when an obvious threat was brought to its notice. In 1580, for example, ships from Lisbon were stopped in the Thames until their merchandise had been aired, and in 1585 a ban was placed on imports from Bordeaux because of plague there. In the early seventeenth century orders for the restraint of shipping in the port of London and elsewhere became more frequent, but they were still usually applied to specific vessels or specific ports of origin.[16] In 1629 and again in 1635, however, the Council ordered customs officials in all ports to stop goods and men being landed from ships from any infected place abroad. When there was plague in the Low Countries in 1655 more rigorous precautions were taken. The Dutch ambassador was consulted, a twenty-day quarantine was imposed on ships from the Netherlands, in place of irregular periods of isolation earlier, and efforts were made to prevent abuses. The orders were to be enforced in

[15] Reading Corporation Records, box 39, plague rate accounts 1607; Slack, 'Poverty and politics in Salisbury', p. 170; Staffs RO, Q.S.Rolls Epiph. 1609/10, no.57; Hants RO, Jervoise MSS., Box 44M69/012, 30 Oct. 1603; Cheshire R.O., Q.S.File 1604(iii), doc. 18, (iv), docs. 18–21.

[16] *Cal. S.P. Dom. 1547–80*, p. 320; *APC 1580–1*, p. 61; *Analytical Index to the Remembrancia of the City of London*, pp. 329–30; *Tudor Royal Proclamations*, Larkin and Hughes, eds., 2, no. 677; HMC, *Salisbury (Cecil)*, XII, pp. 247, 428–9, 438, 703.

every port and to be extended when necessary to other infected countries.[17] Despite the consequences for trade, the Protectorate Council followed the precedent set by its predecessor under Charles I.

By the time the last outbreak of plague began in England in 1665, therefore, public policies were well-established at every level. When it heard of epidemics in the Low Countries, in 1663, the Council set up a special committee for the prevention of plague and imposed a *trientane* of thirty days' isolation on ships from infected ports, followed, in May 1664, by a full quarantine of forty days. The protests of the Dutch ambassador were ignored, vessels were halted at Tilbury, and the government tried as best it could to impose similar controls in provincial ports.[18] When these measures failed and plague arrived in London, the Council set up another special committee, in May 1665, to recommend further action. It issued orders banning fairs in order to prevent the spread of contagion, and it supported local justices and town councils who were now setting strict watches at their gates and on the roads against travellers from the capital. Boats from London were quarantined outside Whitby. In York, the King's brother, James, ordered all innkeepers to report newcomers to the town to the mayor.[19] Throughout the provinces suspected wanderers were traced and where necessary confined to their houses.

The Council's deliberations produced one important revision of past policies. Since the 1630s there had been doubts in the government as well as outside about the wholesale practice of household quarantine, and suggestions that ideally the infected ought to be separated from their families in pesthouses. These opinions were strengthened by projects which the Council received in 1665 insisting that the rigours of household segregation had led 'the infected to conceal their infection' and had increased contagion and mortality. In the end a new Book of Orders, published in May 1666, recommended the preferred alternative. Wherever possible, the sick were to be removed to 'pesthouses, sheds or huts, for the preservation of the rest of the family'.[20]

In practice, however, this meant little, partly because the change came too late, but also because it could not be implemented in major

[17] *Remembrancia*, pp. 339, 345; *APC 1629/30*, p. 160; *Stuart Royal Proclamations, 1625–46*, Larkin, ed., no. 207; *Cal.S.P.Dom. 1655*, pp. 322–3, 381, 598; Hull Corporation Records, Bench Book 5, fos. 136, 191v.

[18] PRO, PC 2/56, pp. 592, 607, 610–11, 624, 676, 688; 2/57, pp. 89, 93, 104, 126–8, 139, 164, 177, 186, 199–200. Cf. the project of 1664 in SP 29/109/108.

[19] PRO, PC 2/58, p. 135; *Cal.S.P.Dom. 1664–5*, pp. 426, 506–7, 535, 538, 569; *North Riding Quarter Sessions Records*, Atkinson, ed., 6, pp. 90–3, 95; York Corporation Records, House Book 38, fos. 16v, 17, 21v.

[20] Slack, 'Books of Orders', pp. 8–9; Bell, *Great Plague*, pp. 333–5.

epidemics. Several towns, including Oxford, Newcastle, and Windsor, had had pesthouses from the beginning of the century. But most of them were no more than temporary wooden shacks hurriedly thrown up outside the walls, and they could hold only a fraction of the infected poor. In Worcester a quarter of the deaths in a great epidemic in 1637 occurred at the pesthouse; and that was exceptional. The proportion in Norwich in 1665/6 – less than 10 per cent – was more usual.[21] Although many towns built new pesthouses in 1665 and 1666, therefore, household quarantine could not be abandoned once the infection spread to more than a handful of families. It was practised in Southampton, King's Lynn, and Bristol as well as Norwich, where houses were nailed up with their inmates still inside them.[22]

A more practicable novelty in 1665 and 1666 was the imposition of a similar kind of isolation on whole villages and towns. County authorities, who were determined to halt the spread of disease, erected what amounted to local *cordons sanitaires* around infected communities and refused to allow provisions in unless they were maintained. The Norfolk justices had guards placed round Yarmouth to prevent movement out of the port, and they forced the council of Norwich to nominate places outside the city to which food could be brought. When Sherborne was infected, neighbouring parishes in Dorset were 'very much startled' by the unruliness of the inhabitants; the local gentry reacted by arranging food supplies, but only on condition that order was restored and that meant, among other things, no movement of the poor out into the country.[23] The famous tragedy at Eyam in Derbyshire resulted from exactly the same kind of pressures. The Rector, William Mompesson, and his Interregnum predecessor, Thomas Stanley, who persuaded the parishioners to cut themselves off from other villages, have been given credit for courageous self-sacrifice, saving their neighbours at the price of enormous local mortality. An altruistic and pious dedication to the common good is certainly evident in Mompesson's letters, but so also is a hard-headed appreciation that this was the only way of guaranteeing some sort of help from other, more fortunate, parts of the county.[24] The quarantine of villages, like

---

[21] *Oxford Council Acts*, Salter, ed., pp. 153, 186, 387; Welford, *Newcastle and Gateshead*, 3, p. 123; Tighe and Davis, *Annals of Windsor*, 2, pp. 52–3; Tinker, *Worcester's Affliction*; *Records of Norwich*, 2, p. 67.

[22] *Cal.S.P.Dom. 1664/5*, p. 449; *1665/6*, p. 568; Bristol Archives Office, Gt. Audit Book 1665–6, pp. 42, 43; Norfolk and Norwich RO, Mayor's Court Book 24, fo. 5v.

[23] PRO PC 2/58, p. 130; Norfolk and Norwich RO, Mayor's Court Book 24, fo. 8r; 'Plague and Cholera Papers', 12 July 1666; *Somerset and Dorset Notes and Queries*, 24, p. 180, 26, pp. 104–6.

[24] Batho, 'Plague of Eyam', pp. 88–90; Bradley, 'Most famous of all English plagues', pp. 65, 80; Wood, *History and Antiquities of Eyam*, p. 83.

the quarantine of households, was imposed from above and outside, by fear.

Such measures were also imposed with considerable confidence in 1665 and 1666. They did not by any means always work, as we shall see, but local authorities were quick to congratulate themselves on success, even when their optimism was premature. In Beverley, for example, the 'effectual care' of the justices in 'separating the infected from the free' was thought at first to have prevented a major epidemic; and the London newspapers were full of reassuring tributes to the care and vigilance of provincial magistrates at the first suggestion of infection.[25] Despite the suffering they imposed on the victims of plague, despite the costs involved in implementing them, despite the doubts of some critical and concerned observers, public policies against plague were not only usual by 1665; they were trusted by the magistrates and governors who implemented them. We must now ask whether that trust was misplaced.

II

An answer to this question must involve some consideration of the aetiology of plague. Most of the measures taken by governments to control the spread of the disease were obviously directed towards human agents; the important part played by the rat was not appreciated before the end of the nineteenth century, and it was therefore transmission of infection by men or their goods which was attacked by quarantine and isolation. Some effort was made to stop domestic animals, dogs and cats, moving from house to house and carrying plague with them, but this did nothing to stop rodents; rather the reverse. In order to judge the potential of contemporary policies for the control of plague, therefore, we need to define the relative importance of men and rats in the origins of epidemics. If men played the major role, those policies may have had an effect. If rats played the major part, it was unlikely to have been good management and more likely to have been good fortune which protected households, towns or countries from plague.

Unfortunately, there is still considerable uncertainty about several aspects of the epidemiology of plague which are relevant here. In particular there is the problem of whether the disease could be carried by the human flea, *Pulex irritans*, from man to man, as well as by the rat flea, *Xenopsylla cheopis*, normally moving from rat to man and only occasionally from one man to another. Such controversial points

[25] PRO, SP 29129/26; *The Intelligencer*, 14, 21 August 1665, pp. 712, 754; *The Newes*, 27 July, 3 August, 19 October 1665, pp. 647, 672, 679, 1015.

cannot be finally determined by employing evidence from only one country, but for our purposes they can best be approached by examining the normal course of an epidemic in early modern England. Four separate stages can be distinguished: the introduction of plague into England; its movement from town to town; its spread within a single town or village; and finally, its transmission between one member of a household and another. Men and rats played a part in all of these, but their relative significance varied from stage to stage.

Human agency was vital at the first stage. Plague was always imported into Britain. Each epidemic wave began in a port, commonly London but sometimes Hull, Yarmouth, or Plymouth. The disease might linger for several years afterwards, as it spread from one town to another; but in the end it normally disappeared and had to be reintroduced from outside. There is no reliable evidence of plague anywhere in England between 1616 and 1624 or between 1654 and 1664, for example.[26] The origins of English plagues are therefore to be found in ships from infected ports overseas, often in the Low Countries; they brought infective fleas, either in their merchandise or on infected rats or, conceivably, in the clothing of infected passengers and crew, into English harbours.

It is probable that men were also important at the second stage, in the long-distance movement of plague from ports to other towns, though there can be less certainty here. There may have been cases, like those documented in modern outbreaks, in which wild rodents carried the disease from field to field in haphazard fashion across the countryside.[27] This would be consistent with the evidence of local studies, of Devon and Essex, for example, which show that odd villages were stricken when their neighbours were not. However, infected villages tended to lie along major routes of human transport, on rivers and roads; and plague often spread very quickly from one town to another, much more quickly than one would expect if wild rodents had been the carriers.[28] Moreover, there is ample contemporary reference to particular individuals or bundles of merchandise being responsible for initiating a local outbreak.[29] In these cases it is probable

---

[26] In 1624 plague arrived in Scarborough and in 1664 in Yarmouth before an outbreak in London: Shrewsbury, *Bubonic Plague*, p. 313; *Cal.S.P.Dom.1664–5*, pp. 78, 90, 92, 95, 196.

[27] Baltazard, 'Déclin et destin d'une maladie infectieuse', pp. 247–62. Cf. Norris, 'East or West?', p. 16.

[28] Slack, 'Mortality crises', pp. 44–7.

[29] For examples, see *ibid.*, p. 46; Bradley, 'Most famous of all English plagues', p. 80; Polwhele, *History of Devonshire*, 1, pp. 327–8; Sheffield City Library, Strafford Correspondence, 12/236; Kent AO, QM/SB 926 (Peter Clark kindly drew my attention to this reference to plague being caught from the coat of an infected man).

that fleas on the backs of men, in bales of cloth or trunks of clothes, first brought infection to the rats of a village or town. The black rat itself is known to be reluctant to move far from its nest, and the balance of the evidence suggests that men, their carts, boats, and baggage formed the vital link between one rat population and another.[30] Wild rodent transmission was not a necessary part of the chain, and there is as yet no reason to suppose that it was a common one in the sixteenth and seventeenth centuries.

Rats were much more important at the third and fourth stages, in sustaining a major epidemic and in spreading plague within a household. This is emphatically not to say that they were solely responsible. Work on modern epidemics of plague in North Africa and elsewhere has reinforced the view that the human flea, *Pulex irritans*, can transmit infection directly from one man to another, provided that it is present in sufficient numbers and provided that the first human host has sufficient plague bacilli in his blood-stream.[31] Both conditions must often have been satisfied in Tudor and Stuart England, and the movement of fleas from man to man was easy in a society in which the poor were short of beds and bedding as well as of clothes, and in which even the rich often slept together in crowded inns. In these circumstances, indeed, *Xenopsylla cheopis* might also readily spread plague directly between one man and another. There is no reason to doubt contemporary observations that people caught plague when they stayed in inns and found themselves sharing beds with unsuspected plague victims.[32]

Nevertheless, there is persuasive indirect evidence that major epidemics in towns had an epizootic foundation. The heavy incidence of plague in suburbs and back alleys, away from main thoroughfares and market-places, suggests that it was not frequency of interpersonal contact which created an urban epidemic, but rather the close proximity of rodents and humans in the poor tenements of these

---

[30] Cf. Pollitzer, *Plague*, pp. 300–1; Hirst, *Conquest*, pp. 303–9. There is some disagreement among medical authorities on plague as to whether the transport of fleas or of rats is the more important: Hirst, *Conquest*, pp. 320–9; Pollitzer, *Plague*, pp. 294, 385–91, 490–9; but this does not affect the point that men were responsible for the transport itself.

[31] Cf. Hirst. *Conquest*, pp. 238–46; Pollitzer, *Plague*, pp. 378–81; Bradley, 'Some medical aspects of plague', pp. 13–15. A recent argument for the importance of human fleas in medieval epidemics, which also summarises the available medical literature, is Ell, 'Interhuman transmission of medieval plague', pp. 497–510.

[32] For example, Kent AO, transcript of Cranbrook register, 1597; Willis, *Medical Works*, pp. 124, 131. On the dangers from infected bedding, see *Cal.S.P.Dom. 1664–5*, p. 548; HMC, *Bath (Longleat)*, 4, p. 255; *Plague Pamphlets of Thomas Dekker*, Wilson, ed., p. 113.

neighbourhoods. A similar conclusion might be drawn from the way in which plague often missed out odd houses in its progress along a street; close contact between neighbours did not guarantee infection. Even at the fourth stage, within a household, it seems likely that rats played an important role. Although the common occurrence of multiple cases of plague in single households might seem to indicate transmission between humans, it has been noticed that there was no correlation between the level of mortality and household size. The number of people present in a house does not seem to have determined the extent of infection. The number of rats, and the opportunities available for their fleas to find human hosts, probably did.[33]

Both inter-human and rat-human transmission should therefore be granted a role in English epidemics. When there were only a few sporadic cases of plague in one or two households, as in Leicester and Reading in 1578, rodents may well not have been involved.[34] Fleas had not moved from men to rats, or if they had, they had not sparked off an epizootic. The transmission of infection then depended on close contact between men; and once the presence of plague was recognised, that was more easily avoided than contact with the unseen and unsuspected danger of dead and dying rodents. In major epidemics in large towns like London or Bristol, on the other hand, when there were clearly separate foci of infection in different widely spaced parishes, there can be little doubt that the human disease had a rodent base. It might be communicated directly between members of a family and perhaps between neighbours, but plague was also moving irregularly from house to house with rats searching for food; and the epidemic could not end until the rat population had been largely destroyed by it.[35]

This is a tentative, not a definitive picture of the origins of plague epidemics, and it may be amended by future study of particular outbreaks. Speculative as in parts it is, however, it suggests two firm conclusions which are supported by all the available evidence, and which are indeed applicable to some degree to all epidemic diseases.

[33] Appleby, 'Disappearance of plague', p. 164; Slack, 'Local incidence of epidemic disease', pp. 55–7; Schofield, 'Anatomy of an epidemic', pp. 104–8. The importance of rats in serious urban epidemics has been admitted even by the foremost French authority who advocates the role of human fleas: Biraben, *Les hommes et la peste*, 1, p. 335 and note.

[34] *Records of the Borough of Leicester*, Bateson, 3, p. 179; Berkshire RO, parish register of St. Giles's Reading. For a similar modern incident, see Laforce, 'Outbreak of Plague in Nepal', pp. 693–706.

[35] Finlay, *Population and Metropolis*, pp. 121–2; Bell, *Great Plague*, map opposite p. 158; Slack, 'Local incidence of epidemic disease', pp. 52–5. Cf. Norris, 'East or West?', pp. 16–17, and 'Geographic origin of the Black Death', pp. 117–19.

First, it was much easier to prevent the introduction of plague in the first place than to control its spread once it had gained hold in epizootic or epidemic form. If ships from infected ports overseas or passengers and goods leaving infected English towns could be stopped, those epidemic waves which swept across Europe and then across England might be cut short. Secondly, when infection did arrive, an epidemic of plague depended on the conjunction of a whole set of circumstances, and therefore to an extent on chance. It required initial transmission by infective fleas – and not all infected fleas are infective – not just to one man or one rats' nest, but to several. It needed an environment where rats and men were crowded together and where fleas were common and taken for granted. There must be the warm climate necessary for the survival and reproduction of the fleas themselves. And all these conditions would need to be met in each successive town visited by plague if there was to be a series of major epidemics.

This explains some of the haphazard features which can be observed in the incidence of plague in the sixteenth and seventeenth centuries. Mortality rates varied enormously from one infected community to another, and in every epidemic wave some towns and parishes escaped entirely. This might sometimes be because rodent populations had not had time to re-establish themselves after an earlier epizootic. It is notable that plague mortality was relatively low in London and Norwich in 1630 and 1631, probably because their rat populations had been decimated in 1625, while it was heavy in the North, in Cambridge, and in Shrewsbury, areas of the country which had not been seriously affected five years before.[36] But towns might also escape simply because infective fleas happened not to arrive, or having arrived not to find new human or animal hosts; or because plague invaded so late in the year that cold weather snuffed it out before more than a handful of cases had developed. Even without government intervention, there was a large range of possible outcomes once the plague bacillus had been introduced into an English town.

III

These epidemiological considerations make it plain that the historian can never be certain whether it was good management or good fortune which prevented a serious outbreak of plague in any particular instance. There were simply too many variables involved in mortality and morbidity differentials. Neither can the historian reconstruct a

---

[36] Slack, 'Disappearance of plague', p. 471.

convincing controlled experiment, comparing the epidemic experience of towns where public controls were imposed and those where they were not. Again the variables are too many; the records often fail us when no administrative action was taken; and even when it was, we can never judge how efficiently the regulations were enforced. They were certainly often evaded. People slipped past the watches or bribed them. Goods from London were smuggled into other towns. Infected people broke out of their houses.[37] The historical record and historical experience are not tidy enough for precise scientific analysis.

What we can do, however, is examine probabilities, on the assumption that some kinds of human action could raise the threshold which plague had to surmount, and so reduce the limits within which mere chance operated. While never wholly effective, efforts to prevent the movement of people and goods from infected places restricted mobility to some degree. Watch and ward cut down the number of infective fleas arriving in a town and thus reduced the risk that one of them would spread plague to native rodent and human populations. It was not infallible, but it could be decisive; and the more rigorous the measures taken, the more likely they were to succeed.

We can see examples both of obvious failure and of apparent success in 1665 and 1666. Once plague was known to be rampant in London in the early summer of 1665, local authorities elsewhere cancelled fairs and arranged watches against men and merchandise coming from the capital. In Exeter these precautions appear to have succeeded: there was no plague in the city.[38] In Norwich, however, they conspicuously failed. A ban on imports and immigrants from infected towns was first imposed in July 1665, but by August there were cases of plague just outside St. Benedict's gate and by September the number of burials was rising in St. Margaret's parish, just inside it. No major epidemic developed before the end of the year, however, and the watch was disbanded in November, only to be tightened up again early in 1666 when mortality increased once more. By then it was too late. The disease had probably already taken hold of the rat population, there were sporadic human cases of plague in February, and from June to September it ravaged all the poorer parishes of the city. In all, 2,251 people died of plague.[39]

---

[37] For London examples, see Kempe, *Historical Notices*, pp. 169–70; PRO, SP 16/175/3, 22, 24.

[38] Exeter Corporation Records, Act Book 11, fos. 31–9r. One suspect from an infected town did get into Exeter, however: Strangers' Book 1621–68, p. 183.

[39] Norfolk and Norwich RO, Mayor's Court Book 23, fos. 253, 257–61r, 268v, 276v; Court Book 24, fo. 6v; Assembly Book 1642–68, fo. 267v; city parish registers; *Cal.S.P.Dom. 1665/6*, p. 252; *Records of Norwich*, 2, p. 67.

There were several reasons for Norwich's misfortune. It was threatened from more directions than Exeter: there had to be orders against travellers from Yarmouth and then from Colchester, as well as from London. The corporation records suggest that the watchmen were more negligent than those in Devon. Most important of all, perhaps, the city was physically less easy to defend than Exeter against an invasion by disease, just as it had been less easy to defend against peasant revolt in 1549: its walls did not extend round the whole perimeter, and guards at the gates could be circumvented without much difficulty.[40]

Even well-walled cities often had problems in preventing the introduction of plague since their extra-mural suburbs remained vulnerable. Exeter's suburban parish of St. Sidwell had proved its Achilles' heel in earlier epidemics;[41] and it was perhaps good fortune rather than the watch which prevented the development of infection there in 1665 and 1666. Walls still remained a useful barrier, however, hindering the passage of domestic rats across them, and presenting opportunities for the control of human movement too. The case of Bristol suggests that energetic action could sometimes confine plague to extra-mural suburbs and protect the inner-city.

The council there imposed a strict watch against Londoners in June 1665, both at the gates and on main roads at the outer limits of the built-up area. It failed. By the end of 1665 there were cases of plague in Pile Street and St. Philip's parish, both outside the walls, and the outer watch was abandoned in February, 1666, leaving only guards at the gates. In the spring there were more plague cases, and the council had to isolate and support their families. Yet there was no epidemic disaster like that in Norwich. Less than one hundred people appear to have died of plague, and the vast majority of them lived outside the walls, in St. Philip's and St. James's parishes. There was only a handful of cases in the inner city: five suspected plague-deaths in St. Nicholas's and St. Stephen's parishes and two or three more certain victims in Tucker Street in St. Thomas's.[42] The fate of Bristol was probably balanced on a knife-edge in the spring of 1666; if fleas had spread plague from men to many of the rats in St. Thomas's and St. Nicholas's there would no doubt have been a serious epidemic. But continuous watches at the

---

[40] Cf. Cornwall, *Revolt of the Peasantry*, pp. 100–2, 151.
[41] Pickard, *Population and Epidemics of Exeter*, pp. 35–6.
[42] Bristol AO, Orders of Mayor and Aldermen 1660–66, 19 June 1665, 13 January 1666; Sessions Minute Book 1653–71, fo. 64r; Common Council Proceedings 1659–75, pp. 130, 133–4; Gt. Audit Book 1665/6, pp. 42–3; registers of St. James, St. Nicholas, and St. Stephen; Latimer, *Annals of Bristol in Seventeenth Century*, p. 333; *Cal. Treasury Books 1660–7*, p. (731).

walls and the isolation of the few infected households within them had reduced the number of occasions on which that might happen.

A still better-documented example of plague being held at bay is provided by York in 1631, where Sir Thomas Wentworth, President of the Council in the North, took firm control. There, as in Norwich in 1665, plague could be seen approaching from more than one direction, from Lancashire as well as from Lincolnshire. There, as in Bristol and Norwich, the disease could not be prevented from infecting outlying villages like Huntington and then the suburb of Walmgate. But it was kept outside the walls by magisterial intervention. As Wentworth told the mayor and aldermen, plague 'may be the easier prevented in the beginnings than hereafter', and 'the greatest pity' they could show its victims, actual and potential, was to take 'severe and strict courses' from the start. Goods coming from infected parts of London were traced and burnt. Suburban houses were shut up when infected, and so were the houses of people who had been in contact with them. When cases of plague were suspected within the walls, their houses were also shut up and in some cases, though not in all, the suspects were quickly removed to extra-mural pesthouses. We do not know how many victims there were altogether, but there cannot have been many in the centre of town, since the parish registers show no sign of an abnormal increase in mortality.[43] The evidence suggests that plague had not reached the rats of the inner city.

York was in many respects exceptional, and not only because of Wentworth's foresight and drive. Throughout the sixteenth and seventeenth centuries its council was unusually, possibly uniquely, active against the threat of infection. The close tracing of contacts which was undertaken in 1631, and again in 1637/8, cannot be paralleled in any other town at this date.[44] It was helped too by its still intact walls and by its geographical position, further removed from London and the continent than many towns. All these factors worked together to ensure that the city had fewer serious epidemics than any other town of comparable size in Tudor and Stuart England.

Even so, York's case does suggest that contemporary mechanisms for the control of plague were not without empirical justification. They could keep it from penetrating a town's defences, and their widespread use in the national alert of 1665 and 1666 may well explain why

---

[43] York Corporation Records, House Book 35, fos. 105–13, 115v–17r (Wentworth's letter), 118–52; PRO, SP 16/200/14; parish registers of St. Michael-le-Belfrey, Holy Trinity, and St. Martin cum Gregory, published by the Yorkshire Parish Register Society.

[44] York Corporation Records, House Book 35, fo. 335r; Book 36, fo. 10r (1637/8).

many English towns and villages escaped serious epidemics then, although they had not done so in earlier waves of infection beginning in 1603 and 1625.[45] Furthermore, we can see that the isolation of the infected could also be useful in the early stages of an epidemic. It was clearly better to move the sick and their contacts away from their homes, to locations outside the walls, than to shut them all up together with domestic rats; the government's final preference in 1666 for pesthouses over household isolation was eminently sensible. But even the more common practice of shutting up houses would be likely to reduce the risk of further infection to some degree when there were only a few cases. It limited the number of human and rodent hosts available to infective fleas. Plague might be confined to one or two households or even, though this could not be guaranteed, to one or two rats' nests.

If these measures failed, however, as they very often did, there could be little point in persevering with them. Once plague had spread to several streets and gained a hold among rats in different parts of a city, household segregation could not hold it back. There were too many opportunities for rat-flea-rat and then rat-flea-man transmission. In any case, the practice usually broke down at the height of an epidemic when scores of families were stricken. In London in 1665, for example, it was reported from St. Giles Cripplegate that 'all have liberty lest the sick poor should be famished within doors, the parish not being able to relieve their necessity'.[46] The only recipe for self-preservation in the middle of an epidemic, as contemporaries well understood, was flight. The question to be asked in the circumstances of established infection was not whether household quarantine was useful, but whether it was counter-productive, as some contemporaries argued. 'Infection may have killed its thousands, but shutting up hath killed its ten thousands', alleged a tract of 1665.[47]

Exaggerated as this indictment was, there is reason to suppose that it contained some truth. Even without quarantine, the household incidence of plague was conspicuous. Infected rats in a house, and the common use of beds and clothes, put all members of a family at risk. But compulsory isolation prevented wives and children being sent away, as they otherwise often were, and turned the risk of infection into a near certainty. It is again difficult to test this assertion

---

[45] Among towns, Worcester, Shrewsbury, Chester, Leicester, Lincoln, and Hull, besides Exeter, Bristol, and York, provide examples. Cf. Wrigley and Schofield, *Population History*, p. 653, which shows a smaller proportion of the Cambridge Group's sample parishes affected in 1665/6 than in 1603/4 or 1625/6.
[46] Brit. Lib., Harl. MS. 3785, fo. 31.   [47] *Shutting Up Infected Houses*, p. 8.

statistically. A comparison of mortality rates in places where isolation was practised and where it was not would tell us little, since there might be many other reasons for local variations. It is notable, however, that the household incidence of plague was unusually high when people were forcibly restrained from escaping from infection. The available English evidence suggests that between one-third and two-thirds of all burials during an epidemic of plague occurred in families which had three or more deaths; and the proportions were highest in towns where we know that some form of quarantine was practised. In Salisbury, for instance, it is likely that most of the families which received support during the epidemic of 1604 stayed at home in return for relief: 61 per cent of the deaths in these households occurred in family groups of three or more. Even more strikingly, the figure was as high as 72 per cent in Eyam when the whole village was isolated in 1666.[48] It is hard to believe that the proportions would have been as great if people had been able to move away.

In the Eyam instance, the slaughter of whole families would have been defended by contemporaries with the argument that it helped preserve neighbouring villages. There was some justification for that view, even if one doubts whether controlling one potential source of infection among many was worth the price which had to be paid. There was much less foundation for the argument that household isolation in the poorer parts of cities protected the more prosperous quarters. Once an epidemic had begun, the rich had more potent defences than that: their relative freedom from fleas, their more frequent changes of clothing and bedding, their distancing from rats in large houses, and, of course, their flight. And the costs, in human suffering, were again enormous. In one London parish in 1593 the clerk tersely recorded the burial of a man who 'died of grief, being now shut up in his house this sickness time'. When the astrologer, Simon Forman, was shut up in the same city in 1603, he was 'left destitute' and 'much abused' by his neighbours: 'They would say that it was better that I and my household should starve and die than any of them should be put in danger'.[49]

It would be both patronising and anachronistic simply to condemn Forman's neighbours, however. We can now see that both the proponents and the opponents of public policies had cases which were intelligible and defensible. Each position was given an emotional

---

[48] Calculated from: Salisbury Corporation Records, S161, compared with the parish registers; Bradley, 'Most famous of all English plagues', p. 92, Table 3. For other figures, see Schofield, 'Anatomy of an epidemic', p. 106; Slack, 'Some aspects of epidemics in England', p. 203.

[49] *Registers of the Parish of All hallows London Wall*, Jupp and Hovenden, eds., p. 120; Bodl. Lib., Ashmole MS. 1436, fo. 72.

charge by the personal tragedies and public horrors of an epidemic. Each involved fundamental moral issues to which there were no simple solutions, as Defoe's graphic *Journal of the Plague Year* among other contemporary sources makes clear. Above all, each could claim to be supported by experience. In the early stages of an epidemic, household segregation, like watch and ward, sometimes paid off; and that supported the hypothesis that 'infection' between men explained plague. At the same time, along with watch and ward, isolation often failed: and then the alternative explanation that the roots of an epidemic lay in 'miasma', in the polluted air of certain localities, seemed justified. As long as the role of the rat was unacknowledged, people could scarcely be expected to distinguish clearly between the circumstances which favoured success and those which did not: between the importance of human transmission in the introduction of plague in the first place, and the equally vital and far more intractable part played by rats and a congested and unhygienic urban environment in sustaining a major epidemic.

IV

This distinction between, as it were, first cause and necessary conditions is also useful when we come to consider the part played by public policies in the final disappearance of plague from England. Many of the explanations which have been put forward to account for that remarkable event refer to the local circumstances which provided the tinder for an epidemic. They would postulate increasing resistance to the bacillus among rats or humans, a change in the main rodent species, or improvements in public and private hygiene or in housing. It can be argued, however, that these developments worked, if at all, only in the long-term, and that they had little impact before the end of the eighteenth century.[50] If we wish to account for the absence of epidemics in England between 1670 and 1800, we should consider the possibility that it was the initial spark which was missing, and ask whether the quarantine precautions taken by governments may not have kept the plague bacillus out of the country.

We have seen that English defences against ship-borne infection were rudimentary before 1620, and they failed at least twice after that. In 1635 and 1664 the disease reached England from the Low Countries, with disastrous consequences for London immediately afterwards. It did not arrive in 1655, however, and quarantine, along with the

---

[50] For such an argument, see my 'Disappearance of plague'.

commercial disruptions caused by the Dutch and Spanish wars, may help to account for that. There may also have been local successes. The measures taken in Hull against ships from the Netherlands and London between 1663 and 1665 helped to prevent an epidemic in that vulnerable east-coast port.[51] Similarly, between 1667 and 1669, while the last embers of the epidemic of 1665 were still flickering in London, precautions against shipping from northern France and the isolation of Frenchmen suspected to have died of plague in Dover and Yarmouth may have stopped the introduction of a new and more virulent strain of the bacillus.[52] As a general rule, however, once plague had reached north-western Europe from the Mediterranean, and particularly when it had reached Amsterdam, whose trade with English ports was so continuous, it was difficult to keep it out of Britain.

After 1670 that dangerous proximity never recurred. The sophisticated quarantine procedures adopted elsewhere in Europe, and especially in Italy and France, kept plague at a safer distance, usually in the eastern Mediterranean. The voyage from the Levant to England, for example, was long enough for many infected fleas in cloth or cotton to have died on the way,[53] and certainly long enough for the government to be warned of the danger in time to take appropriate action. Orders were issued against shipping from Malaga in 1680, from the Baltic ports between 1709 and 1713, from Marseilles and the Levant between 1720 and 1722, and from various Mediterranean harbours in the 1730s and 1740s. Quarantine was even enforced against ships from the West Indies when, as in 1692, infectious disease seemed to threaten from there.[54] With each fresh emergency, the government sought advice on how the policy had worked in the past and how it was enforced in foreign countries, including the Netherlands.[55] Administrative practice was given the support of statute law in 1710, and a ship was forfeited to the Crown in 1713 for failing to comply with it. Further statutes, in 1721, 1722, 1728, and 1753 added the death penalty for those refusing or escaping quarantine, and confirmed the erection of a

---

[51] Hull Corporation Records, Bench Book 6, pp. 545, 548, 591–2; Book 7, pp. 21–5.

[52] *Cal.S.P.Dom. 1667/8*, p. 580; *1668/9*, pp. 409–10, 413, 555, 577; PRO, PC 2/60, pp. 444–5, 2/62, p. 29; Wellcome Historical Medical Library, MS. 3109, 3 September–5 October 1668, 1 July 1669.

[53] It took at least twenty-five days; fleas have been shown to be able to transmit plague after periods of starvation lasting up to twenty-nine days: *Parl. Papers*, 1824(VI), *Minutes of Evidence, Quarantine*, p. 74; Pollitzer, *Plague*, p. 381.

[54] *Cal. Treasury Books 1679/80*, p. 536; *1689–92*, pp. 1708, 1762; *1709*, pp. 357–8, 410, 425, 445; *1710*, p. 233; *1713*, p. 329; *Cal. Treasury Papers 1720–8*, p. 435; PRO, PC 2/87, pp. 15–16, 313–17; *Cal. Treasury Books and Papers 1729–30*, p. 206; *1731–4*, pp. 89, 141; *1739–41*, pp. 471–3; *1742–5*, pp. 295, 307–8.

[55] *Cal. Treasury Books 1681/2*, p. 256; PRO, PC 1/2/232, 2/87, p. 324.

quarantine station at Standgate Creek, at the mouth of the Medway, for ships intending to enter the Thames.[56]

The most public test of this machinery came in the great panic of 1720 to 1722 caused by plague in Marseilles. Customs officials in the provinces urgently insisted that troops or frigates were needed to enforce quarantine properly; they could be provided only in the neighbourhood of Portsmouth, at Milford Haven, and off Standgate Creek.[57] In the event, however, that proved to be enough, since the few suspect vessels from infected ports could now be closely monitored. The government was rightly told that there was no need for precautions against ships from Italy, thanks to the model regulations enforced there. On the other hand, it was quickly informed by the British consul in Venice that two ships were approaching London from Cyprus, where there was plague; that one of them had been turned away from Messina and Leghorn because it was suspect; and that they carried cotton which experience had shown could often harbour infection (and, modern epidemiologists would note, fleas). The ships were isolated when they arrived and finally burnt by order of the King in Council under authority of the statute of 1721, parliament voting £24,000 as compensation to the owners.[58]

Public awareness of the danger of imported infection was also productive. Forewarned by newspaper reports of plague in foreign towns, local officials in Channel ports turned away vessels coming from the Mediterranean. When goods were smuggled into Canterbury from the two ships which were soon to be burned, the Council was told immediately.[59] People rushed to report suspected cases of plague in the Isle of Man, in Portsmouth and Hartlepool, and the government responded with advice on how to isolate them if the cases were confirmed.[60] They were not. A combination of public awareness, relatively rapid government action, and quarantine in other countries seems to have worked.

Chance played a part in the success of such endeavours, of course. Quarantine was no less fallible than the watch and ward erected around towns like Bristol and York. Some ships would always penetrate even the most imposing defences, and merchandise be smuggled ashore from those which were caught. Maladministration could have led to an epidemic in London after 1665 as it did in

[56] Mullett, 'Century of English quarantine', pp. 527–45; Cal. Treasury Books 1713, p. 186.
[57] PRO, SP 35/23/124, 126, 127, 133, 145, 153; PC 2/87, pp. 24–5, 391.
[58] PRO, SP 35/23/90; PC 1/3/89.
[59] PRO, SP 35/23/126, 35/28/26, 33, 36. Cf. London Gazette, 16–20 April, 30 April–4 May 1668; Lee, Defoe, 2, pp. 142, 277–8, 464–5.
[60] PRO, SP 35/24/3, 6–8; 35/25/101, 102, 107; 35/28/85, 86. Cf. PC 2/87, p. 167.

Marseilles in 1720.[61] As with watch and ward, however, the more often the machinery was employed, the more likely it was to prove effective. It is not stretching the evidence to argue that the risks of initial infection were gradually reduced between 1650 and 1750 until in the end they were negligible; and the much more difficult problem of controlling a plague epidemic once it had begun could be shelved, and shelved, as it turned out, for good.

So sanguine a conclusion could not be established beyond dispute at the time. Neither could the reasons for it be understood until the epidemiology of plague had been fully worked out, at the end of the nineteenth century. Until then the relative importance of human transmission and local environmental conditions, and the relative merits of 'infection' and 'miasma' as explanatory hypotheses, could not be precisely determined. Hence it was easy for eighteenth-century writers to reject the argument which has been presented here and to suggest alternatives. From the 1720s to the 1820s defenders of free trade and critics of the quarantine laws denied the efficacy of the latter. They argued that Britain's trade with the Levant, where plague was still rampant, was simply too voluminous to be monitored effectively. Quarantine was not responsible for the absence of outbreaks in England, therefore.[62] Some writers attributed it instead to social improvement. They pointed out that in the seventeenth century the disease had largely been confined to the 'squalid classes', and they concluded that 'improved habits of life' in the eighteenth century had produced a 'continued diminution of susceptibility' to it. Others could find no satisfactory explanation for the end of the plague apart from divine providence.[63]

Edward Gibbon was an exception. Less insular in his historical perspective than most of his contemporaries, armed with all the secular self-assurance of the Enlightenment, he could refer coolly and confidently to 'those salutary precautions to which Europe is indebted for her safety' from plague.[64] This chapter has tried to show that Gibbon was right; but it will have failed if it has not also demonstrated why many Englishmen in the seventeenth and early eighteenth centuries could not be so certain.

[61] Biraben, *Les hommes et la peste*, 1, pp. 231–2.

[62] For early examples, see Pye, *Discourse of the Plague*, p. 37; Anon., *Doctor Mead's Short Discourse*, pp. 33–4.

[63] *Parl. Papers*, 1824 (6), *Minutes of Evidence, Quarantine*, pp. 47, 51; Short, *New Observations*, pp. 240–1. For further diverse views on the nature of plague, see Howard, *Lazarettos in Europe*, pp. 32–41; Mullett, *Bubonic Plague and England*, chapters 13, 14.

[64] Gibbon, *Decline and Fall*, 4, p. 373.

5

Demographic crises and subsistence crises in France, 1650–1725

JACQUES DUPÂQUIER

In his essay, 'Grain prices and subsistence crises in England and France, 1590–1740', Appleby

attempts to explain why England had no food crises from 1650 to 1725, a period when France was unusually vulnerable to famines. During this time, oat and barley prices in England did not always increase following a failure of the wheat crop. In France, however, all grain rose in price simultaneously, leaving the poor with no affordable substitute grain when the wheat and rye harvests failed.

He argues

that in those regions where both winter and spring grains were grown – that is, northern France and most of England – a symmetrical price structure, in which prices of all grains increased significantly at the same time, and famine went hand in hand.[1]

Appleby's arguments are impressive and the graphs accompanying his article show clearly that while the market price of spring grains at Norwich and Reading in the 1690s rose much less than the price of winter wheat, at Pontoise (thirty kilometers from Paris) the market prices of all grains remained closely correlated during the crises of 1661, 1693, 1709, and 1740.[2]

[1] Appleby, 'Grain prices', pp. 865–87, the quotations come from pp. 865 and 887, respectively.
[2] Oats have been omitted since they were almost entirely reserved for horse feed. The following percentage increases in prices (at Christmas) were observed for four crises:

Crisis	Reference Period	Wheat	Barley	Rye
1661	1654–7	172	174	108
1693	1687–90	330	384	387
1709	1704–7	475	623	355
1740	1732–5	309	362	300

We have absolutely no intention of challenging Appleby's general thesis. Rather, in this chapter we propose to examine whether there were any significant differences between France and England in their experience of major mortality crises between 1650 and 1725, and whether the correlation between mortality crises and high prices in France was absolutely clear, as supporters of the 'subsistence crisis' theory claim was the case.

We now know the course of births, deaths, and marriages for England since 1539, thanks to the magnificent work of Wrigley and Schofield.[3] For France the national sample data collected by INED are, unfortunately, only available from 1740,[4] but we can draw support from the following complementary series:

1 aggregate data for a representative sample of sixty-one villages in the period 1670 to 1739.[5]
2 partial data for the *Bassin parisien* (comprising 28 per cent of the current area of France) from 1671 to 1720.[6]
3 some scattered statistics relating mainly to small towns in the Ile de France from 1650 to 1670.[7]

At a colloquium held at Montebello in Canada in October 1975 several indices were proposed as measures of the intensity of crisis mortality, each with its advantages and disadvantages.[8] In the absence of any general agreement I shall use the index I proposed myself, because it is easy to calculate, and because it does not require a knowledge of the size of the population, being based solely on the annual numbers of deaths:

$$I_x = (D_x - M_x)/S_x$$

where

I_x = Standardised index for year x
D_x = Number of deaths in year x
M_x = Mean number of deaths during the previous ten years
S_x = Standard deviation of the annual totals of deaths during the ten year reference period.

Since the index refers to a calendar year, and mortality crises often extended over several years, an index value for a multi-year crisis is calculated by adding to the index of the first year, the amount by which the index for any subsequent year exceeded unity. For example, in

[3] Wrigley and Schofield, *Population History*.
[4] Blayo, 'Le mouvement naturel', pp. 15–64.
[5] Rebaudo, 'Le mouvement de la population', pp. 589–606.
[6] Dupâquier, *La population rurale*.   [7] *Ibid.*
[8] The conference papers and discussions are reported in Charbonneau and Larose, *The Great Mortalities*.

England the index reached 5.580 in 1657 and 4.547 in 1658. The crisis of 1657–58, therefore, scores 5.580 + (4.547–1.000) = 9.127.

Of course, one should not rely on the apparent precision of the index, because its level is affected by the choice of the reference period. Furthermore, in evaluating the severity of crises, it would seem preferable to adopt a ranked scale comprising five levels as follows:

Level	Severity	Index values in range
1	minor	1.00– 1.99
2	medium	2.00– 3.99
3	serious	4.00– 7.99
4	major	8.00–15.99
5	catastrophic	16.00–

On this basis it appears that in the period 1650 to 1725 the English population experienced eight mortality crises, spread out over fourteen years:[9]

1 major crisis (level 4), in 1657–8
2 serious crises (level 3), in 1679–81 and 1719–21
3 medium crises (level 2), in 1665, 1705, and 1711–12
2 minor crises (level 1), in 1654 and 1723.

It is more difficult to establish the chronology of crises in France, because the three sets of data do not yield exactly the same results.

The scattered statistics (1650–70) show serious crises (level 3) occurring in 1652 and 1661/2, but the former is mainly confined to the area around Paris, and probably did not exceed level 2 on a country-wide basis.

The data for the *Bassin parisien* (1671–1720) indicate crises in 1675–6 (level 2), 1679–80 (level 1), 1691–4 and 1705–12 (level 5), and 1719 (level 1).

According to the sample of sixty-one villages (1670–1725), the country as a whole probably experienced the crisis of 1676 as more serious, and the crisis of 1691–4 as less serious (level 4). Also the crisis of 1705–12 splits into three peaks: a crisis at level 2 in 1705, one at level 1 in 1707, and one at level 3 in 1709–10. Unfortunately the method of calculating the index erases the crisis of 1719 because, although the number of deaths rises by 28 per cent, the reference period includes the crisis of 1709–10 and so the index for that year only reaches 0.774. Finally, there is a crisis at level 1 in 1724.

In summary, one might suggest the following inventory of mortality crises for the whole of France between 1650 and 1725:

[9] Based on calendar year totals from Wrigley and Schofield, *Population History*, table A2.3, pp. 498–9.

1 crises at level 4: in 1693–4
2 crises at level 3: one in 1661–2, the other in 1709–10
3 crises at level 2: in 1652, 1676, and 1705
4 crises at level 1: in 1680, 1707, 1719, and 1724.

Let us say a total of ten crises, extending over thirteen years. The balance sheet is not noticeably different from the one we drew up earlier for England; in both countries the years 1650–1725 were a difficult period, characterised by frequent bouts of excess mortality.[10]

What is most remarkable is the way in which the chronology of crisis mortality differs in the two countries, as shown in figure 1. Before 1705 there is only one year of coincidence (1680), and even that is doubtful. The great English crisis of 1657–8 had no echo in France, and the great French crises of 1661–2 and 1693–4 had no repercussions in England. On the other hand, after 1705 the two countries marched in step: the

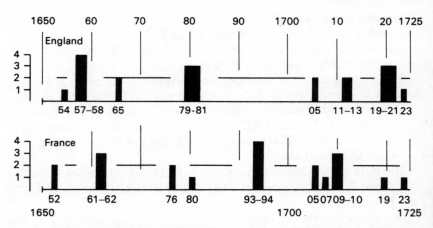

Figure 5.1 Comparative chronology of mortality crises in England and France, 1650–1725

[10] Wrigley and Schofield arrive at a similar result by a different route; they work with deaths grouped in years running from July to June and use as a reference period a centred twenty-five year moving average. They classify as a crisis year any year in which the death rate was at least 10 per cent above the moving average, and distinguish three levels of intensity: (1) when the annual rate is between 10 and 20 per cent, (2) when it is between 20 and 30 per cent, and (3) when it is above 30 per cent higher than the moving average. In the period 1650–1725 they find eleven crisis years (three at level 3, one at level 2, and seven at level 1), the years concerned being 1657–8, 1678–82, 1684, and 1719. Wrigley and Schofield, *Population History*, pp. 332–4. Applying the same method to French data for 1650–1725 we obtain twelve crisis years (five at level 3, one at level 2, and six at level 1), the years concerned being 1676, 1678–9, 1693–4, 1705, 1707, 1709–10, and 1725. For France the two methods yield similar chronologies, while for England the Wrigley and Schofield method finds less severe crises in the seventeenth century and fewer crises in the eighteenth century.

crisis of 1705 was common to both of them; the French crisis of 1709–10 was followed closely by the English crisis of 1711–12; the severe crisis which struck England in 1719–21 was echoed in France; and the crisis of 1723 was similar in the two countries.

Might one conclude from this that seventeenth century crises were 'national', and eighteenth century crises 'international' (or at least Anglo–French)? That would be too hasty. In fact, so far as one can judge from the available evidence, which limits the analysis to the period from 1670 to 1725, the French crises were not 'national'. The crisis of 1676 affected mainly the northern half of France, the crisis of 1693–4 spared the east and south–east, and the crisis of 1705 was clearly evident only in the west. Finally, in 1709–10 the regions affected were the north, the east, and the whole of central France; the whole of the south escaped.

If the eleven parishes studied by Rebaudo can be taken as representative of the *bocage* areas of western France, the only crises that are indicated for this region in the period 1680–1725 are those of 1693–5 and 1705 (level 3), 1707 and 1719–21 (level 2), and 1725 (level 1).[11]

Similarly, in England, according to Wrigley and Schofield, contemporary mortality crises were also regional:

For example, in the heavy mortality associated with fever (with some outbreaks of plague) in 1638 . . . local crises were almost entirely confined to the south-east; very few occurred north-west of a line running from the New Forest to the Wash. In the national 3- and 2-star crisis years 1657/8 and 1658/9 local crises were more widespread, with the south-east midlands and Yorkshire particularly badly affected, but once again the far north and the west of country escaped almost completely. A rather similar pattern obtained during the years 1678/9 to 1680/1 which ushered in a six-year period of very heavy mortality . . . local crisis mortality was fairly widespread, though on this occasion the areas of greatest intensity were Kent and Sussex, the east midlands, and the far north-east. But once again the west of the country was relatively little affected.[12]

II

This comparison of England and France in turn raises questions about the theory of subsistence crises, according to which all the major mortality crises of the seventeenth and early eighteenth centuries were directly linked to dearth, that is to say, to substantial increases in the price of grain.

[11] Rebaudo, 'Le mouvement annuel'.
[12] Wrigley and Schofield, *Population History*, pp. 679–81. See, especially, the maps on pp. 678–9 which show the geographical distribution of parishes affected by the crises of July 1657–March 1659, and July 1678–June 1681.

The theory of subsistence crises, in its contemporary guise, was first formulated by Meuvret in 1946.[13] As an economic historian and specialist in price history Meuvret was struck by the coincidence between high prices and the increase in the number of deaths in the region of Gien in 1709–10. He then posed the problem of the nature of demographic crises, very tentatively at first, since he thought it a hopeless quest

to try to distinguish statistically between phenomena that were so closely associated: namely, mortality through simple inanition; mortality caused by disease, though attributable to malnutrition; and mortality by contagion, which in turn was linked to the scarcity that helped both spawn diseases and spread them through the migration of poor beggars.[14]

In the twenty years which followed, the theory of subsistence crises enjoyed a considerable success, thanks to Goubert who popularised it in his famous thesis on Beauvais and the *Beauvaisis*.[15] However, not every historian accepted it: Chaunu observed that there were mortality crises without high prices, and high prices without a mortality crisis.[16] And Baehrel challenged the causal influence of an increase in prices on mortality:

Often the two peaks coincide, but both could have a common cause of which we are unaware, perhaps connected with the weather . . . Scarcity, consequently famine, and lethal diseases were both produced by bad weather. If the year is a healthy one, and the shortage of bread is due to some other cause, only the peak in prices will be observed.[17]

In response, the supporters of the subsistence crisis theory adopted a more intransigent attitude. To make their arguments clearer they have been represented schematically in figure 2, which can be supplemented by five propositions

1 There is a close correlation between high prices and crisis mortality; it is subsistence crises, not wars or epidemics, which explain mortality crises in the past.
2 Demographic crises are caused by poor harvests which are produced by climatic shocks (a rainy spring as in 1693, a 'Siberian' winter as in 1709).
3 Scarcity is linked to high prices much more than to the physical absence of food.
4 Scarcity also causes a reduction in the number of marriages, and in the number of births after a lag of nine months.

---

[13] Meuvret, 'Les crises des subsistances'.   [14] *Ibid.*, p. 644.
[15] Goubert, *Beauvais et le Beauvaisis*.
[16] Chaunu, *La civilisation de l'Europe classique*, p. 229.
[17] Baehrel, *La Basse-Provence rurale*, p. 293.

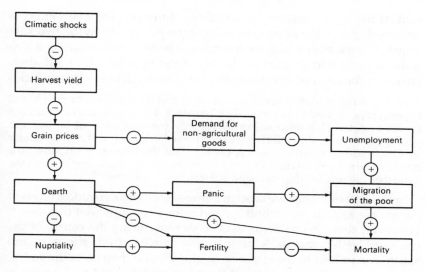

Figure 5.2 A model of subsistence crises

5 Epidemic disease is triggered by scarcity, and spread by the subsequent migration of the poor; it is a secondary phenomenon.

Of course, these propositions cannot be entirely dismissed. It is quite true that in France prices erupted in the wake of the deficient harvests of 1693 and 1709 and, at the same time the number of deaths rose, marriages and conceptions fell, and a large number of migrants took to the road, helping to spread infectious disease.

Nevertheless, if the theory were to be accepted in its entirety, the following features should be observed

1 The mortality peak should always occur at the end of spring, when the supply of grain is at its lowest.
2 The crisis should affect all parishes without exception in every region suffering the climatic shocks.
3 The mortality crises should occur immediately and simultaneously. But what do we observe in England and France in the period 1650–1725?

For England, Wrigley and Schofield's maps reveal a very complex situation: during the crises of 1657–59 and 1678–81 one can find some parishes which were spared, even in the regions most affected.[18] During subsistence crises the correlation between grain prices and crisis mortality seems undeniable, but overall it explains only 16 per

[18] See note 10, above.

cent of the total variation in mortality. Moreover, the main effect is observed, not in the same year as the high prices, but in the two subsequent years, after which the mortality echo becomes negative. It is as if the scarcity had shaken the health of the population, or left aftereffects in the form of infectious disease. The English study concludes

Analyses of the mortality–grain price relation that do not allow for distributed lag effects are bound to be seriously misleading. Furthermore, one could not expect to detect this relationship by visually scanning plots of burials and prices; it is weak, and its effects are too dispersed in time. It will be shown later that there are non-linear effects operating; that the pattern of response to a large increase in price is different from the response to a small one; and that the nature of the relationship changed substantially over time.[19]

In the case of France we lack such fine-scale data: Rebaudo's totals of events are annual, not monthly, and refer to regions, not parishes.[20] However, they do enable us to observe that during the course of the crisis of 1691–5 the peak of mortality moved: from the east and south-east in 1691 to the south-west in 1693, and then on to the south, the centre, the Paris region and the north in 1694, and to the west in 1694–5. One gets the impression of a slow diffusion like a drop of oil, not of a sudden and simultaneous crisis. Similarly, during the crisis of 1709–10, we can observe that the east suffered in 1708–9, the southeast, the centre, the Paris region and the north in 1709–10, and the south and the south-west only in 1710.

We are better informed about the *Bassin parisien*, widely construed.[21] At Pontoise during the first crisis the price of corn reached its maximum, as expected, when grain stocks were at their lowest, in May and June 1694; but the peak of mortality did not occur until December 1694 and January 1695. On the other hand, in 1709–10, both the highest prices and the greatest number of deaths occurred during September and October, with the crisis extending until January 1710. The discrepancy between the seasonal incidence of the two crises is doubtless partly to be explained by a difference in the nature of the causative agents of the epidemics.[22] But, in the case of the second crisis, recourse was also had to a substitute grain. In fact, as soon as the farmers of the *Bassin parisien* discovered that the autumn-sown grains had frozen in the ground and that the whole crop would be lost, they re-sowed the land with spring grain and obtained a harvest so

[19] Lee in Wrigley and Schofield, *Population History*, p.372.
[20] Rebaudo, 'Le mouvement annuel'.
[21] Dupâquier, *La population rurale*.
[22] During the crisis of 1693–4 it was mainly adults who were affected; in the crisis of 1709–10 it was mainly very young children and those aged fifty and above.

bountiful that the year 1709 would live in folk memory as 'the barley year'. However, despite this abundance, the price of barley remained very high from March 1709 until January 1710 (at more than twenty *livres* a *setier*, compared with eight *livres* earlier). This episode would appear to contradict Appleby's thesis that the severity of subsistence crises in France was produced by the lack of a sufficient recourse to substitute grains.

Furthermore, it is evident that even in the areas which suffered most a number of parishes remained unaffected in the mortality crises of 1693/4 and 1709/10. And these crises, far from appearing suddenly in a simultaneous outbreak, were preceded by a progressive rise in the number of local crises. For example, in the *Bassin parisien*, for which about eighty parish register series are available, the annual frequencies of local crises observed during the period 1688 to 1697 were as follows (expressed as a percentage of the villages in observation)

Year	Crisis %	Year	Crisis %
1688	13	1693	57
1689	14	1694	79
1690	19	1695	28
1691	36	1696	9
1692	37	1697	3

Similarly, for the crisis at the beginning of the eighteenth century, when a hundred parish series are available, the annual frequencies of local crises ran

Year	Crisis %	Year	Crisis %
1703	7	1709	51
1704	11	1710	44
1705	38	1711	20
1706	40	1712	26
1707	38	1713	15
1708	32	1714	10

This leads to the conclusion that the weather was not the only cause of the mortality crises; epidemic diseases, probably accompanied by epizootic and fungus infections, were also at work.

In order to discover whether the variations in nuptiality, fertility, and mortality were produced solely by subsistence crises, an investigation was made of the demographic effects of twenty local epidemic crises which struck a number of villages in the *Bassin parisien* in a period of low prices.[23]

It was observed that the number of deaths rose by 17.5 per cent, and the number of baptisms fell by 5.5 per cent in the year following the crisis. However, the number of marriages rose by 17.0 per cent in the crisis year itself, no doubt because many of those who were widowed remarried without delay, and because the disappearance of many older couples gave young people the chance of forming a household. If one also takes into account the year which followed the crisis, the increase in marriages reached a level 48 per cent higher than in the pre-crisis reference period. Thus epidemics appear to have had little effect on fertility, but to have stimulated both mortality and nuptiality.

A reciprocal test was also made, in order to discover whether there were any periods of high prices without mortality crises. The following example was taken from the *généralité* of Paris, where the price of corn at Pontoise in 1699 rose 120 per cent above its average for the years 1695–98. Mortality rose by 10 per cent, which is probably not significant in view of the very low level of the reference period after the crisis of 1693–4. At the same time nuptiality fell by 28 per cent, and the numbers of baptisms fell by 7 per cent in 1699, though in 1700 they exceeded their usual level.

Thus periods of high prices, when they did not coincide with periods of epidemic disease, seem to have had little effect on mortality. On the other hand, they caused a noticeable reduction in nuptiality and, when there was also a scarcity, a reduction in fertility.[24]

It seems that the major demographic crises of the seventeenth century, with the exception of those connected with plague, resulted from a conjunction of scarcity and epidemic disease. The latter comprised a series of independent events with a random periodicity, while the former resulted not only from climatic shocks, but also from fungal infections which may have followed a periodicity of their own.

Figure 3 shows how, in my view, the classic model of subsistence crises can be completed by taking into account the role of epidemic and fungal infections.

There are many puzzles still be to solved: as yet we know very little

---

[23] Dupâquier, *La population rurale*, p. 265.
[24] Without going so far as to provoke widespread amenorrhoea. See Le Roy Ladurie, 'L'aménorrhée de famine'; Frisch, 'Nutrition, fatness and fertility'.

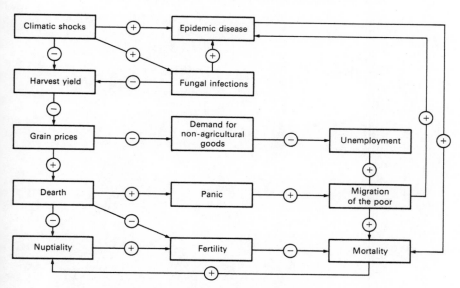

Figure 5.3 A model of demographic and subsistence crises

about the relationships which may exist between the causal agents of epidemic and fungal infections, and we have only an imperfect understanding of biological rhythms. Nor are economic phenomena themselves always self-evident: for example, why did the prices of secondary grains in France in the seventeenth century remain closely linked to the price of wheat, whilst in England they already showed a certain independence? As we have seen, it was not the effect of a different pattern of production, since French peasants were widely engaged in the cultivation of both barley and rye. Perhaps, in the last analysis, one is forced to invoke the organisation of the market: in France there was little movement of grain, and it was difficult to compensate for the effects of a poor regional harvest, whilst in England this could be done, thanks to the strategic role played by coastal shipping. In the seventeenth century there was no unified national market on the continent, while on the other side of the Channel everything was organised around London. To conclude in the words of the well-known headline: 'Fog in Channel – Continent isolated'.

6

Markets and mortality in France, 1600–1789

DAVID R. WEIR

Quantitative studies of subsistence crises provided an early meeting ground for economic history and historical demography. French scholars must be considered pioneers in the field: following the studies of economic crises and price history by Labrousse, Sée, Simiand, and others in the interwar years,[1] Jean Meuvret opened the modern study of prices and mortality with a famous article in *Population*.[2] The topic gained even wider recognition with the publication of *Beauvais et les Beauvaisis* by Pierre Goubert, a student of Meuvret, and has since become a staple of regional and urban histories.[3]

Andrew Appleby was instrumental in bringing the study of prices and mortality to England,[4] and remains one of the few scholars to have attempted a comparative history of France and England.[5] Ronald Lee introduced greater econometric sophistication into the topic.[6] In his study of the Paris Basin, Jacques Dupâquier notes that Meuvret expected that more and better data on prices and deaths would demonstrate the phenomenon more and more clearly.[7] The accumula-

The author gratefully acknowledges many helpful conversations with Ronald Lee and Patrick Galloway of the Graduate Group in Demography at the University of California at Berkeley. Financial support was provided by a grant from US NICHD number RO1–08–R:1 HD18107, obtained by Ronald Lee. Roger Schofield and Larry Neal provided useful comments on an earlier draft.

[1] Simiand, *Le salaire*; Labrousse, *Esquisse du mouvement des prix*, and *La crise de l'économie française*.
[2] Meuvret, 'Les crises de subsistances', pp. 643–50.
[3] A thorough review of the literature can be found in Lebrun, 'Les crises démographiques', pp. 205–34. Important recent additions include Dupâquier, *La population rurale*; Perrenoud, *La population de Genève*, and Bardet, *Rouen*.
[4] Appleby, *Famine in Tudor and Stuart England*.
[5] Appleby, 'Grain prices'.
[6] Lee, 'Methods and models', in Lee, ed., *Population Patterns in the Past*. Lee, 'Short-term variations', in Wrigley and Schofield, *Population History*.
[7] Dupâquier, *La population rurale*, p. 28.

tion of *mercuriales* and parish registers is rapidly bringing his dream to reality. But it appears that now, just as the data are beginning to accumulate and the statistical procedures become more exacting, the usefulness of the topic is being called into question. The arguments stressing the limitations of studies of subsistence crises, many of which are cogently expressed by Jacques Dupâquier in this volume, are quite persuasive but from only one perspective; that of the demographer. Whatever its significance for demographic analysis, the topic remains an important one for the economic historian.

The demographic logic is inescapable: prices explain only a minority fraction of mortality variations which themselves explain only a minority fraction of variations in population growth rates, so the impact of prices on population growth must have been minimal. Subsistence crises cannot have been the prime mover of Malthusian equilibrium. Recent accumulations of demographic evidence have provided convincing proof for both assertions. Epidemic disease, sometimes very localised, was capable of producing large mortality variations quite independently of price variation. More surprising, perhaps, is the finding that nuptiality not only provided a steady brake to population growth in early modern Europe through delayed marriage,[8] but also was responsive to economic and mortality variations.[9]

Economic historians and historical demographers have somewhat different interests in the relation of mortality to grain prices. Both should recognise that the effects might not be fully visible in a contemporaneous correlation of the two series. Subsistence crises are to the history of prices and mortality what wars are to the history of politics: dramatic events arising from a structural problem. Even more than in political history, *histoire événementielle* is inadequate for understanding the underlying causes of mortality's dependence on prices. A comparative *histoire structurelle* is needed. We can begin by improving statistical measurement.

As Ronald Lee has shown for England, distributed-lag regressions allow one not only to see the effects of prices on mortality in crisis years, but also to chart the progress of recovery as mortality dips below average later on.[10] For demographers concerned with population size and growth the rebound effect is particularly important. A measure

[8] Hajnal. 'European marriage patterns'.
[9] Wrigley and Schofield, *Population History*, pp. 417–35.
[10] Distributed-lag regressions estimate the effect on deaths of prices in current and previous years. For a discussion of specifications, see Lee 'Short-term variations', pp. 357–9, 371–3; and Weir, 'Life under pressure', pp. 36–9.

like the cumulative effect of a price shock on deaths after five or more years is an appropriate summary statistic of the regression analysis for the purpose. Economists might not be so concerned with the extent of recovery. Evidence of a strong effect of prices on deaths, even if it is later negated by compensating effects, suggests a serious shortcoming in the food supply system. Long-run population size may have been indifferent to a modest rearrangement of the timing of deaths (more now, fewer later), but people surely were not. An appropriate statistic from a welfare viewpoint, then, is the number of early deaths occasioned by a rise in grain prices. The extent to which they are compensated for by a shortage of deaths later is a separate phenomenon.

In the next section, some of the economic connections between markets and mortality will be elaborated. But prices and deaths may be correlated for reasons having little to do with economics. Omitted variables like weather conditions, mobilisation for war, or disruptive epidemics could create 'spurious' correlations. Put another way, high prices never directly 'cause' deaths: the statistical association alerts us to the existence of a relationship whose nature must then be an object of informed speculation. The *structure* is the fact to be explained; the estimated coefficients tell us what, not why. Although the statistical apparatus used to describe the structure of the relationship between mortality and grain prices is complex and similar in form to causal hypothesis testing, it remains essentially a descriptive exercise. Hypotheses are more an output than an input into the examination of aggregate time series of deaths and prices. Until data become available to test more fully-specified models of the determinants of mortality, our only recourse is to be cautious and broad-minded in interpreting results. Differences in the magnitude and timing of the impact of prices on deaths in different regions and time periods may help us to discern the nature of the relationship and direct research to areas where hypotheses can be tested.

In an earlier paper using national data, I reported confirmation of Meuvret's observation that subsistence crises had faded after the first quarter of the eighteenth century.[11] This chapter will disaggregate the analysis to explore regional differences in the response of mortality to prices. Urban–rural comparisons within market regions are sorely needed. Recently published data permit such a comparison for the Paris Basin and some other cities. We begin with a description of grain markets in France and a consideration of their possible connection to mortality.

[11] *Ibid.*, p. 42.

Markets

Economic explanations of the price–mortality connection have traditionally emphasised the development of markets. Regional expansion of grain markets, or market integration, is the most familiar explanation for the disappearance of price-linked mortality crises.[12] Wider markets spread risk and reduce the variability of prices. They can also prevent the extreme deprivation most likely to lead to excess mortality. Appleby proposed an alternative hypothesis to explain French crises: the close correlation of prices for wheat and substitute grains.[13] In his view, a resource-constrained French agriculture was unable to expand the (spring) oat crop in response to a failed (winter) wheat crop.

Grain markets were political as well as economic phenomena in early modern Europe. Their management was a major preoccupation of governments,[14] and their operation often invoked political response from below.[15] Government intervention could distort the historical record of the price–mortality link. Two common forms of intervention were price ceilings (the *maximum*) and subsidies (in cash or grain) to the poor. A price ceiling alone would lead to quantity rationing on some basis that would not necessarily provision the most needy. Recorded prices would vary relatively little while deaths might respond strongly. A policy of buying grain at free market prices for redistribution, or giving cash to the poor, would have the opposite effect. Prices would fluctuate widely (reflecting the increased effective purchasing power of the poor) while the extension of 'entitlements' to the needy ought to reduce the mortality response.[16] Longer-term effects could include different incentives for migration during crises. Because most welfare policies were local, their effects can only be studied at a local level.

Markets other than grain may be involved in the price–mortality connection. Labour markets are implicated by Meuvret's suggestion that high prices induced migration which in turn brought disease to regions of destination. Capital markets influence the cost of storing grain and therefore the extent of inventories.[17] They may be involved in other ways, as well. Grain represented a large share of total national

[12] Appleby, *Famine*; Meuvret, 'Les crises de subsistances'.
[13] Appleby, 'Grain prices'.
[14] Tilly, C. 'Food supply' provides a general overview of the issues. Kaplan, *Bread, politics and Political Economy* treats French developments in greater depth.
[15] Tilly, L. A., 'The food riot'.
[16] The role of entitlements in famine has been analysed by Sen in *Poverty and Famines*.
[17] McCloskey and Nash, 'Corn at interest'.

product in early modern Europe. Demand for grain was traditionally inelastic – implying that total expenditures on grain rose when the size of harvest fell. There is no evidence that declining expenditures on other commodities were sufficient to offset the increase in expenditure on grain. In other words, aggregate nominal income may well have gone up when real income fell during a harvest failure. A temporary increase in the price level could only have been accomplished through an expansion of lending and the resulting increase in the velocity of circulation of money. One consequence was the concentration of land-ownership when indebted farmers were unable to pay off their loans in subsequent 'good' years.

Economists propose several empirical tests for market integration. A simple test is the equality of price in different regions. Different units of account make this an awkward test in practice, and there are good theoretical reasons to avoid it. Tariffs (natural, like transportation costs, or politically imposed taxes) can keep mean prices apart when regions trade regularly. Another test involves correlations of prices across regions over time. They should be higher the better-integrated are the regional markets. The danger here is that shared monetary trends (inflation or deflation) will create positive correlations among even perfectly disjoint wheat markets. Louise Tilly's evidence for a national market is of this kind.[18] After detrending, however, correlations offer a potentially useful measure of the degree of price synchronisation across regions.

The remaining limitation of correlations of detrended prices is important and applies not only to regional patterns but also to cross-grain correlations such as wheat and oats examined by Appleby. There will be two sources of covariation between two price series: correlated variations in quantities supplied and substitutability between the two products. Take the example of Paris wheat and Toulouse wheat. If climatic shocks to quantities supplied are perfectly correlated, then prices will be perfectly correlated no matter what the connection between the two markets. If the markets are perfectly integrated (in effect, one market), then prices will also be perfectly correlated even if harvests vary independently of one another. We can never be certain, from price data alone, whether a strong correlation is due to correlated harvest volumes or to strong substitutability in demand (integrated markets). On the other hand, a weak correlation implies both that supplies are weakly correlated and that the products are weakly related in demand.

<hr/>

[18] Tilly, L. A., 'The food riot', pp. 35–9.

To assess the extent of price synchronisation across many markets, it will be useful to have one summary measure rather than an entire matrix of correlation coefficients for each time period. Ideally, it should not be sensitive to the number of markets considered so that it can be used to compare different times and places for which different amounts of data are available. To reinforce the analogy with a simple correlation coefficient, it can be scaled to vary between zero and one as the extent of integration increases.

The measure described here exploits the fact that the variance of a variable constructed as the mean of several component variables, holding constant the number of components and their variances, will be larger the higher are the correlations among the components. In this case the component variables are the local price series and their mean is the national average price. The year-to-year variance of the national average price will increase when the variances in the local market series increase, fall when the number of local series rises, and increase with greater correlation across markets. We are interested only in the third effect, so we need to control for the effects of the other two in constructing the measure.

For simplicity, let us assume momentarily that the variance of each local series is the same: Var (X). If the variables are perfectly independent, then the variance of their mean will be:

$$\text{Var}(X) \,/\, n, \qquad \text{where n is the number of series}$$

Like the sampling error of a mean of a random sample, it will go to zero as n goes to infinity.

On the other hand, if the variables are perfectly correlated, there will be no offsetting effects (prices would be high everywhere simultaneously), and the variance of their mean will be the same as the variance of each series, i.e. Var(X). Under perfect integration, then, variance of the average is n times as large as under perfect autarky. The observed variance will lie somewhere between the two extremes.

To control for the effect of variances in the components, we can form the ratio of the observed variance of the composite national average to the variance expected in the absence of any correlation across regions. It will be:

$$\frac{\text{Var (Nat)}}{(\text{Var}(X) \,/\, n)}$$

This ratio will range from one (zero correlation) to n (perfect correlation). Now we need to control for the effects of sample size (the number of local series under study). To rescale the measure from zero to one, subtract one from the ratio and divide by $n-1$. Finally, we must relax our assumption of identical local variances. If we estimate Var(X) by the average of the local variances, the final version of the measure of price synchronisation becomes:

$$R = \frac{\dfrac{\text{Var(Nat)}}{\sum_i \text{Var(i)} / n^2} - 1}{(n-1)}$$

The measure can, with some loss of statistical precision, be interpreted as the average correlation coefficient across regions. To recapitulate how it is calculated: compute a national series as the average of the detrended local series; calculate for a fixed time period the variance of each (detrended) local series and of the national average; divide the national variance by $1/n$ times the average of the variances; subtract one; and divide by $n-1$.

Eight market series have been selected for France to provide wide geographical dispersion and continuous coverage from the late sixteenth century. They are: Paris, Douai, Strasbourg, Grenoble, Aix, Toulouse, Poitiers, and Angers. Sources for these and other markets are given in the appendix, and their locations are shown in figure 6.1. Some available series were excluded from the national market integration measure because they were very close in included markets. Other areas, notably Burgundy and Gascony, are under-represented because no published price series could be found for Dijon or Bordeaux.

The measure was calculated for overlapping fifty-year periods (1575–1625, 1600–50 . . . 1750–1800) with the results plotted in figure 6.2. A steady rise in the extent of price synchronisation is apparent throughout the seventeenth century, with a peak in the period 1675–1725. After that time there appears to have been a 'dis-integration' of markets for wheat. Nothing in the economic history of eighteenth-century France would prepare us to believe that such a phenomenon actually occurred following the reign of Louis XIV.[19] A more plausible explanation is that the late seventeenth-century rise in price synchronisation came from the supply side (highly-correlated climatic shocks) and not from the demand side. Indeed, a wide variety of long-run climatic indicators bottom out in the 'Little Ice Age' of the

[19] Usher, *The History of the Grain Trade in France*, ends his chronicle on a mildly optimistic note, concluding that the newly developed wholesale markets continued to spread and improve (albeit slowly) through the eighteenth century, pp. 41–4.

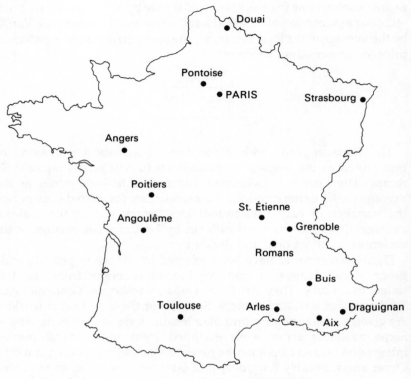

Figure 6.1 Location of markets with grain price series

late seventeenth century and recover significantly by the middle of the eighteenth.[20]

It is impossible to disentangle the effects of correlated harvest shocks from the effects of market integration. We might, however, wish to exclude years in which prices were exceptionally high or low. This will probably eliminate years not only of major climatic variation, but also those in which exceptional regional price differentials were sufficient to induce trade and therefore drive up prices elsewhere. We are interested in the decline of the margin within which grain prices could fluctuate locally without inducing trade (market integration) and not

[20] Lamb, *Climate*, summarises the evidence. Galloway, 'Long term fluctuations', relates climate trends to productivity and population growth. A more critical view can be found in Appleby, 'Epidemics and famine', pp. 643–4 or de Vries, 'Measuring the impact of climate'.

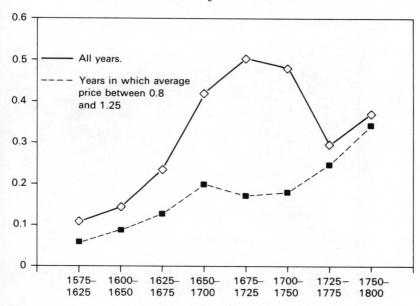

Figure 6.2 Price synchronisation

Note: for definition of measure, see text. The eight wheat price series used were: Paris, Douai, Strasbourg, Grenoble, Aix, Toulouse, Poitiers, and Angers. All were detrended by division by a centred eleven-year moving average.
Source: see appendix 1.

changes in the frequency with which prices exceeded some fixed gap sufficient to induce trade.

As figure 6.2 reveals, prices were much less closely synchronised in calm years than in all years taken together. More importantly, a gradual trend toward market integration appears in place of the enormous rise in price synchronisation at the end of the seventeenth century. Whatever the extent of political and economic catharsis occurring under Louis XIV, it appears that his reign coincided with a dramatic and temporary, if unwitting, nationalisation of harvest failures.

Further support for the supply-side explanation and the hypothesis of poorly integrated markets comes from Labrousse's data on wheat prices for thirty-two *généralités* of France between 1756 and 1790.[21] For each and every series, the pattern of correlation with the other series is very similar: extremely high correlations with neighbouring districts, high correlations at one and two districts away, some weak correla-

[21] Labrousse, *Esquisse du mouvement*, pp. 106–14.

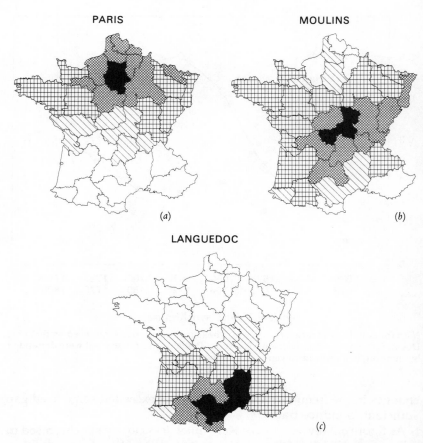

Figure 6.3 Price correlations with three regions (a) Reference region = Paris (b) Reference region = Moulins (c) Reference region = Languedoc

Note: shading indicates the statistical significance of the correlation of prices (deviations from moving averages) between the reference region and the shaded region. The solid shade is the reference *généralité* to which correlations refer. Cross-hatched regions are correlated at p<.001. Box-striped regions are correlated at p<.01 and diagonal regions are correlated at p<.1. After detrending, the years in observation are 1761-84.
Source: Labrousse, *Esquisse* for wheat prices by *généralité*.

tions at greater distance, and insignificant correlations with prices in the most distant regions. Figure 6.3 illustrates the pattern for three relevant cases: Paris, Moulins, and Languedoc. *Généralités* at the extremes (Provence, Bretagne) had the broadest range of uncorrelated regions at the opposite ends of the country, while central regions showed some correlation with nearly all areas. No decisive borders can

Table 6.1 *Price correlations: wheat and oats by market, time period*

Market	Years 1501–99	1600–69	1670–1739	1740–89
Paris	n.a.	.54	.65	.72
Douai	.63	.52	.57	.44
Strasbourg	.54	.89	.92	.54
Grenoble	.88	.67	.86	.65
Aix	.84	.60	n.a.	n.a.
Toulouse	.77	.84	.80	.53
Angoulême	n.a.	.75	.80	.77
Angers	n.a.	.58	.72	.44
Coutances	n.a.	n.a.	.79	.79

Notes: Prices are for calendar years, detrended by division by a centred eleven-year moving average, except for Angoulême which is harvest year data.
Sources: As given in the appendix for each market. Paris wheat and oat prices are from Hauser, *L'histoire des prix.*

be drawn between distinct regions, nor can central places be identified in this highly aggregated data. Whether the geographical range of correlations reflects transportation costs or the increasing dissimilarity of climatic shocks over greater distances cannot be determined. The evidence is clear enough, however, to establish that it would be premature to speak of a national market in the eighteenth century. By the same token, the distances (and populations) over which strongly significant correlations did extend are comparable to most of the other nations of Europe. France may well have had several grain markets as broad as any of the integrated national markets of Europe.

Proper controls for long-term trends lead one to reject Louise Tilly's overly optimistic evidence for a national market. But that by no means invalidates her central observation that a trend toward increasing market involvement led to new forms of protest around grain movements in early modern France. Nor does it deny the importance of national policy in promoting such involvement via taxation of the peasantry and support of merchants. The Bourbons of the *ancien régime* may not have constructed a national market but they did help to forge a market nation. That they did so during a period of unusually severe climatic stress may help to account for the especially virulent form of anti-capitalist protest in early modern France.

Oat and wheat price correlations for urban markets reflect many of the same conditions. As shown in table 6.1, for most of the markets the period around the turn of the eighteenth century was a high point for cross-grain price correlations. On the other hand, the fall in the correlation after that period is so modest and so variable that it is unlikely to be able to account for the great change in mortality in the eighteenth century. It is worth noting that Douai, a market in the Flemish region where mixed husbandry originated, showed consistently the lowest correlation of wheat and oats. The presence of large animal populations could reduce the degree of substitutability between wheat and oats and thereby reduce their price correlation through demand rather than supply.

Mortality

Mortality by region, 1670–1739

Rebaudo provides data on mortality in eight regions of rural France.[22] For each region a regression was used to identify the effects of current and (four) lagged prices in the appropriate market on current deaths, controlling for deaths in the preceding two years. The estimated coefficients were used to simulate the effects of a price shock in a single year on deaths in that year and future years.[23] The simulated effects for individual years can be added together to construct useful summary statistics. The *demographic* impact of prices can be measured by the cumulative impact after five years, while the *human welfare* impact can be summarised by the maximum cumulative impact attained before deaths begin to recover from the price shock.

Table 6.2 presents data and results for each region, using two price series for regions where there was not an obvious single choice based on size, location, or availability. The regions are rank-ordered by the extent to which the timing of deaths was affected by fluctuations in prices (column 6 of the table). This number is the product of the maximum cumulative impact of prices on deaths as estimated in the regressions (column 5) and the historically observed standard deviation of prices over the period (column 4). Its two components each represent one side of the structural dependence of mortality on prices.

[22] Rebaudo, 'Le mouvement annuel', pp. 589–606.
[23] In the year of the price shock (year 0) the effect is equal to the coefficient on current prices from the regression. In the year following the price shock (year 1) deaths deviate from the trend by an amount equal to the coefficient on lag 1 prices plus the carry-over from the previous year (year 0) effect times the coefficient on deaths lagged one year. The next year (year 2) combines the direct effect of lag 2 prices with the carry-overs from year 0 (year 0 deviation times the coefficient on deaths lagged two years) and year 1 (year 1 deviation times the coefficient on deaths lagged one year). And so on.

Table 6.2 *Prices and mortality by region, 1677–1734*

(1) Region	(2) Market	(3) Deaths s.d.	(4) Prices s.d.	(5) Impact	(6) Weighted impact	(7) National impact	(8) Lag	(9) Five-year impact
North	Douai	.366	.497	.487	.242	.241	1	.127
Centre	St. Etienne	.365	.231	.898	.207	.200	1	.062
Southwest	Toulouse	.388	.232	.813	.189	.230	0	.073
Midi	Aix	.336	.183	.920	.168	.221	1	.087
Paris	Paris	.362	.299	.500	.150	.185	0	−.013
Southeast	Geneva	.305	.230	.568	.131	.091	0	.001
	Grenoble		.274	.401	.110		0	−.062
East	Geneva	.338	.230	.487	.112	.105	0	.011
	Strasbourg		.336	.145	.049		0	−.012
West	Coutances	.197	.254	.043	.011		2	−.062
	Angers		.303	−.044	−.013	.030	—	−.081

Notes: Deaths are deaths above age five only. Standard deviations (s.d.) are calculated on detrended variables. Prices are calendar year wheat prices in the market indicated in column (2).

(1) Region as described by Rebaudo 1979.
(2) Market from which price data were taken.
(3) Standard deviation of detrended total of deaths (above age five only).
(4) Standard deviation of calendar year wheat prices.
(5) Impact is the maximum cumulative increase in deaths following a price shock, prior to beginning of recovery.
(6) The impact as in column 5 weighted by the standard deviation of prices as in column 4.
(7) The impact of national prices weighted by its standard deviation.
(8) The number of years after the price shock in which the largest single-year effect occurred.
(9) The cumulative effect of prices on deaths after five years, weighted by the standard deviation of prices.
Sources: Rebaudo, 'Le mouvement annuel' for deaths. Price sources by market are discussed in the appendix.

High price volatility itself indicates instability in the markets for essential grains. The estimated impact of prices on deaths measures the responsiveness of mortality to a price shock of a given size. In fact, the rank order of regions is similar whether or not the volatility of prices is taken into account, as a comparison of columns 5 and 6 will show.

A notable exception is the top-ranked North in which the unweighted impact of prices appears much smaller than in the regions appearing just below it on the table (Centre, Southwest, and Midi). However, because the price series for Douai was so much more volatile than that for the other regions it would be incorrect to say that price fluctuations had less of an impact there than elsewhere. While an equal-sized price shock had less effect in the North than in the Centre or Southwest, the shocks were on average larger in the North. The combined measure has the virtue of standardising for regional differences in the volatility of grain prices, without providing any insight into why such differences exist.

Possible explanations for higher volatility of wheat prices would include better credit markets, fewer government controls, fewer substitute foodstuffs, and, of course, more volatile harvests. If regional differences were purely nominal, i.e. unrelated to differences in the magnitude of quantity variation, then the adjusted coefficient is a measure of mortality's response to quantity variations. To the extent that the differences are real, the adjusted coefficient combines the size of shocks and the magnitude of response. Even though price volatility was not the major determinant of the force of subsistence crises during this period, we may wish to consider regional differences. Price variation was lowest in the South and Centre of the country and highest in the North. This is consistent with the greater reliance on wheat in Northern agriculture. A more polycultural system in the South could have kept wheat prices within a narrower band by providing more substitutes in consumption. Alternatively, stronger local authority in regions distant from Paris may have led to greater use of price controls. Clearly there are important questions for local studies.

Several other measures confirm the consistency of the regional orderings derived from the regressions on local prices. The volatility of death totals, shown in column 3, tended to vary with the extent to which deaths were dependent on prices. In other words, a strong price–mortality connection increased the variance of mortality. Identical regressions using a single national average price series in each region yielded generally similar estimates of the weighted maximum impact (column 7, table 6.2). A different measure based on the local price regressions – the cumulative effect after five years (weighted by the standard deviation of prices) – does not suggest a greatly different pattern (column 9, table 6.2), though it does distinguish sharply between the top four in which compensation was not complete and the bottom four in which the effects of a crisis were more than compensated for by later mortality declines. Finally, note that in three of the four top regions the year of maximum impact was one year after the price shock (though there was in all cases a positive effect in the year of the shock). Simple inspection of plots or the use of contemporaneous correlations might well have masked the magnitude of the relationship.

With the exception of the West, where deaths and prices both moved in ways substantially different from the rest of the country and not particularly in step with one another, the main conclusion must be on the essential similarity of experience. In all regions, price shocks created surplus deaths in the same year and often in the next. Since price shocks were closely correlated across regions, most of France experienced the consequences at roughly the same time. Regions differed somewhat in the magnitude of the impact and somewhat more in the degree of recovery after five years.

Mortality by region 1740–89

The *enquête anonyme* of the Institut National d'Etudes Démographiques (INED) adopted a ten-region partition of rural France that does not correspond exactly with the eight regions constructed by Rebaudo.[24] A rough attempt at matching will be made later in this section. Table 6.3 shows the results of distributed-lag regressions in the INED regions, again sorted in descending order of severity. The first thing to notice is that even the top-ranked regions of this period would rank at the bottom of the table constructed for the earlier period in terms of the extent to which price fluctuations induced mortality fluctuations. The decline was due both to a decline in price volatility and a fall in the impact of prices on mortality. Four of the ten regions show a weak negative effect of prices on deaths even at the point of maximum cumulative impact. Only three of the ten regions retained any positive effect after five years.

In addition to the dramatic fall in the magnitude of mortality's response to prices came a change in the timing of the response. Only in the Centre and South-east was the effect greatest in the current year;

---

[24] Blayo, 'Le mouvement naturel', pp. 15–64.

Table 6.3 Prices and mortality by region, 1747–84

(1) Region	(2) Market	(3) Deaths s.d.	(4) Prices s.d.	(5) Impact	(6) Weighted impact	(7) National impact	(8) Lag	(9) Five-year impact
Southeast	Geneva	.245	.185	.811	.150	0.76	0	.098
	Lyon	.245	.157	.758	.119		0	.055
	Grenoble	.245	.105	.562	.059		1	−.019
Centre	St. Etienne	.207	.193	.478	.088	.094	0	.031
Southwest	Toulouse	.303	.171	.450	.077	.082	2	.069
Midi	Aix	.167	.142	.507	.072	.015	1	−.021
East	Geneva	.150	.185	.330	.061	.012	2	.011
	Strasbourg	.150	.153	.124	.019		2	.013
West	Angers	.239	.198	.116	.023	.114	3	−.009
North	Douai	.141	.164	−.030	−.005	.040	2	−.021
Normandy	Paris	.164	.142	−.063	−.009	−.003	1	−.071
Centre West	Angoulême	.281	.186	−.086	−.016	−.003	2	−.226
Paris	Paris	.150	.142	−.162	−.023	.019	2	−.083

Notes: Columns are as defined in table 2. Deaths have been adjusted to remove the expected number of infant deaths in each year using the formula:
adj. deaths(t) = deaths(t) −0.74*0.25*births(t)
−0.26*0.25*births(t−1)

Sources: Deaths by region from Blayo, 'Le mouvement naturel'. Prices by market are discussed in the appendix.

for most regions it was one or two years later. In a sense, then, France was becoming more like England where the relationship between prices and deaths had established this pattern of small magnitude and delayed impact sometime earlier.[25]

Recall that the local price series were less closely correlated in the mid eighteenth century than they had been earlier. One might expect, then, to find that the national average price performed less well relative to local prices in this period than in the preceding period. That was not always the case. National prices often explained more of the variance in mortality and in several regions had a larger impact (column 7, table 6.3). One might be inclined to think that perhaps France was a national market, with local variations arising from measurement error and not from meaningful differences. But the geographical pattern of correlations in Labrousse's data for the *généralités* rules out pure random error as the only source of cross-sectional variation. A logical next question is whether the local urban market data capture the same geographical patterns of price movements as Labrousse's *généralités*. The comparison led to some still more puzzling discoveries and a possible interpretation.

For the period of overlap with the Labrousse data (1761–84 after detrending), the local urban price series were compared with the individual *généralités* and with regional averages corresponding to the INED regions. With the exception of Brittany-Angers the highest correlations were found between the regional averages and the corresponding local series. In other words, variation in the local series represented true local price variation. All the price series were then matched to the regional death series, with the expectation that the correlations between current deaths and current and lagged prices would be highest for regionally matched death and price series. Although there was some tendency in that direction, the local price series for St. Etienne showed the highest correlation with virtually all the regional death series. Randomness being what it is, one might expect to find a distant price series performing better than a local one on occasion, but certainly not one particular series out-performing most local series in their own regions. Aix and the *généralité* of Provence also showed high correlations with deaths in other regions (though not with prices). It would appear that national prices predicted Northern and Western deaths better than local prices because of the inclusion of Southern and Central prices. That leaves the question of why prices in St. Etienne influenced deaths in faraway regions through some mechanism that circumvented local prices.

[25] Lee, 'Short-term variations'.

To explore the association, distributed-lag regressions were run using St. Etienne prices as an explanatory variable for each regional mortality series. The results were sufficiently different from both the local and national price findings to suspect some other influence. For nearby regions (Centre, Southeast, Midi, and East) there was a strong positive contemporaneous effect, no effect at a lag of one year and a recovery after that. In the Western regions (Southwest, Centre West, West, and Normandy), there was a small to negative contemporaneous effect, followed by a larger effect at a lag of one year and then a recovery. Normandy was an exception in that there was an even larger effect after two years. In that respect it was more like the Paris region and the North where the effects (though smaller) were concentrated at lags 1 and 2. The pattern certainly suggests some sort of geographical diffusion away from the centre.

Baehrel has argued that deaths in Provence depended on prices only because of an omitted variable influencing both: drought.[26] Certainly that is consistent with a weak correlation of prices in the normally wet North and the normally dry South. A dry year would help crops in the North and hurt the South. One still wonders how a Southern drought could influence Northern and Western deaths with a year or more lag. Two mechanisms suggest themselves: one human, one geological. Grain shortages in the Centre and South could have promoted out-migration and the spread of disease to regions of destination. Alternatively, poor rainfall in the Central mountains will lower the water table of the run-off regions of the North and West in subsequent years. The effect may not damage crops enough to affect prices but could lead to lower quality of water sanitation and increased incidence of water-borne disease. Data on rainfall or on the heights of rivers in the plains might permit a test of the hypothesis.

Patterns of change

Although all regions (except the mysterious West) showed marked declines in the force of subsistence crises, not all changed equally or in quite the same way. Table 6.4 illustrates some of the differences. Regions have been matched in the two periods according to the local price series used. Normandy and the Centre-West have no easy correspondence with a region from the earlier period. The statistic used to summarise the impact of prices in the previous tables was the product of the standard deviation of prices and the maximum

---

[26] Baehrel, *La Basse-Provence rurale*, pp. 292–8.

Table 6.4 Patterns of change by market region

(1) Region	(2) Market	Index 1747–84/1677–1734				
		(3) Prices s.d.	(4) Impact	(5) Weighted impact	(6) National impact	(7) Percent of change due to impact
Paris	Paris	.475			.103	
North	Douai	.330			.170	
Southwest	Toulouse	.737	.554	.407	.357	65.7%
Centre	St. Etienne	.835	.532	.425	.470	73.8%
Midi	Aix	.776	.551	.429	.068	70.4%
East	Geneva	.804	.678	.545	.114	64.0%
	Strasbourg	.455	.855	.388		16.5%
Southeast	Geneva	.804	1.428	1.145	.835	263.1%
	Grenoble	.383	1.401	.536		−54.1%

Notes: Index numbers are the ratio of values in table 6.3 to those in table 6.2. The price series are identical in the two periods, but the regions are not. Percentage of change due to impact (6) was calculated as the natural logarithm of column 4 divided by the natural logarithm of column 5; times 100. For Paris and Douai, maximum cumulative impact was below zero in the second period.

cumulative impact on deaths. Change in it can be decomposed into changes in the two parts.

The regions fall easily into three groups. In the region around Paris and north to the Belgian border mortality lost all connection with local wheat prices. Price variation fell considerably, as well, from very high levels in the earlier period. In the South and Centre price variation fell by only 20–30 per cent while mortality retained about half of its earlier dependence on prices. Combined, these changes lowered the extent of price-driven mortality variation by nearly 60 per cent. In the Eastern portion of the country there was less progress. Genevan prices changed about as much as prices in Aix or St. Etienne. Strasbourg and Grenoble, on the other hand, resemble the Northern cities. Whichever price series is used, mortality retained more of its connection with prices; actually increasing in the Southeast (Burgundy–Rhone) region, as it did in the West.

It is worth examining in closer detail, then, the changing relationship between deaths and prices. These are displayed graphically in figure 6.4. The Northern regions around Douai show what might be described as the 'classic disappearance' pattern of change (panel a). From the pronounced current and one-year effect of the earlier period emerged an insignificant pattern of fluctuations close to the mean during the second period. The Paris region was similar, although the

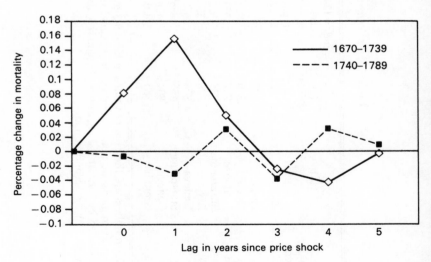

Figure 6.4 Proportional effect on mortality of a price shock: three regions and two towns
(a) North region (Douai)

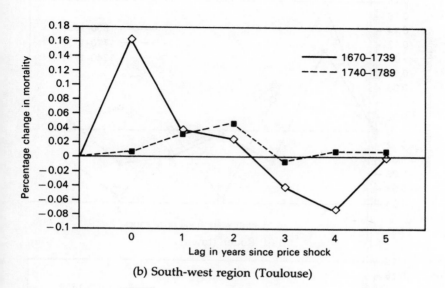

(b) South-west region (Toulouse)

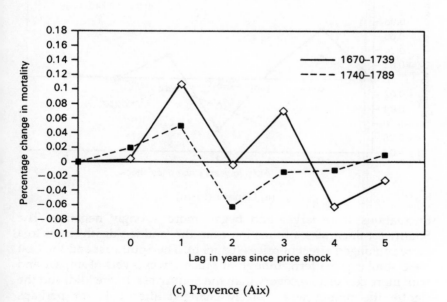

(c) Provence (Aix)

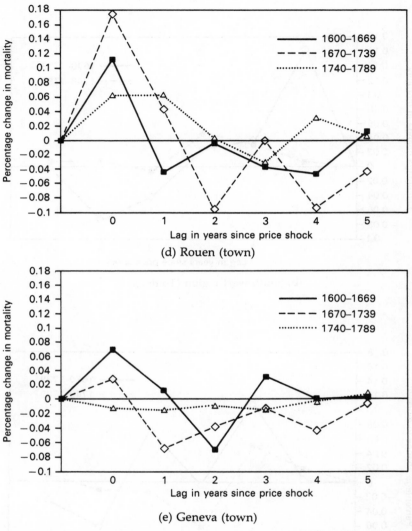

(d) Rouen (town)

(e) Geneva (town)

fluctuations were larger and began more strongly negative. The Southwest illustrates a transition from the 'sudden-death' crisis to a more prolonged effect of prices (panel b). The Southeast and the East were similar in pattern, though at much lower levels of impact and with more complete recovery than the Southwest. In the Midi and the Centre the timing was scarcely changed after 1740, or perhaps accelerated, but the effects were smaller and recovery more complete than in the earlier period (panel c).

Mortality in urban areas

Urban–rural conflicts over food supplies and terms of trade are a standard theme of early modern European economic history. Yet very little has been done to compare the effects of harvest fluctuations on mortality in cities and countryside. If grain markets first developed as 'one-way' streets to provision cities but without the capacity to bring grain to rural supply areas, then we might expect to find urban mortality to be less responsive to price fluctuations than the surrounding countryside. On the other hand, since cities were known to have food-distribution networks during crises, there might have been an influx of migrants from starving rural areas to spread disease in urban areas. The topic can only be studied adequately at a regional level, with close attention to urban rules regarding the regulation of grain markets and the handling of migrant beggars. Nevertheless, some aspects can be illuminated by looking at simple comparisons.

The most promising region for study in the seventeenth century is the Paris Basin. Rural and small-town series have been constructed by Jacques Dupâquier for time periods between 1600 and 1720.[27] The major city of Rouen has been the subject of an important study by Jean-Pierre Bardet.[28] He has published vital event totals covering 1600–1850. Perrenoud's study of Geneva provides an interesting contrast to Rouen for the same period.[29] For the whole of the eighteenth century, we can add a comparison between Toulouse and its rural hinterland.[30] Not only are local data more voluminous for the eighteenth century, but the INED *enquête* provides separate series of deaths from national samples of small, medium, and large cities beginning in 1740.

We turn first to the early seventeenth century in the cities of Rouen and Geneva, a set of towns in the Ile-de-France, and a collection of rural parishes from the same region. Regression results are reported in table 6.5. All four regions showed some responsiveness to prices, though Genevan mortality was far-less sensitive than the Northern regions. The large city of Rouen was evidently better-suited to cope with price fluctuations at that stage of development than were the smaller towns and rural parishes of the Paris region. Recovery after five years was also more complete in the urban centre.

[27] Dupâquier, *La population rurale*.
[28] Bardet, *Rouen*.
[29] Perrenoud, *La population de Genève*.
[30] Frêche, *Toulouse* sets up the contrast and provides data for the hinterland. Toulouse data were more easily obtained from Coppolani, *Toulouse*, and Rives, 'L'évolution démographique'.

Table 6.5 *Prices and mortality: local studies*

(1)	(2)	(3)	(4)	(5)	(6)	(7)	(8)
Locality	Market	Death s.d.	Prices s.d.	Impact	Weighted impact	Lag	Five-year impact
1600–70							
Rural Ile-de-France	Paris	.521	.237	1.148	.272	0	.044
Urban Ile-de-France	Paris	.521	.237	1.129	.268	0	.174
Rouen	Paris	.306	.237	.445	.105	0	−.022
Geneva	Geneva	.325	.219	.360	.079	0	.041
1670–1719							
Rural Rouen	Paris	.497	.335	.959	.321	0	.154
Rouen	Paris	.395	.335	.648	.217	0	−.003
Rich Districts		.395	.335	.475	.159	0	−.054
Poor Districts		.395	.335	.481	.161	0	−.014
Urban Ile-de-France	Paris	.331	.335	.586	.196	0	.014
Rural Paris	Paris	.337	.335	.573	.192	0	.030
Bassin Parisien	Paris	.283	.335	.447	.150	0	.004
Geneva	Geneva	.138	.266	.106	.028	0	−.131

1720–84						
Rouen	Paris	.176	.229	.576	.132	1	.130
Rich Districts		.175	.229	.445	.102	1	.101
Poor Districts		.195	.229	.424	.097	1	.057
Dole	Dole	.282	.197	.514	.101	1	.013
Paris	Paris	.123	.229	.363	.083	0	.009
Strasbourg	Strasbourg	.174	.146	.094	.014	2	−.004
Geneva	Geneva	.089	.219	−.057	−.012	n.a.	−.058
1747–84						
Dôle	Dôle	.282	.177	.527	.101	1	.013
Rouen	Paris	.164	.142	.470	.067	1	.044
Caen	Caen	.192	.190	.174	.033	0	.005
Paris	Paris	.094	.142	.134	.019	0	.014
Strasbourg	Strasbourg	.174	.148	.094	.014	0	−.004
Grandes villes	France	.086	.114	.117	.030	0	−.026
Petites villes	France	.132	.114	.096	.011	1	−.047
Moyenne villes	France	.100	.114	.096	.011	0	−.025
Rural France	France	.096	.114	.264	.030	2	−.051

Notes: Deaths adjusted to remove infant deaths as described in table 3. For Geneva, deaths under age five were eliminated directly.

Sources: Deaths are from Dupâquier, *La population rurale* for Ile-de-France, Paris Basin, and rural areas in the *généralités* of Rouen and Paris; from Bardet, *Rouen* for the city of Rouen; from Perrenoud, *La population de Genève* for Geneva; and Perrot *Genèse d'une ville moderne* for Caen.

In the next period, 1670–1720, our regional scope remains narrow, but we can look in more detail. When comparing sub-regions to their aggregate, it should be remembered that estimated effects will be smaller in each sub-region if the true model is the same simply because measurement error will be a larger fraction of total variance in the (smaller) sub-samples and measurement error will tend to bias coefficients toward zero. In the markets from which Baulant constructed her series for Paris, price fluctuations were 40 per cent larger in this period than the preceding one. In the city of Rouen mortality responsiveness also increased, so the impact of an 'average' price change more than doubled. It is possible to separate richer and poorer districts within the city. Somewhat surprisingly, the better-off districts (Centre, North, and West) were virtually identical to the poorer districts (East, Faubourgs). The price–mortality mechanism, at least in its urban form, does not appear to have been dependent on average levels of standard of living, in contradiction to Malthus's intuition. Since wealth is protection against starvation but not against disease, this finding suggests that migration and disease may have been important links between high prices and early death in cities.

Turning to the rural districts, Dupâquier's aggregate Paris Basin, while responding sharply to prices, was not nearly so sensitive as the localities collected for the period 1600–70. When examined separately, however, the parishes of the *généralité* of Rouen reveal much stronger responses than those under the *Intendant* of Paris. Its coefficients rival those of the earlier period, and, coupled with the greater price volatility, reveal Rouen's rural hinterland as the region where prices dictated demographic movements to the greatest extent. Rural regions near Paris were slightly less sensitive than the city of Rouen, implying a substantial contrast between Normandy and Ile-de-France. Norman villages may have been more dependent on grain imports to support their dairying and proto-industrial workforces than the grain lands around Paris.[31]

Meanwhile, Geneva had virtually eliminated any dependence of mortality on prices. Referring back to the regional analysis for this period in table 6.2, we see that the rural areas bordering Geneva (East and Southeast) were not among the leaders in the impact of prices on deaths, but were more strongly influenced by Genevan prices than was the city itself. Again, urban populations were better-insulated than rural. The *généralité* of Rouen falls within Rebaudo's North region

---

[31] Chaunu, 'Malthusianisme économique'.

where prices had a stronger impact than in her Paris region–a consistency that suggests regional differences within the Paris Basin might be explored still further with interesting results.

Dupâquier's data end in 1720, but we gain some new urban series, including data on Paris itself.[32] Rouen preserved a strong link between prices and mortality which declined in magnitude from the reduction in price volatility and from a fall in the response of mortality. The recovery, however, was less complete than in earlier periods. As shown in figure 6.4(d) the timing of the response changed in the now-familiar pattern toward a flatter and more prolonged effect. In terms of immediate impact, Rouen was rivalled by Dôle, a small city in Burgundy. Paris emulated Rouen in timing, but with smaller responses. Finally, Strasbourg and Geneva show very little effect. Figure 6.4(e) depicts the elimination of subsistence crises from Genevan mortality. The urban contrasts are all the more remarkable in light of our earlier finding that rural areas around Paris became much less responsive to prices in the eighteenth century, while the East and Southeast did not. Rural–urban interactions must have been very different in the two regions; tending to favour large cities in the East and rural areas in the Paris Basin. Our finding that death did not spare the richer districts of Rouen suggests that the difference may have more to do with migration and disease than with starvation.

The rural–urban comparison is biased somewhat by different periodisations. The Northern subsistence crisis of 1740/1 is excluded from the regressions using the INED data, but included in the local series studied here. If it was the last gasp of the old price–mortality structure, then perhaps the post-1740 period should be analysed separately. Regressions run on Rouen and Paris for years comparable to the INED data show clearly that the effects of prices were declining in the first half of the eighteenth century, but did not disappear. The conclusion that subsistence crises disappeared more completely in rural areas than in cities appears to be robust. Nevertheless, an extension of Dupâquier's data to 1789 would be extremely useful.

Table 6.6 presents results of similar analyses for the Toulouse region. In addition to the rural–urban contrast and the comparison across time periods, table 6.6 explores the differential dependence of mortality on millet and wheat prices. Millet prices become maize prices as that crop expands in the Southwest. Before interpreting the results, some comments on the data must be made. Deaths in the city were read from

---

[32] Charlot and Dupâquier, 'Mouvement annuel'.

Table 6.6 *Prices and mortality in Toulouse and its hinterland*

Locale	Grain	Deaths s.d.	Prices s.d.	Impact	Weighted impact	Lag	Five-year impact
1704–45							
Urban	wheat	0.207	0.242	0.940	0.228	0	0.228
Urban	millet	0.207	0.371	0.513	0.190	0	0.190
Rural	wheat	0.225	0.242	0.927	0.224	0	0.224
Rural	millet	0.225	0.371	0.567	0.210	0	0.207
1740–84							
Urban	wheat	0.340	0.174	2.244	0.390	2	0.390
Urban	millet	0.340	0.273	1.756	0.479	0	0.479
Urban*	millet	0.340	0.273	0.897	0.245	0	0.245
Rural	wheat	0.180	0.174	0.737	0.128	1	0.128
Rural	millet	0.180	0.273	0.641	0.175	1	0.175
1704–84							
Urban	wheat	0.292	0.211	1.492	0.315	1	0.315
Urban	millet	0.292	0.329	0.980	0.323	0	0.323
Rural	wheat	0.207	0.211	0.822	0.173	0	0.173
Rural	millet	0.207	0.329	0.583	0.192	0	0.192

Notes: Columns are as defined in previous tables. Deaths have not been adjusted for the timing of births. Urban* was estimated with a dummy term in the regression for the crisis year 1752.
Source: Frêche '*Les prix des grains*' for prices of wheat and millet in Toulouse; Coppolani, *Toulouse*, p. 103 for a graph of deaths in Toulouse, 1699–1789, supplemented by Rives, 'L'évolution démographique', p. 118 for 1750–89; and Frêche, *Toulouse*, p. 68 for deaths in rural parishes near Toulouse, 1688–1789.

graphs in several sources, while deaths in a sample of rural parishes were available in tabular form.[33] Any random error due to misreading of graphs will reduce the measured impact of prices in the urban regressions. Neither set of data was adjusted for the timing of births, so all the estimates of table 6.6 will be biased downward relative to those of earlier tables using adjusted deaths.[34]

[33] Frêche, *Toulouse*, p.68 for rural parishes. Coppolani, *Toulouse*, p. 103 for Toulouse deaths 1699–1749; Rives 'L'évolution démographique', p. 118 for deaths 1750–89. The latter two in graphical form only.

[34] There are two reasons for the upward bias of adjustment on the estimated effects of prices on deaths. Infant deaths are generally not as sensitive to price shocks (see, e.g. Rives, 'L' évolution démographique' or Perrenoud, *La population de Genève*, so removing them increases the measured response of the rest. Secondly, the adjustment only approximates the true time path of infant deaths and therefore acts like a constant deduction from each year. Deducting a constant from all values raises the variance relative to the mean.

In light of the special qualities of the data, the results are impressive. Both urban and rural show strong dependences on prices in the early period. There is no great difference between the two grains in total impact, but closer examination of the regressions shows that millet prices have a slightly stronger immediate impact. In the second half of the eighteenth century, the rural parishes show less responsiveness and the city more. Millet prices had a slightly stronger impact in the second period than did wheat. A simple plot of the time series of deaths in the city and outside it would show that the main difference was the enormous spike in deaths within the city in 1752, following four years of high prices. An alternative regression for urban deaths, using a dummy term for 1752, reveals a structure much more like the earlier period for urban deaths. The persistence of a strong structural dependence in Toulouse, stronger even than in Rouen, was therefore not entirely due to one crisis year. The large coefficient on the dummy for 1752, and the effect on other coefficients when it is included raise the possibility that the simple linear structure used to identify the effects of prices on deaths may not be adequate.

Figure 6.5 shows the changing timing of the mortality response in urban and rural settings. The rural areas were clearly moving in the direction of a lower, more delayed response to price shocks, while the city was not.

Conclusion

Wheat prices were an important determinant of the timing of deaths in France in the seventeenth century and the first quarter of the eighteenth. That ceased to be true after mid century in much of northern France and was less true everywhere. Price fluctuations had a relatively small impact on long-run population growth, but an 'average' price increase in an 'average' region during the early period was associated with the premature deaths of about eight per thousand of the population over a period of two or three years.[35] By contrast, America's war in Vietnam occasioned the premature deaths of perhaps 0.25 per thousand Americans and her bloody Civil War probably no more than five per thousand.[36] To be sure, deaths during subsistence

---

[35] From tables 2 and 4 it appears that a 'weighted impact' (standard deviation of prices times maximum cumulative impact of prices on deaths) of about 0.2 was typical of many areas of France during the long seventeenth century (before 1740). Assuming an annual crude death rate of forty per thousand, this implies 0.2(40) = eight per thousand premature deaths.

[36] Vietnam produced 47,000 American battle-related deaths from a population of about 190 million, while the Civil War had 140,000 deaths out of a population of 31.4 million.

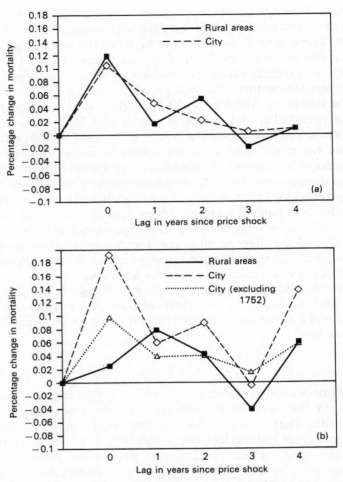

Figure 6.5 Proportional effect on mortality of a price shock: Toulouse, urban and rural (a) Toulouse, 1704–45 (b) Toulouse, 1740–84

'crises' were spread more evenly through the age–sex pyramid and set against a background of much higher mortality. Fewer years of life were lost for each premature death. Nevertheless, the phenomenon has great historical importance and its disappearance is a triumph for modern economic development.

In seeking the economic origins of the change, however, there were some surprising results. Most economic improvements should reduce the volatility of prices. That clearly happened in all regions and especially in the north after 1720. But better-integrated markets should also increase the degree of correlation across regions. Just the opposite actually occurred. The reduced volatility of prices, therefore, probably had little to do with improving national markets. Since price fluctuations are the reflection of quantity fluctuations through the demand function, we can look for an explanation of calmer prices either in a reduction of quantity fluctuations or an increase in the elasticity of demand for wheat. On the 'supply' side, the hypothesis that an improving climate reduced variability has much to commend it. Decreased correlation across regions would also be consistent with the elimination of major climatic shocks. Improved productivity might have the same effect as better weather, but has been strongly questioned by Morineau.

On the side of increased elasticity of demand, we have already ruled out any major improvement in the marketing of grain across large regions. Better markets within the large regions studied here remain a possibility. Now that the myth of a national market has been dispelled, perhaps subsequent research can document the rise of integrated regional markets through an intensive use of *mercuriales* from a single region. Appleby's hypothesis regarding the availability of substitutes is an intriguing one. More substitutes will raise the elasticity of demand for wheat. It is far from clear, however, that 'more' substitutes necessarily implies weaker correlations between the prices of different crops, as asserted by Appleby. Indeed, the strength of correlations between oat and wheat prices showed no particular relationship to the strength of mortality effects in the regions analysed here. Douai, for example, had the worst mortality responses 1677–1734 but the lowest correlation of wheat and oats. On the other hand, in the Toulousain millet (maize) and wheat prices were strongly correlated and deaths responded strongly to both. Other foodstuffs will need to be examined: maize and chestnuts in the South and Centre, rye in the East and buckwheat in the West, to name only the most obvious.

The reduction of mortality's dependence on prices was not only a result of the decline in price volatility. The impact of price movements also declined in most regions. From the limited evidence presented here it also appears that the two components tended to move together. In considering hypotheses for the structural change in the equation linking deaths to prices we will want to emphasise those that are also consistent with declining price volatility. Ruled out are hypotheses in which price volatility was determined solely by credit availability or government controls. If differences in price volatility were merely a statistical artifact one would expect to find them compensated for by opposite movements in the estimated magnitude of price effects on mortality. This did not occur. Increases in average product might have moved the French population out of the danger zone to a point where quantity shocks were smaller (thereby reducing price fluctuations) and did not venture into starvation levels (thereby reducing the mortality impact of any given price movement). This could have been the result of improved technique or of milder climate.

Climatic changes could have affected the relationship of mortality and prices even without affecting average output. To the extent that prices act as a proxy in the estimated equations for the effects of climate on disease, a change in climate might alter the observed price–mortality connection. The warming trend of the eighteenth century may well have reduced the combination of cold, wet years, poor harvests, and high winter mortality, especially in the North. The South continued to suffer occasionally the effects of hot, dry years, poor harvests, and high summer mortality. The surprising finding that high prices in St. Etienne were followed in later years by high mortality in Normandy and the Paris region suggests a climatic connection through water-borne disease that left no trace in Northern grain prices. More could be learned by matching seasonality patterns with the force of subsistence crises, or by using monthly data directly in the analysis of price effects.

Government activity could also have played a part. Distribution of grain and control of prices in some French cities could have reduced price variability, drawn off the starving rural population, and exposed the augmented urban populations to increased risk of disease. That would explain why Rouen and Toulouse continued to feel the effects of price movements while rural areas did not, and why social class did not shield the richer districts. Cities in the East, on the other hand, may not have provided the same service to their hinterlands; protecting themselves while leaving rural areas at risk.

Our goal in this chapter was to add to our knowledge of the regional diversity of 'subsistence crises' in France and thereby to promote informed speculation as to its causes. There is no shortage of interesting hypotheses remaining after this investigation. As the data on deaths and prices continue to accumulate it will be possible to match more closely regional mortality and local markets. Urban–rural interactions should be studied more intensively. We may never know the full story of how subsistence crises were eliminated. We can discover more about the relative importance of the forces of nature, the impersonal human forces of economic growth, and the direct actions of a concerned society.

Appendix. Local market series of grain prices

Wheat price series

1 Paris (Baulant)	1500–1788	
2 Paris (Hauser)	1520–1789	
3 Pontoise	1670–1790	
4 Douai (1329)	1500–1789	
5 Strasbourg	1501–1792	
6 Grenoble	1501–1790	
7 Buis (1501)	1670–1792	
8 Romans (1501)	1670–1792	
9 St. Etienne	1643–1789	
10 Aix	1570–1789	
11 Arles	1651–1789	
12 Draguignan	1616–1790	
13 Toulouse	1512–1792	
14 Poitiers	1548–1792	
15 Angoulême	1643–1792	
16 Angers	1580–1789	
17 France (CEL)	1700–1790	
18 Paris (HY: B&M)	1521–1698	
19 Angoulême (HY+1)	1643–1792	

Oat price series

20 Douai (1329)	1500–1792	
21 Aix	1570–1681	
22 Angoulême (HY1)	1643–1792	
23 Paris (Hauser)	1601–1774	
24 Strasbourg	1531–1792	
25 Grenoble	1501–1781	
26 Toulouse	1512–1792	
27 Angers	1580–1789	
28 Coutances	1678–1778	
29 France	1726–1789	

Other series

30 Coutances wheat	1678–1778

Sources

Aix   Baehrel, *Croissance*, pp. 535 (wheat), 558–9 (oats).
Angers   Hauser, *L'histoire des prix*, pp. 258–69.
Angoulême   George, 'Les mercuriales'. Annual data are for harvest years.
             Monthly data used to convert to calendar years.
Caen   Perrot, *Genèse d'une ville moderne*.
Coutances   Hauser, *L'histoire des prix* (wheat and oats, 1678–1778).
Dôle   Lefebvre-Teillard, *La population de Dôle*, pp. 76–7 (wheat: 1710–89).

Douai   Mestayer, *'Les prix du blé,'* pp. 167–76. (wheat and oats, 1329–1793).

Geneva   Perrenoud, *La population de Genève,* pp 403. Prices read from a graph of deviations from a nine-year moving average.

Grenoble   Hauser, *L'histoire des prix,* pp. 365–71 (wheat 1501–1790, oats 1501–1781).

Lyon   Garden, *Lyon,* p. 761. Prices read from a graph of annual wheat prices 1700–89.

Paris   Baulant, *'Le prix du blé',* pp. 538–40. Published annual prices computed from data on nearby rural markets (wheat 1431–1788).
             Hauser, *L'histoire des prix,* pp. 107–20. (wheat 1520–1774, oats 1600–1774).

Poitiers   Raveau, *'Essai',* pp. 360–5. (wheat 1548–1792).

Pontoise   Dupâquier, *La population rurale,* pp. 40–99. Simple annual mean of published quarterly data. (wheat 1676–1789).

St. Etienne Gras, *Histoire du commerce,* pp. 230–70. (wheat 1643–1789).

Strasbourg   Hanauer, *Etudes économiques,* pp. 94–101. (wheat 1501–1792, oats 1531–1792).

Toulouse   Frêche, *Les prix des grains,* pp. 85–91. (wheat, oats, and millet 1512–1789).

7

Some reflections on corn yields and prices in pre-industrial economies

E. A. WRIGLEY

King and Davenant

Playing with figures fascinated Gregory King. His notebooks bulge with calculations about the chief economic and demographic preoccupations of the day. Nothing King wrote was published until long after his death, but some of his estimates and speculations were published by Charles Davenant (who repeatedly made clear the extent of his debt to King).[1] Given the nature of pre-industrial society, it was to be expected that one of the topics that would attract King's attention was the scale of agricultural production and the price of the foodstuffs produced.

It had long been high in the consciousness of men and of governments that when the harvest failed the price of food was affected disproportionately and Davenant attempted to set out the relationship quantitatively. How far Davenant's discussion of this issue was directly his own work and how much it was a summary of King is unclear, but his analysis has been immensely influential and it is convenient to refer to the 'model' under Davenant's name. He specified the degree to which price was increased by harvests which were successive deciles below the average. His estimates were widely quoted and broadly confirmed by a number of later examinations of the same issue. Jevons, for example, accepted the general accuracy of the formula which Davenant published and sought an expression which would generalise the relationship between quantity and price. Having determined the general form of the function from a consideration of the behaviour of price in very extreme conditions of supply, he suggested

This chapter was originally published in E. A. Wrigley *People, Cities and Wealth: The Transformation of Traditional Society*, Blackwell, Oxford (1987) chapter 5.
[1] Davenant, *Essay upon the Balance of Trade*.

Table 7.1 *The results of the formulas of*
Davenant and Jevons compared

	Price of grain	
Quantity of grain[a]	Davenant	Jevons
1.0	1.0	1.06
0.9	1.3	1.35[b]
0.8	1.8	1.78
0.7	2.6	2.45
0.6	3.8	3.58
0.5	5.5	5.71

Note: [a]Quantity of grain in an average
year = 1.0.
[b]Jevons gives a figure of 1.36 but in doing
so slightly miscalculated the result
obtained by his formula.

that the price of corn would be approximated by the formula $y = 0.824/(x - 0.12)^2$ where x is the ratio of the quantity currently available to that normally available. He showed the closeness of fit between Davenant's results and those obtained by his formula in a table reproduced as table 7.1.[2] Jevons added that, 'roughly speaking, the price of corn may be said to vary inversely as the square of the supply, provided that this supply be not unusually small'.[3] In support of the obvious implication of the formula, he noted that Tooke had made estimates of the extent to which farmers in the bad harvest years of 1795, 1796, 1799, and 1800 had benefited from the shortfall and enjoyed incomes above the average. 'If the price of wheat', he concluded, 'varied in the simple inverse proportion of the quantity, they would neither gain nor lose, and the fact that they gained considerably agrees with our formula as given above.'[4]

Jevon's discussion of the issue occurred in the course of his general discussion of price variations and forms part of the wider thesis that 'the variation of price is much more marked in the case of necessaries of life than in the case of luxuries'.[5] He initiated his discussion by a quotation from Chalmers which includes the following passage, 'let

---

[2] Jevons, *Theory of Political Economy*, p. 182.
[3] *Ibid.* The presence of a negative constant in the squared term of the denominator of Jevon's formula has the effect, of course, of producing a more violent increase in price when the quantity harvested falls below average by a given proportion than reduction in price when there is a harvest which exceeds the average by the same proportion.
[4] *Ibid.*, p. 183.   [5] *Ibid.*, p. 176.

the crop of grain be deficient by one third in its usual amount, or rather, let the supply of grain in the market, whether from home produce or by importation, be curtailed to the same extent, and this will create a much greater addition than one third to the price of it. It is not an unlikely prediction that its cost would be more than doubled by the shortcoming of one third or one fourth in the supply.'[6] Very similar observations were made by many men with practical experience of the corn trade in the eighteenth and nineteenth centuries and by those who commented upon it, notably Thomas Tooke.[7]

This view of the behaviour of corn prices in relation to supply is intuitively attractive as well as firmly grounded in theoretical considerations, but will bear some re-examination since it is a more complex matter than might appear at first blush. The quotation from Chalmers is instructive in this regard. In certain circumstances much hangs upon the distinction between overall yield and market supply over which he hesitated.

Davenant himself was well aware of the difference between gross yield and the quantity of grain that could be marketed. Earlier in his essay, in presenting some of King's estimates of arable production in 'years of moderate plenty', he gave a table of output exclusive of seed-corn and then discussed how greatly its inclusion would have raised the output figure. But the phrasing of his introduction to the table showing the relationship between the extent of the 'defect' of the harvest and its effect in raising the price of corn 'above the common rate' is ambiguous and the rest of this passage in his essay contains no explicit clarification of the point. In commenting on his table, for example, he wrote that 'when corn rises to treble the common rate it may be presumed that we want one third of the common produce; and if we should want five tenths, or half the common produce, the price would rise to near five times the common rate'.[8] Such remarks leave his intention unclear. In referring to 'common produce', had he in mind

---

[6] *Ibid.*

[7] Economic historians from Thorold Rogers to Slicher van Bath have also had resort to the ideas of Davenant (and/or King) in seeking to relate harvest quantities to price movements. Thorold Rogers, who worked so extensively on the subject, is especially warm in his praise: 'Gregory King has rarely, even in modern times, been surpassed in the special and very exceptional power of understanding what is meant by statistical figures. King discovered the law which regulates the price of the necessaries of life on the occasion of a scarcity, and formulated a geometrical proportion which experience has proved, with some minor modifications, to be a rule of safe action.' Thorold Rogers, *Work and Wages.* p. 465. See also Thorold Rogers, *Economic Interpretation of History.* pp. 250–3 for his elaboration of King's law and the implications which flow from it. For Slicher van Bath, see below, pp. 249–51.

[8] Davenant, *Essay upon the Balance of Trade*, p. 83.

Table 7.2 *Gross and net yields (average yield = 10 bushels)*

Gross yield (bushels per acre)	Net yield (a)[a]	Net yield (b)[b]	Value (Bouniatian's formula) Gross	Value (Bouniatian's formula) Net (a)	Value (Bouniatian's formula) Net (b)	Value (Average year = 100) Gross	Value (Average year = 100) Net (a)	Value (Average year = 100) Net (b)
10	7.5	6.5	10.00	7.50	6.50	100	100	100
9	6.5	5.5	11.49	8.30	7.02	115	111	108
8	5.5	4.5	13.49	9.27	7.59	135	124	117
7	4.5	3.5	16.31	10.48	8.16	163	140	126
6	3.5	2.5	20.56	11.99	8.57	206	160	132
5	2.5	1.5	27.65	13.82	8.30	277	184	128

Note: [a]Gross yield less 2.5 bushels for seed-corn.
[b]Gross yield less 2.5 bushels for seed-corn and 1 bushel for fodder for draught animals.

The following table shows how the quantity of grain available affects its price using Bouniatian's formula [$y = 0.757/(x - 0.13)^2$] where 1.0 is the quantity of an average harvest.

Quantity	Price
1.0	1.000
0.9	1.277
0.8	1.686
0.7	2.330
0.6	3.427
0.5	5.530

the gross yield of corn, or what remained for consumption after setting aside seed-corn and any other necessary deductions from the quantity of grain initially harvested?

The importance of the distinction between net and gross output in relation to price may be seen in table 7.2. In it farmers' incomes at varying crop yields are set out, using Bouniatian's formula for estimating price from quantity rather than that of Jevons. It is an inconvenient characteristic of Jevons's formula that in a year of average harvest, taken to be a quantity of 1.0, the implied price is not 1.0 but 1.06 (see table 7.1), which means that the price in a year of deficient harvest can only be expressed as a percentage of the price in an average year after a further calculation (thus table 7.1 shows the price of grain in a year when the harvest is only 80 per cent of normal as 1.78; this is, however, not 78 per cent above normal but only 68 per cent above (100 × 1.78/1.06 = 168). Bouniatian's formula avoids this inelegance but otherwise produces results closely similar to those of Jevons.[9]

Table 7.2 sets out two illustrative cases. In both I have assumed an average gross yield of 10 bushels per acre and that 2.5 bushels of corn were needed as seed for each acre sown, but case (b) differs from case (a) in that I have also assumed that a further bushel has to be set aside to supply 'fuel' for draught animals. The available evidence suggests that from medieval times until the nineteenth century a figure of 2.5 bushels per acre for seed must be approximately correct for wheat: it would be higher for other grains.[10] Animal fodder needs varied more

[9] Bouniatian set out his own formula after noting the difficulty with Jevons's formula. Bouniatian, *La loi des prix*, p. 64. His discussion of King's law was both well informed and judicious. He began by noting that, although normally attributed to King, it was probably due to Davenant. He was well aware that the comparative simplicity of earlier centuries had been much altered by international trade and by the development of major substitutes for grain, especially the potato. And he explained clearly how the carry-over of grain from one year to the next could blur the impact of good or bad harvests, using French data for 1815 and 1816, and for 1819 and 1820 to illustrate the point (p. 66). Nevertheless, he argued that the relationship of price and quantity for Prussian rye in the mid nineteenth century and for American maize between 1866 and 1911 both showed the basic soundness of King's law, and concluded by asserting, in a passage which he italicised, that King had succeeded in expressing '*la loi de formation du prix du blé lorsque la récolte de l'année représentait la quantité disponible du blé comme moyen presque unique d'alimentation de la population pour l'année à venir*'.

[10] See, for example, Bowden, 'Agricultural prices', p. 652; or Slicher van Bath, *Agrarian History*, p. 173. A figure of 2.5 bushels is more appropriate for wheat than for barley. With the latter a substantially higher quantity of seed-corn was used: 4 bushels was a normal figure. Beveridge also discussed this point. He gives the following average quantities of seed in bushels per acre for nine Winchester manors over the period 1200–1450, and for comparison included the comparable figures for England 1895–1914 (given in brackets): wheat 2.48 (2.72); barley 3.76 (3.04); oats 4.32 (4.80). The related yields per acre were 9.36 (31.36); 14.32 (32.96); 10.56 (40.72). Beveridge suggested that the contrast between modern and medieval yields was more

widely. They were affected by the type of animal used and by local agricultural practices, and were far more likely to fluctuate from year to year according to the scale of the preceding harvest. But they could not be altered substantially without penalty in the subsequent harvest since the amount of useful work obtainable from draught animals was strongly affected by both the quantity and type of fodder given to them.[11] Animal 'fuel' was needed for many aspects of arable farming, but especially for ploughing, other forms of cultivation and carting. It could be very costly in grain. One of the most original of all writers on agricultural economics, von Thünen, provides a vivid instance of the very large requirements of draught animals for grain 'fuel' if they were to perform efficiently. He had the inestimable advantage of practical experience in running a big agricultural estate to guide him in quantifying farming operations. His estate lay at Tellow, 23 miles from the market town of Rostock. He noted that a four-horse team was used to take grain to market and that the round trip took four days. The team's normal load was 2,400 Hamburg pounds weight but the team needed 300 pounds of grain in fodder to perform the round trip (the Hamburg pound was slightly heavier than the English pound).[12] The assumption that one bushel of corn per acre is an appropriate allowance for animal fodder in pre-industrial agriculture is entirely arbitrary, but it may well represent a closer approach to reality than the assumption that seed-corn alone need be deducted to derive a net from a gross figure. Even if animal fodder needs are treated as zero, it is still useful to consider the two alternatives. For example, the second might stand for the seed requirement of barley where the first represents wheat.

In Davenant's day average yields of both wheat and barley were probably somewhat higher than 10 bushels per acre, but 10 bushels is a reasonable, if not indeed a generous, estimate for earlier centuries or

pronounced even than his statistics suggested because medieval yields were for the areas actually cultivated. If they had been reckoned 'as they lie' to include various forms of wasted space, the area would have been nearly doubled whereas this consideration did not apply to nineteenth-century data. Beveridge, 'Yield and price of corn', pp. 158–9. Bairoch has summarised his findings from a large body of wheat yield data for continental Europe in the nineteenth century. He concluded that, excluding Russia, yields rose on average by just over 50 per cent between 1800 and 1910 from 11.9 to 18.3 bushels per acre (converting from quintals per hectare, and assuming 60 lb to the bushel), but that the quantity of seed sown per acre increased by only 8 per cent, from 1.84 to 1.99 bushels. Bairoch, 'Rendements agricoles', p. 9.

[11] Slicher van Bath, Agrarian History, p. 22. Smith, Western Europe, pp. 204–10, especially figure 4.5, p. 206.

[12] Von Thünen, The Isolated State, p. 13. Unlike ploughing and cultivation, carting whether within the farm or from farm to market was not, of course, a fixed overhead but varied with the size of the harvest.

for pre-industrial western Europe as a whole.[13] In any case, the purpose of the exercise is to expose the implications of the distinctions between gross and net yields under certain assumptions rather than to exemplify conditions at a particular point in time. Table 7.2 shows that if prices are obtained by applying Bouniatian's formula to gross yield as a proportion of its own average level, and it is assumed that the whole crop is sold, the value of the crop rises steeply with successively more severe harvest failure until when the crop is only half its normal level its value approaches three times that of a normal year. On this basis, the substantial farmer appears to have good reason to prefer a poor harvest to a plentiful one. If, however, price is calculated in the same way but it is assumed that only the net yield can be marketed, then the picture changes substantially. The quantity of grain which can be released into the market falls proportionately very much faster than gross output. In consequence, the total value of the crop rises more moderately and the farmer has far less reason to hope for a bad or fear a good harvest. Even on assumption (a), there is already a substantial contrast in value compared with the gross yield value figure, and the contrast is greatly accentuated on assumption (b). In the latter case, the value of the crop varies only modestly over the whole range of yields shown in table 7.2.

If, therefore, Davenant in framing his table was relating gross output to price, it does not necessarily follow that agriculture derived a bumper income from bad years, nor suffered such a serious drop in income when harvests were exceptionally good. (Bouniatians's formula implies that a harvest 20 per cent above normal would reduce income from grain to only 79 per cent of its normal level if the marketable quantity varies with gross yield, whereas a calculation equating the

---

[13] There is a convenient summary of estimates of wheat yields in England for the later seventeenth and eighteenth centuries in Turner, 'Agricultural productivity', table 5, p. 504. Grigg has assembled estimates of wheat yields in Europe in about 1850 which suggest that even at that date in Spain, Greece, and Russia yields were about 7 bushels per acre, and that in several other countries including France, Italy and Spain they were between 7 and 10 bushels per acre. (I have taken 1 bushel of wheat to be of 60 lb weight.) Grigg, *Dynamics of Agricultural Change*, table 25, p. 175. Titow's work suggests that medieval English wheat yields were probably slightly less than 10 bushels per acre. Titow, *Winchester Yields*, table 2b, p. 13. In converting the frequency distributions of yield given in Titow's table, I have assumed that the yields in each yield category were at the midpoint of the range except for the category 0 to 7.9 bushels where I have assumed that the average was 6 bushels. This procedure gives an overall average of 9.6 bushels. See also Bennett, 'British wheat yield', pp. 12–29; the article by Lennard, 'Statistics of corn yields'; and Jones and Healy, 'Wheat yields', table 1, p. 189. Overton's analysis of probate inventories suggests that wheat yields in East Anglia rose from about 8 to about 13 bushels per acre between the 1580s and the 1660s, and had increased still further to perhaps 15 bushels per acre by the 1720s and 1730s. Overton, 'Estimating crop yields', figure 1, p. 371.

marketable surplus with net yield suggests figures of 84 and 86 per cent respectively for assumptions (a) and (b) of table 7.2.)

From the farmer's point of view, the balance of advantage between good and bad harvests is further affected by any consumption of grain by his household. Because of household needs, the quantity available for sale in poor years will be even more sharply depressed than is implied by the distinction between gross and net yield in table 7.2. For example, a farmer devoting 50 acres to corn would harvest 500 bushels in an average year. On assumption (b) of table 7.2 he would need to set aside 175 bushels for seed and fodder. He might also have to reserve 75 bushels for the use of his household, making a total of 250 bushels as a fixed deduction from total production. In these circumstances, a fall of 20 per cent in gross output, from 500 to 400 bushels, would mean a fall of 40 per cent in output available for sale from 250 to 150 bushels. The resident farm family, which, together with any living-in servants, was also the prime farm workforce, took a substantial part of its 'payment' in the form of food. Grain used for this purpose falls into much the same logical category as animal 'fuel'. Maintenance of something approaching the normal level of food supply was a condition of the efficient working of the farm. If output for sale fell by 40 per cent, and if the price of corn changed in the manner set out in table 7.2, the farmer's income would be almost exactly the same in the deficit year as in an average year. Equally, he would have less to fear from a bumper harvest than might be thought at first blush since his net surplus would rise very much faster than his gross output. An increase of 20 per cent in gross output, on the same assumptions used in the previous calculation, would increase the quantity of grain for market by 40 per cent, and would reduce the farmer's income by only 7 per cent. The bigger the farmer and the higher the average output per acre, the less the force of the considerations just advanced, of course, but for many centuries and for wide tracts of territory they are relevant to the assessment of the farmer's interest in the face of fluctuating harvest fortunes.[14] The example considered is an arbitrary selection, of course. Other assumptions about farm size would lead to different relative fortunes in the wake of generous or niggardly yields, but to explore in full the interplay of the many factors that could affect the outcome is an enterprise beyond the scope of this chapter.

The validity of the arguments used in connection with the distinction between gross and net yield retains its full force, of course, only to the

---

[14] Abel provides some numerical illustrations of the importance of farm size in this connection. Abel, *Agricultural Fluctuations in Europe*, pp. 9–13. Abel was also conscious of the 'leverage' exerted by low yield/seed ratios (p. 41).

degree that it is proper to assume that the absolute quantity reserved from sale was invariant, or to phrase the point differently, that the price elasticity of the farmer's demand for corn was zero. The assumption that the quantity of grain used as seed-corn did not vary from year to year whatever the scale of the previous harvest is especially important since, at the levels of yield under discussion, this would be in many cases the weightiest element in deciding the matter. The issue appears to have attracted little historical attention. For many periods and places the evidence needed for empirical study is lacking,[15] and it may be thought that it is unreasonable to suppose that a constant quantity of corn was always reserved for seed (or, where seed was customarily obtained from other areas, bought through the market). Yet it is also true, that even if the price elasticity of the farmer's demand was greater than zero but much below the price elasticity of other demands, much of the effect would remain, though less starkly than under the assumptions used above. Nor should it be overlooked that a bad harvest might often result in *more* seed than usual rather than less, being sown for the next crop. For example, at a public meeting of the 'principal inhabitants' of the county of Aberdeenshire held in the December following the disastrous oats harvest of 1782, it was held to be essential, in spite of the desperate shortage of grain, to reserve thirty bolls for seed rather than the customary twenty-five because the seed was of poor quality.[16]

Price runs and yields

Suggestive indirect evidence exists, however, which lends plausibility to the view that usage of seed-corn may not have varied significantly from year to year. Agricultural historians command far more evidence about prices in the past than about aggregate output or about yield, so that their picture of harvest fluctuation is often based principally upon a knowledge of the behaviour of prices. One of the most striking features of grain price series for earlier centuries is that they display 'runs' of years when prices were either above or below the local average. It has been common to interpret such runs as evidence that there were parallel sequences of good and bad harvests when corn was comparatively scarce or plentiful for several successive years. Sometimes the phenomenon is attributed to runs of years of favourable or

[15] Manorial grange accounts are a promising source for the medieval period, perhaps superior to later materials before the nineteenth century.
[16] Flinn *et al.*, *Scottish Population History*, pp. 11–12. I am grateful to John Walter for drawing my attention to this evidence.

unfavourable weather conditions, but it has also been attributed to the
'knock-on' effects of individual good or bad harvests due to seeding
practice. Hoskins, for example, in two influential articles, suggested
that the reason for successions of years with prices above or below the
long-term moving average was to be found in the quantity of seed
sown. He stressed the low level of yield/seed ratios and added

This means that a large part of the arable land had to be kept for growing next
year's seed. It also meant that a bad harvest, by reducing the yield ratio to a
dangerously low level, almost automatically ensured another bad harvest from
a sheer deficiency of seed. In very bad years, the rural population must have
staved off the worst of their hunger by consuming part of next year's seed
corn . . . So one bad harvest tended to generate others . . . Conversely, of
course, one good harvest tended automatically to produce another through the
abundance of seed corn.[17]

Hoskins' hypothesis is difficult to test effectively for the period from
the late fifteenth to the mid eighteenth century, the period whose price
data he was discussing, for lack of suitable sources of information, but
some light is thrown on the matter by nineteenth-century French data.
From 1815 onwards information on cereal acreage, production, and
therefore yields, was collected and published in France.[18] Such data for
wheat, used in conjunction with a wheat price series, enable the
behaviour of yield and price fluctuations to be examined, and the latter
to be compared with similar English data from the medieval period
onwards. These exercises are described in detail in the appendix to this
essay, but the patterns they reveal lend themselves to a simple
summary.

During the century from 1815 to 1914 wheat yields in France varied in
a random fashion. There was no tendency for years of exceptionally
good or bad harvests to be followed by further years of above- or
below-average yield. Nor were runs of good or bad harvests any more
frequent or more prolonged than would be expected to occur by
chance. Moreover, there was no relationship between the yield in one
year and the area sown in the next. The die was thrown afresh each
year and the result of the cast was not biased by the number produced
by the throw of the previous year. If the quantity of corn retained for
seed did vary with the scale of the harvest, it was not enough to
influence the yield in the following year systematically, even to the
limited extent of keeping it on the same side of the average yield. On
the other hand, the *price* of wheat did not vary randomly from year to

[17] Hoskins, 'Harvest fluctuations 1480–1619', pp. 32–3.
[18] Mitchell, *European Historical Statistics*, tables D1 and D2.

year, and runs of high and low prices did occur.[19] Clearly, although the quantity of the harvest varied randomly, grain prices did not follow suit.

The French data show unambiguously that it is dangerous to argue from the behaviour of a wheat price series to the pattern of annual fluctuations in the wheat harvest. Moreover, comparison with English price data reveals a striking similarity between the characteristics of wheat price fluctuations in nineteenth-century France and those of comparable wheat price series in England from medieval times onwards.

The absence of any evidence in French yield data that there were runs of good or bad years tells against the Hoskins hypothesis since he envisaged a shortage of grain in one year causing less seed than usual to be sown in the next and a smaller than average harvest to result. The proximate cause of runs in the price series, in other words, was held by him to be runs in the production series. If they are not visible, his explanation does not carry conviction. It is more plausible to assume that the scale of the carry-over from one harvest to the next was the cause of price runs. A bumper harvest in year *t* will mean that supplies in year *t* + 1 will also tend to be above average if yields vary randomly from year to year. Equally, a bad harvest, by restricting the carry-over, will produce an opposite effect. In this way random 'shocks' in the production series can give rise to runs in the price series, and the effect, *ceteris paribus*, need not be confined to the year next following.

The presence of very similar patterns in medieval and early modern English price series to those found in the nineteenth-century French series does not, of course, prove that an English yield series, if it existed, would display characteristics like the French, but it does suggest great caution in supposing that there were runs in the yield series in parallel with those in the price series. Moreover, there are other features of the Exeter wheat price series when the very long series (1316–1800) is broken down into sub-periods which are consonant with the hypothesis that variations in the carry-over of grain from year to year were the prime cause of the patterns in the price series.[20]

A priori one might doubt whether nineteenth-century evidence is relevant to the understanding of earlier times. For example, radical improvements in communications, and the consequent concatenation of producing areas, might be expected to have greatly reduced the

---

[19] Price data for harvest years were taken from labrousse *et al.*, *Le prix du froment*, pp. 13–14.
[20] See appendix, pp. 276–8.

pressure to trench upon seed-corn after a poor harvest. Only further empirical research can adequately resolve this question, but it is worth noting that eighteenth-century French wheat price series behaved in a very similar manner to those in the nineteenth century down to at least 1860; and also that the level of wheat yields in France after the Napoleonic wars was very low by the standards of contemporary England. At about 13 bushels per acre, it was no higher than in England two centuries earlier.[21]

It is an added complication that Hoskins' assertion about variation in seed usage in response to harvest fortune might be true, but the inference which he drew might be mistaken. Bad harvests might cause seed-corn to be consumed and lead to thinner sowing before the next harvest, and good harvests might be followed by an unusually liberal use of seed, without this variation having a significant effect on the succeeding harvest. For example, the high price of grain after a poor harvest might encourage the employment of an abnormal amount of labour in tillage, weeding, birdscaring, gleaning, etc, sufficient to offset the decline in yield per acre that might otherwise have occurred. Or again, yield may have been only very weakly responsive to seeding density even with unchanged cultivation practices. More widely spaced seeds, for example, encourage freer tillering. Against this, it is reasonable to suppose that normal seeding rates represented optimal practice in the circumstances of the day, and that any major change in the rate must have involved some penalty in output. If, however, to take an extreme position, changes in the seeding rate had little or no effect on yield, this fact, by increasing the probability that the yield series was random, would increase the likelihood that the presence of runs in the price series was attributable to the effect of carry-over.

At present, therefore, it is difficult to assemble sufficient evidence to specify unambiguous conclusions either about the invariability of the difference between gross and net yields, or about the question of the existence of runs in yield series comparable to the demonstrable runs in price series, or about the causes of such runs if they existed. But the French evidence lays the burden of proof upon those who have assumed that yield series were other than random and undermines any argument about yield runs which depends upon the existence of price runs.

Harvest yield and price

On the first point, the invariability of the quantity reserved from the market by consumption on the farm, whether for seed, self-consump-

---

[21] See note 56 below.

tion or animal fuel, Davenant's formula should be considered in relation to consumption by market purchase as well as to production requirements. If his formula were understood to mean that when the supply available in the market was reduced to half the normal level, its price rose more than fivefold, this would imply that almost three times the usual quantity of money was expended on corn. This interpretation is fraught with problems. For example, it is not easy to square with the fact that family budgets in pre-industrial times suggest that perhaps as much as three-quarters of all income were devoted to the purchase of food even in ordinary years, and that the bulk of food purchases consisted of grain. Since most families had little or no reserve of cash to call upon in hard years and were unlikely to be able to borrow, it is scarcely conceivable that they, who formed the bulk of the purchasers of corn, could raise their expenditure to the degree implied by the formula.[22] If, on the other hand, his formula for estimating price, though based on variations in gross output, should be related to the quantity available to be marketed, which was subject to much more violent fluctuations, the additional expenditure on grain even in a very bad year is relatively moderate on the assumption that the farmer's reservation from the market changed little from year to year.

The pressure towards higher prices in the wake of a bad harvest will vary not just, or even mainly, as a function of the extent of the harvest shortfall, but also as a function of the ability of purchasers to afford higher prices. For some men times of famine presented few problems. The wealthy spent relatively little of their income on food and were not greatly inconvenienced by grain price rises. Others enjoyed a sharply enhanced income in times of dearth because they had grain to sell. But many of those who depended chiefly upon wages were exposed to double jeopardy. The price of their main item of expenditure rose while at the same time employment was more difficult to find. Journeymen in the textile trades, for example, were notoriously vulnerable. Since others would always, when the pinch came, put food ahead of clothing in their domestic budgets, demand for the products of the textile industry, and hence employment within it, fell back just when it was

---

[22] It is often held that prices of other foodstuffs tended to move in unison with that of wheat, leaving no means of escape for most purchasers. Lee recently tested this point: 'As a first step it needs to be shown that wheat prices are a good proxy for food prices in general. Numerous statistical analyses were carried out relating short-run variations in wheat prices to those of other grains, livestock, animal products such as eggs and milk, and a general food price index, using the annual price series for the period 1450 to 1650 published by Bowden. There were no systematic leads or lags, and changes in the series were closely associated with one another.' Wrigley and Schofield, *Population History of England*, p. 357. It is to be noted, however, that Bowden himself came to a rather different conclusion. Bowden, 'Agricultural prices', p. 629.

most vital to those who made a living from it. In extreme cases, the lack of purchasing power on the part of those most in need might be so acute that famine conditions might prevail with few indications in price behaviour that a grave situation existed.[23] The scale and nature of transfer payments to those in poverty, and the sensitivity of any such payments to prevailing circumstances, played a significant part both in determining how successfully exposed members of the community could weather the storm, and in deciding how much prices rose. In bad times, high food prices may paradoxically be a favourable sign rather than the reverse. They are evidence that additional purchasing power has been placed in the pockets of those in greatest need. It is likely that Davenant's law only applies where the worst-off members of the community can tap a wider pool of resources than that of the family.

This point was well understood by some observers in the past. Thomas Tooke, who had an exceptional familiarity with the operation of European grain markets in the late eighteenth and early nineteenth centuries, wrote 'supposing a given deficiency, the degree in which the money price may rise, will depend upon the pecuniary means of the lowest classes of the community'. Where these were very limited, as in Ireland and much of the continent, Tooke argued, 'the rise in price may not be very considerably beyond the defect of quantity', but where, as in France by the intervention of the government or in England by the operation of the poor laws, great efforts were made to alleviate the miseries of the bulk of the population, backed by public funds, 'the price would rise very considerably beyond the ratio of the deficiency'. In the former case it was likely, he argued, that some would perish and many suffer disease and malnutrition; in the latter, the effect was to 'limit the consumption and to apportion the privations resulting from scarcity over a larger part of the population; thus diminishing the

[23] Sen notes that in the province of Wollo in Ethiopia during the Ethiopian famine of 1973 there were many deaths from famine even though the price of grain did not rise in that year in the main market at Dessie. Wollo peasants had no income source which could enable them to enter the market as effective purchasers. He also showed that large-scale mortality occurred during the Bengal famine in 1943 when the overall supply of rice available was little different from that of the years immediately preceding, principally because of the acute inflation in the wartime economy of Bengal which caused a very sharp increase in prices while wage labour rates increased only modestly. Thus, depending on local circumstances, it is possible for there to be heavy mortality from starvation without any shortfall in normal supply or, equally, for the level of supply to fall far below normal and to produce widespread deaths without leaving any trace in price statistics. Sen, *Poverty and Famines*, pp. 63–78, 94–6, 101–2. It may be of interest to note that Malthus noticed and analysed the 'Wollo' phenomenon in a modified form, contrasting conditions in the Swedish province of Värmland with those in England, and drawing the same inference as Sen. Malthus, *The High Price of Provisions*, pp. 2–3, 18–20.

severity of the pressure upon the lowest class, and preventing or tending to prevent any part of it from perishing, as it might otherwise do, from actual want of food'.[24]

Tooke's remarks represent a gloss upon a very familiar theme. The sufferings induced by famine were not spread uniformly in pre-industrial societies. Just as in animal societies one of the functions of the hierarchical ordering of individuals appears to be the identification of those who will die first when food runs short in order to safeguard the health of those higher up the pecking order,[25] so the market may perform a similar role in a monetised economy. Where little was done to assist those most exposed, more died but the spasm was reflected only in a muted form in the record of prices. Where transfer payments were substantial and well suited to need, fewer if any died but prices rose with greater apparent savagery.

The consistency with which Davenant's formula 'saves the phenomena' in pre-industrial European economies deserves much more extensive investigation than it has so far received. In pursuing the topic, it is important to be aware of the potential significance of the distinction between gross and net yield when analysing harvest information. An example may be taken from the writings of Slicher van Bath. He was in general very much alive to the importance of the distinction between gross and net yield, and provided a particularly cogent exposition of the topic in the opening section of his *Agrarian History of Western Europe*.[26] When, however, he later turned to a discussion of Davenant's formula and those of Jevons and Bouniatian, he used an illustration which demonstrates how easily confusion can arise. The top two panels of table 7.3 reproduce the material that Slicher van Bath published. Drawing on Farmer's work on the Winchester pipe rolls, he set out the relative size of the wheat and barley crops and their prices in 1315 and 1316, which as a pair were perhaps the worst famine years in English medieval experience. In the second panel he showed the expected prices using Jevons's formula. He noted that the data were of dubious accuracy but made no comment on the poor fit between the actual price and the expected price in three of the four cases, other than to suggest that prices were kept down in 1315 by imports and by wheat stored up in previous years, and to make

---

[24] Tooke, *History of Prices*, 1, pp. 13–14.
[25] Wynne-Edwards has written much on this and related themes. See, e.g. his recent essay, Wynne-Edwards, 'Populations of red grouse'. For an illuminating study of a similar process at work in human populations, see Derouet, 'Une démographie différentielle'.
[26] Slicher van Bath, *Agrarian History*, p. 18–23.

Table 7.3 *An illustration of the significance of the distinction between gross and net yields in calculating an implied price*

	Size of wheat crop (1.00 = average)	Price (1.00 = average)	Size of barley crop (1.00 = average)	Price (1.00 = average)
Farmer's data from the Winchester pipe rolls				
1315	0.57	2.40	0.59	2.33
1316	0.62	2.37	0.77	2.13
Expected prices using Jevons's formula				
1315	0.57	4.07	0.59	3.73
1316	0.62	3.30	0.77	1.95
Expected prices after conversion to gross yield basis and using Jevons's formula (Bouniatian's formula)				
1315	0.68	2.63 (2.50)	0.71	2.37 (2.25)
1316	0.72	2.29 (2.17)	0.84	1.59 (1.50)

Note: For details of conversion see text.
Source: For top two panels, Slicher van Bath, *Agrarian History*, p. 120.

reference to a possible switch in demand to the cheaper grain, barley in 1316.[27]

It appears to have escaped Slicher van Bath's notice, however, that Farmer's estimates were of *net* yield.[28] The information Farmer gave was not sufficient to convert the data back to the original gross yields, but if we assume that in an average year the gross yield exceeded the net in the ratio 4 : 3 for wheat and 3.5 : 2.5 for barley (yield ratios for barley were normally lower), then the ratio of each year's crop to the average level can be recalculated on a gross yield basis and the expected price re-estimated. If this is done, as may be seen in the bottom panel of table 7.3, the expected price and the actual price agree quite well in both years for wheat and in 1315 for barley, while the discrepancy for barley in 1316 may plausibly be attributed to the shift of demand in the second year to the cheaper grain as Slicher van Bath suggested. This evidence also strongly underwrites Tooke's view, implicit in the application of the formula to gross yields, that the total amount of money spent on grain in a year of harvest disaster could not massively exceed that of an average year unless some source were available other than their own pockets to assist the poor in their plight. For example, assuming that the top panel of table 7.3 roughly reflects the net quantity of grain available for consumption and the price paid for it, multiplying the two together gives an estimate of the total expenditure on grain. In the case of wheat, this suggests that in 1315 and 1316 total expenditure was 37 and 47 per cent above normal respectively, and in the case of barley 37 and 64 per cent – substantial, but not sensational, increases.

Intriguing as such particular illustrations are, however, only the collection of much more empirical data can clarify the question of the degree of applicability of any model of price behaviour in times of grain surplus or shortage in the past. Table 7.2 was designed to enable one extreme, though not necessarily unlikely, possibility to be examined. At the other extreme, if the amount set aside for seed, instead of being a fixed quantity, could be shown to have been reduced in proportion to the deficiency or excess of the previous harvest, the assumptions leading to the construction of table 7.2 would be proved to be unjustified and the argument based upon it would be nugatory.[29] In

---

[27] Farmer, 'Grain price movements'. Slicher van Bath, *Agrarian History*, p. 120.

[28] Farmer's wheat yields were expressed as yield/seed ratios after deducting one unit for seed, 'as the resulting net yield gives a more accurate impression of the disposable harvest surplus'. Farmer, 'Grain price movements', p. 217.

[29] It may be of interest to note that Robert Loder appears to have sown a relatively constant quantity of seed per unit of area on his farm in the early seventeenth century. He expressed the area he sowed each year in 'lands' and it is clear that he regarded

connection with the pressures to reduce sowing rates for seed-corn, incidentally, it may be important to note that wheat was a winter-sown grain, but barley was spring-sown. Immediately after harvest, even if the harvest were bad, the temptation to skimp on seed usage must have been less strong than after a further five months had elapsed.

Pending the assemblage of fuller information about the pre-industrial past, it may be of interest to touch upon another implication of the Bouniatian formula which is of potential importance when price data are so much more abundant than yield data. To the extent that the formula succeeds in capturing the relationship of quantity and price, it can of course be used to calculate quantity from price as easily as the reverse, though, because prices were not affected solely by the scale of the previous harvest, the estimation of harvest variations from price data must be subject to substantial margins of error. If $y = 0.757/(x - 0.13)^2$ then $x = 0.13 + 0.757/y$. An example may illustrate the use to which the reverse formula can be put, and once more suggests the value of distinguishing gross and net yields. The year 1596 is commonly held to have been the worst harvest year of the early

them as of a fairly constant size. The following table shows the number of 'lands' of wheat sown over a period of nine years, the quantity harvested, the number of bushels of wheat produced per 'land', the yield/seed ratios and the quantity of seed sown per 'land' for the following year. There is no evidence here that a poor harvest tended to cause seed to be used more sparingly. Loder normally kept aside a part of his previous harvest to serve as seed, though occasionally he also bought in a little seed. He was, however, a farmer on a fairly large scale and not necessarily, therefore, typical of the majority of his contemporaries.

Year	No. of 'lands'	Production (bushels)	Production per 'land' (bushels)	Yield/seed ratio	Seed per 'land' sown for next harvest
1611	26.0	167	6.4	—	1.28
1612	23.5	238	10.1	7.9	1.41
1613	27.0	209	7.7	5.5	1.45
1614	20.0	381	19.1	13.1	1.43
1615	23.0	241	10.5	7.3	1.07
1616	20.5	444	21.7	20.2	1.19
1617	37.0	362	9.8	8.2	1.15
1618	62.0	942	15.2	13.3	1.08
1619	96.5	1054	15.2	14.1	—

Note: The yield/seed ratios given here are in general closely similar to those given by Fussell (table 3. p. xvii), except for 1616. Fussell calculated a figure of only 7.8 for that year because he appears to have mistaken the quantity of seed sown. Loder himself referred to the 1616 wheat harvest as 'a most marveylous yield' when the lord had made 'the cloudes to drope fatnes' (p. 110).
Source: Fussell (ed.), Robert Loder's Farm Accounts.

modern period, and indeed in the Exeter wheat price series, the price of wheat rose higher relative to its own twenty-five year moving average than in any other year (though 1556 runs it fairly close).[30] In 1596 wheat stood at 2.21 times its moving average. Where y is 2.21, x is 0.72, suggesting that the gross yield of wheat in that year was 72 per cent of its normal level. This is substantially below average, of course, but if the quantity of wheat available for human consumption had fallen by only a little over a quarter it is perhaps unlikely that it would have caused the degree of distress that occurred in the wake of the harvest of 1596. However, that the net figure of food available after providing for seed-corn may have fallen by a significantly larger fraction may be seen by consulting table 7.2: a gross yield of 72 per cent of an average yield of 10 bushels per acre, implies a net yield of only 63 per cent of normal on assumption (a), or 57 per cent of normal on assumption (b). It is interesting to note that these figures are not greatly dissimilar from the comparable estimates of harvest shortfall for wheat and barley on the Winchester estates in 1315 (57 and 59 per cent respectively).

Coping with risk

In order to examine various aspects of yield and price in the past, I have used figures relating to wheat and barley or more generally to corn as if all types of corn were essentially similar in their characteristics. In many contexts, this may be legitimate, but not in all. 'Corn' was not a uniform product. Wheat, rye, barley, and oats were not used for the same purposes, nor did their fluctuations in yield run in parallel to one another. Whereas wheat was chiefly used for bread in England, oats were principally fodder for horses in most parts of the country. If all grains were perfectly substitutable for one another, their predominant usage in an average year would not affect an argument couched in terms of 'corn' in a year of harvest failure. But if men always ate wheat or barley and horses always ate oats, then human nutrition would be unaffected by the availability of animal fodder and vice versa. Probably the former is a better paradigm than the latter. 'Trading down' into cheaper grains was a very frequent concomitant of hard times, but different types of grain were not completely interchangeable in use.

The lack of parallelism in harvest fluctuations in the yields of different grains is worthy of emphasis. A disastrous year for a winter-sown cereal, such as wheat, for example, might be a moderate

[30] It is important to note that the Exeter wheat price series rose exceptionally sharply in 1596 and in other English wheat price series it does not stand out quite so strikingly.

year for a spring-sown cereal, like barley, or vice versa. This may be seen either on the scale of the individual farm or on that of a whole country. The year 1619 was a good one for wheat on Robert Loder's farm. The yield/seed ratio was 14.1, 22 per cent above the average for the nine years 1612–20. Barley, in contrast, yielded only moderately well: its yield/seed ratio was 7.9, only 6 per cent above the average of the same nine years. And in 1616, an *annus mirabilis* for wheat, Loder's yield/seed ratio for that grain was 74 per cent above the average though the barley ratio was almost exactly at its average level.[31] On a national scale the contrasts could be just as striking. In France, for example, 1830 was a poor year for wheat but a very good year for barley; whereas in 1832, when there was a bumper wheat crop, barley yields were only a little above average. (Expressed as percentages of the average yields over the eleven years 1825–35, the wheat yield in 1830 was 85 when the figure for barley was 115, while in 1832 the two comparable figures were 126 and 108, when compared with the local eleven-year average.)[32] The varying fortunes of different cereals at harvest time is both of interest in itself, and has related implications. For example, inasmuch as the different types of cereal were interchangeable in use, an index of 'corn' yield based on the yield of only one cereal can be a misleading guide to the availability of grain.

As an illustration of the importance of bearing such points in mind, consider the argument advanced by Appleby in one of his most stimulating articles, concerning subsistence crises in England and France. He noted that in England in the 1690s there was no longer a close correlation between price movements in wheat and the cheaper cereals, whereas in France there was still a very strong relationship as exemplified by price movements in the *mercuriales* at Pontoise. The situation in England, he argued, betokened relative sufficiency of overall grain supply and freedom from starvation: that in France meant that the poor still stood at the end of the precipice. Further, he argued that a century earlier in the 1590s the English case was more like the French.[33]

There is clearly a danger in using price data from a single market as if it were typical of the whole of France. Assuming, however, that Appleby's thesis about comparative price movements is fundamentally correct, the patterns he observed may still have been due, at least in part, to other influences. It is striking how largely wheat dominated

---

[31] See note 29 above for yield/seed ratios for wheat 1612–19. The ratio in 1620 was 14.6. The barley ratios are taken from Fussell (ed.), *Robert Loder's Farm Accounts*, table 3, p. xvii.

[32] Mitchell, *European Historical Statistics*, tables D1 and D2.

[33] Appleby, 'Grain prices and subsistence crises'.

other grains in quantity terms in the Pontoise market. Dupâquier, Lachiver, and Meuvret published a large body of price data for seven markets, but information about the quantities sold only for Pontoise in the period 1752–61. For these years the quantities of wheat, maslin, rye, barley, and oats are detailed separately. Over the ten years as a whole wheat formed 64 per cent of the total of *setiers* sold.[34]

Davenant's estimates suggest a very different position in England at the end of the seventeenth century. In a year of 'moderate plenty' he supposed that the national net produce (excluding seed-corn), expressed in millions of bushels, was wheat 14, rye 10, barley 27, and oats 16.[35] The quantity produced and the quantity placed on the market may have been widely different, of course, but it is at least highly likely that, on the assumption of some interchangeability of use between the cereals, there would be a tighter correlation between wheat and other grain prices at Pontoise than in England. Shortages or gluts of wheat at Pontoise must have influenced the demand for other grains to a degree not found where wheat was much less dominant. Nor is it clear that the situation in England in the 1590s was so greatly different from that a century later. It is true that in 1596 and 1597, when wheat was so dear, the prices of other grains were also very high. But grain prices did not move in unison in all dear years. In 1600, for example, wheat was not expensive. Expressed as an indexed figure based on a twenty-five year centred moving average, wheat stood at exactly 100, but barley and oats were 137 and 154 respectively. On the other hand, in 1608 the comparable figures were 136, 83, and 108 (again relating each price in 1608 to the long-term average for that year). For comparison, the ratios in 1596 were 173, 172, and 196.[36] Here once more there is scope for further analysis.

Risk spreading and price behaviour might also repay increased attention. For some communities and in some periods trade links limited the effects of poor local harvests by concatenating supplies over a large area, what might be called geographical risk spreading. Price movements would then be less at the mercy of local harvest fortunes. Similarly, temporal risk spreading took place in all communities to some extent since grain might be stored for quite long periods with only limited loss or deterioration where storage conditions were good. Indeed, just as a large enough dam on a river is capable of dampening out seasonal and annual fluctuations in the volume of flow downstream from the dam, so a sufficiently large and efficient grain storage

---

[34] Dupâquier *et al.*, *Mercuriales du pays de France*, pp. 230–1.
[35] Davenant, *Essay upon the Balance of Trade*, p. 71.
[36] Bowden, 'Statistical appendix', pp. 819–20.

system may in principle largely offset the effects of a poor harvest or even of a run of poor seasons. Such effects were beneficial to the consumer, but could create difficulties for the small producer since they tended to exaggerate the fluctuations in his income by dampening price rises in years of poor harvest and moderating price falls when harvests were plentiful.

Contemporaries were alive to the issue as it might affect the impoverished consumer. Davenant, for example, was concerned about the small margin upon which England operated in his day. He thought that following a good harvest only five months' stock remained when the new harvest was gathered in, and in an 'indifferent' year four months' stock. This he contrasted unfavourably with the prudence of the Dutch in storing grain on a much larger scale so that 'those dearths which in their turn have afflicted most other countries, fall but lightly on their common people'. In this way the Dutch were able to sell 'us our own corn dear, which they had bought cheap'.[37] Food can, of course, be 'stored' by other means than in a granary. Animals kept for meat, for example, form a living foodstore which may be drawn upon in hard times, and in this regard England was probably relatively well provided.

To round off the discussion of gross and net yields in relation to harvest fluctuations, two further points may be mentioned. First, it may be helpful to make explicit something which was implicit in earlier discussion. In a country which consisted exclusively of small husbandmen, each farming an area sufficient only to meet the needs of a single family in an average year, it would be impossible in a bad year to devote an unchanged quantity of corn to usage as seed, animal 'fuel' and family consumption since these between them would have comprised all types of grain usage in an average year. Since the total supply would be smaller, one or more of the usual forms of consumption would also have to be reduced. At the other extreme, where all farmers operated on a large scale and normally disposed of the bulk of their crop in the market, it would have been a relatively straightforward matter to keep the farmer's reservation of corn at a constant level in a bad year, especially as price movements were likely to be such as to enable him to enjoy an increased income even though the quantity reserved for seed and other uses on the farm was unchanged. 'Pure' cases of either extreme seldom if ever arose over wide regions of a country as a whole, but the position of individual countries varied considerably on the spectrum of possibilities. The

[37] Davenant, *Essay upon the Balance of Trade*, p. 84.

assumption of an unchanging absolute margin between gross and net yields is probably more accurate for pre-industrial England than for other countries because of the unusual character of the farming units, and especially so in the later centuries of the early modern period. Large farms were more common; small, 'family' peasant holdings less widespread than elsewhere.

Secondly, inasmuch as the quantity of grain used for seed per acre cultivated appears to have changed very little between the Middle Ages and the nineteenth century, but the yield per acre increased from less than ten to more than twenty bushels per acre for wheat, with similar gains for other cereals, the distinction between gross and net yield became less and less significant to most of the issues discussed above. At a yield of, say, eight bushels per acre the proportion of the harvest needed for seed in the case of wheat was 31 per cent; at a yield of, say twenty-five bushels per acre it was only 10 per cent. Over time, therefore, it ceased to matter greatly for most purposes which measure was employed when studying short-term changes in the relationship of quantity and price.

The significance of secular trends in yields

In other contexts, however, the distinction remains important even though, indeed because, the percentage gap between gross and net yields grew steadily less with the elapse of time and the rise in output per acre. Consider, for example, a comment made by Hoskins when reviewing the whole period covered by his survey of harvest fluctuations from 1480 to 1759. He noted that gross yield ratios appeared to have doubled between 1500 and 1650 and that population had also doubled over the same period, and added, 'Thus the remarkable advance in yields in this period brought no real improvement in basic food supplies for the mass of the population.' Yet what counted in this connection was not what happened to *gross* yields but what happened to *net* yields. If, therefore, it were the case that gross yield ratios had risen from four to eight, or by 100 per cent, as he claimed, the net figure must have risen by 133 per cent, that is from three to seven.[38]

This point has a wider relevance. Suppose that the average yield of corn per acre in England was ten bushels in 1500 and had reached twenty-two bushels by 1800, and assume that there was no change in seed usage per acre. It would follow that net corn output must rise more sharply than gross. On assumption (a) of table 7.2, net yield

---

[38] Hoskins, 'Harvest fluctuations 1620–1759', pp. 17, 25, 27.

would increase from 7.5 to 19.5 bushels. The gross yield rises by 120 per cent, the net by 160 per cent (on assumption (b) the comparable net figure is 185 per cent). It is probable that other changes between 1500 and 1800 may have further increased the differences between the percentage increases in gross and what might be termed effective net yield. Some grain is always lost between harvest and consumption because of spoilage and the depredations of rodents, insects and birds. More effective storage, say in brick or stone-built barns, would tend to reduce this loss, which may be regarded as a percentage toll rather than a fixed quantity per acre as with seed-corn. Suppose that loss under this head fell from 15 to 10 per cent between 1500 and 1800, then on assumption (a) of table 7.2, the final net supply of corn per acre would rise from 6.0 to 17.3 bushels, or by 188 per cent (on assumption (b) by 226 per cent).

Viewed in this way, it is considerably less difficult to account for the success of English agriculture in keeping pace with English population growth over the early modern period. Between 1550 and 1820 the population of England roughly quadrupled, while home agriculture throughout supplied the overwhelming bulk of the corn consumed.[39] If attention is focussed on gross yields the fact that population quadrupled while yields per acre rose by 120 per cent would suggest that about 80 per cent more land must have been devoted to growing corn at the end of the period compared with its start at constant consumption per head. If, on the other hand, net yield is taken as the more relevant yardstick, and if net yields did indeed rise by 188 per cent over the three centuries, then the additional land needed to cater for the increase in population is far more modest. An increase of the acreage of corn of 39 per cent will suffice. Even ignoring the supposition about reduced spoilage, an increase in cereal acreage of 54 per cent would permit a constant level of grain consumption per head to be maintained (or 23 and 40 per cent respectively under assumption (b) of table 7.2). In the light of these considerations it is reasonable to suppose that a relatively modest increase in the cultivated area may have sufficed to meet the needs of the greatly enlarged population.

A further implication of any substantial rise in corn yields is that the significance of the annual fluctuations in yield is reduced. If it is safe to assume that the variations in weather and in the incidence of pests and diseases which affect crops are such as to produce the same *percentage* variations in *gross* yield on average whatever the *absolute* average level of yield, then, in contrast, the effect of weather and pests on *net* yield

[39] Wrigley and Schofield, *Population History of England*, table 7.8, pp. 208–9.

will not be independent of the absolute level of yield. Suppose, for example, that the mean annual percentage variation in gross yield is a constant 15 per cent irrespective of the absolute level of average yields, then with average yields at 10 bushels per acre the mean annual percentage variation in net yield will be 20 per cent on assumption (a) of table 7.2 (where gross yield is ten bushels, net yield is 7.5 bushels, and $100 \times (1.5/7.5) = 20$). If average gross yield were to rise to twenty-two bushels per acre, however, the mean annual percentage variation in net yield would fall to 17 per cent ($100 \times (3.3/19.5) = 16.9$). On assumption (b), the comparable mean annual percentage variations in net yield are 23 and 18 per cent respectively. Inasmuch as short-term fluctuations in real wages in pre-industrial economies were principally a function of short-term movements in food prices and above all in the price of corn, this would mean that, *ceteris paribus*, living standards in a regime of low yields per acre would be inherently more unstable than where yields were higher. An economy which enjoyed high yields per acre would thus be in a better posture to meet the inevitable random shocks of harvest variability without as great a degree of disruption as would attend an economy which also had to cope with the effects of low yield per acre.[40]

Declining marginal returns

Another instance of the importance of distinguishing between gross and net yields may be found in considering the question of the effect of declining marginal returns to labour. An illustration is given in table 7.4. When ten men are engaged in working the 100-acre plot, it yields on average 1,000 bushels and the presence of the tenth man adds an amount equal to the average productivity of the group as a whole, or 100 bushels. At this level of activity average and marginal productivity are equal. If, however, an eleventh man is added to the labour force the gross output is assumed to increase by only ninety bushels; a twelfth would add eighty bushels to gross output, and so on until the sixteenth man adds only forty bushels. Average labour productivity falls continuously and increasingly steeply because the marginal product associated with each additional worker is assumed to fall away very

[40] It may be significant that the mean percentage annual variations of the real wage from its own centred twenty-five year moving average declined fairly steadily from 10.5 per cent in 1550–74 to 5.8 in 1750–74 before rising slightly to between 6 and 7 per cent in the first half of the nineteenth century. The real wage index used in this calculation, that of Phelps Brown and Hopkins, is heavily influenced, of course, by short-term price fluctuations, and these in turn largely reflect the behaviour of cereal prices. Wrigley and Schofield, *Population History*, table 8.7, p. 317.

Table 7.4 Labour inputs and output per head

Area (acres)	Men employed	Gross output (bushels)	Net output (bushels) (a)	Net output (bushels) (b)	Last man contributes (bushels)	Average gross output per man (bushels)	Average net output per man (bushels) (a)	Average net output per man (bushels) (b)
100	10	1000	750	650	100	100	75	65
100	11	1090	840	740	90	99	76	67
100	12	1170	920	820	80	98	77	68
100	13	1240	990	890	70	96	76	68
100	14	1300	1050	950	60	93	75	68
100	15	1350	1100	1000	50	90	73	67
100	16	1390	1140	1040	40	87	71	65

Assumptions (a) and (b) as table 7.2.

rapidly. If we turn to net product, however, the picture is different. Once again, two cases are considered, embodying the same assumptions as were used in table 7.2. The absolute increment to net product as each additional man is employed is the same as the increment to gross product and there is also a declining marginal product per man, but for a time each additional man adds more to the total net product than the previously prevailing average and the average net output per man therefore rises. This holds true up to the point where twelve men are employed under assumption (a), or up to fourteen men under assumption (b). Thereafter, with net as with gross product, the employment of further men will depress the average, but even with as many as fourteen men employed the average net output per man is no lower than where ten men are employed under assumption (a); the same point is not reached until sixteen men are employed under assumption (b). Gross output per man, on the other hand, is 7 per cent lower with fourteen rather than ten men employed, and 13 per cent lower with sixteen men employed. Looked at in another way, the gross output of the 100-acre plot rises only 39 per cent when 60 per cent is added to the labour force, but a part of this product is never available for food and this part is assumed to be a fixed absolute quantity for any given acreage. As a result the net product rises by 52 per cent under assumption (a) or by 60 per cent under assumption (b).

If the exercise is carried out at lower gross yields per acre, the result is, of course, even more striking. For example, if gross output with ten men is 800 bushels, and the proportionate fall in marginal output per man is the same as in table 7.4 (i.e., the eleventh man produces seventy-two bushels, and the twelfth sixty-four and so on), then the average net product per man is only 2 per cent lower with sixteen rather than ten men under assumption (a) and 6 per cent higher under assumption (b).

The general point related to table 7.4 may be put quite simply. Any given acreage in cereal crops must first 'carry' a fixed quantity of output to be used for seed, or for seed and 'fuel', before it can begin to meet other demands for corn. The fixed element remains unaffected by the number of those at work on the land in question. As long as the addition to output achieved by introducing an extra man into the labour force exceeds the *net* productivity per man of the pre-existing labour force (their average output after the deduction of the fixed element), his presence will increase the effective (net) output per head. Similarly, a reduction of one man in an initial labour force will only increase the effective output per head if his presence contributes less than the average *net* productivity per man of the remaining workers.

The fact that, where production per acre is low, there will be a range of intensity of land use over which average output per man will be moving in opposite directions for net and gross figures may have relevance to the interpretation of long-term economic change in pre-industrial societies. For example, suppose that there was a period of falling population, such as took place during much of the fourteenth and fifteenth centuries in wide tracts of Europe, during which the land became less densely settled and less intensively worked. The gross output of cereal agriculture is assumed to have fallen, but less steeply than population. It is tempting to draw the conclusion from such data that living standards and levels of nutrition should improve whatever the other concomitants of a contracting population. But the conclusion may be over-hasty for, whereas average *gross* output would rise, average *net* output might fall. This would be the case where the marginal gross productivity of labour lost was greater than the average net productivity at that point.

In table 7.4, for example, under assumption (b) average gross output per man rises as the number of men employed falls from fourteen to ten but average net product falls. If the marginal gross product of the ninth and eighth man were the same as the tenth (100 bushels), a further fall of two men in the labour force would leave the average gross product per man unchanged but would result in a marked further contraction in average net product per man of 13 per cent as a constant deduction for seed and animals is spread amongst fewer workers. Overall, in moving from fourteen to eight men employed on the 100-acre plot, gross output per man would rise by 8 per cent but net output per man would fall by 17 per cent. No doubt this example is over-simplified to the point of caricature, but it suggests that care is necessary in drawing inferences about living standards from gross cereal output per head.[41]

---

[41] That this possibility is not entirely hypothetical is suggested by the recent work of Campbell on the manor of Martham in Norfolk. He gives details of seed sown and yields per acre in 1300–24 and 1400–24. Net yields of wheat (gross yields less seed) fell from 16.5 to 9.2 bushels, or by 44 per cent; of barley from 13.0 to 11.4 (− 12 per cent); of legumes from 7.5 to 4.0 (− 47 per cent); but net yield of oats rose from 13.0 to 16.4 bushels (+ 26 per cent). Oats in the earlier period had been used as a smother crop with very dense seeding: its gross yield changed only marginally but net yields rose more substantially. Martham was an untypical manor which had used very labour-intensive methods before the Black Death, and seeding levels fell in all four crops so that gross and net yields fell about equally (apart from oats). Moreover, Campbell does not provide sufficient detail about the use of labour and the balance of crops on the demesne to make it possible to determine whether net yields per man-year fell. Nevertheless, his data do suggest that lower population densities may not necessarily connote higher output per man. The number of man-days worked by *famuli* fell by 27 per cent over the century, which seems consonant with a fall in output per man-day given the scale of the fall in yield per acre and the fact that the frequency

Unless labour is so plentiful that marginal gross productivity is already low, falling populations may well be associated with *falling* net agricultural output per head even when gross figures are moving upwards. Indeed, to be provocative, one might imagine the possibility of a low-density, low-living standard equilibrium trap where a population, following a fall in numbers which had led indirectly to a reduced net cereal output per head, would experience a higher mortality or a reduced nuptiality, or both, sufficient to prevent a recovery in population. It is worth repeating in this connection that a lower gross output per acre will tend to increase the mean annual percentage variation in net yield, and therefore, inasmuch as mortality may be raised by the effects of reduced food supply in the wake of bad harvests, the fall in population may indirectly be a cause of higher mortality for this reason also.

Conclusion

Until well into the nineteenth century no other aspect of economic life was consistently of such great concern to private individuals and to public authorities alike as the scale of the last harvest and the prospects for the next year. Jointly, they regulated the fortunes of both agriculture and industry because of the way in which they affected the price of food and the demand for goods of all types. It follows, therefore, that achieving a juster and more exact appreciation of the relationship between the quantity of the harvest and the behaviour of prices must prove of great value in gaining a better understanding of the pre-industrial economy of England.

Speculation is a poor substitute for demonstrable knowledge, yet it may prove to be its forerunner. The bulk of this chapter has been speculative. When confronted by systematic empirical evidence, some of the hypotheses advanced may prove to be sustainable, but others may need to be refined or retracted. My concern, however, has not been with empirical testing so much as with showing how much uncertainty or imprecision still attaches to the treatment of a number of issues relating to the yield and price of corn in the past. In particular, I have laid stress on the importance of the distinction between gross and net yields to several topics: the relationship between yield and price, the variability of prices, the implications of good and bad harvests for the producer and the consumer, the interpretation of long-term trends

of fallowing doubled, but Campbell notes that the fall in casual, hired labour was even steeper than the decline in *famuli* labour. Campbell, 'Agricultural progress in medieval England', pp. 38–9 and table 5, p. 38.

in yields per acre, the returns to increasing and decreasing inputs of labour. Those with specialist knowledge may well be able to call into play evidence to clarify many of these issues forthwith. Other problems should yield to further research and reflection. The purpose of this chapter will have been well served if interest in this range of questions is heightened, for any attempt to understand pre-industrial economies must be strongly coloured by the way in which the functioning of its agriculture is apprehended, and the same is equally true of the transition from an agricultural to an industrial society.

Appendix: The relationship between the yield and price of grain

The purpose of this appendix is to examine a single, limited issue: whether it is safe to argue from the behaviour of grain prices as they varied from year to year to certain characteristics of the grain harvest. Grain price series exist in comparative abundance for pre-industrial Europe, and in some cases a particular series may extend over many decades, even over several centuries, with only minor gaps. In contrast, evidence about the physical yield of harvest is far less abundant. Where it exists it often refers only to a particular farm or manor, and may be frequently broken by substantial gaps. Furthermore, the information may be imprecise and its use is usually complicated by the idiosyncrasies of local measures of volume, area and weight. It is therefore tempting to attempt to make inferences about fluctuations in the size of the harvest from the behaviour of prices, since an abundant supply depresses the price of grain, while a shortage causes prices to rise.

It has often been observed that grain prices display a strong tendency to develop 'runs'; a number of successive years in which prices are either above or below the longer-term average. This characteristic of price behaviour is often supposed to be due to fluctuations in the physical yield of grain from year to year. Indeed, the connection is sometimes seen as so obvious as scarcely to warrant independent argument or empirical investigation. The reason why yields in turn should be high or low for several years in succession has also attracted some comment. Occasional runs might, of course, occur even though yields were randomly distributed through time because chance will produce them occasionally, just as several successive rolls of a die may result in the same number. But a systematic tendency for the bunching of good or bad years must have some other explanation. Environmental circumstances constitute a possible explanation but, though the weather can favour or damage the harvest and pests or diseases can each seriously affect yields, these are factors which are also broadly random in their impact.

A more promising line of attack has been to consider disturbances which, though peculiar to a particular year, might have a 'knock-on' effect, boosting or depressing yields in subsequent years. Hence the attractiveness of Hoskins' argument concerning the strategic import-ance of seed-corn.[42] If the harvest in any year is exceptionally poor due to a 'shock' of a type which may itself be random in its distribution, but the effect of a deficient supply of grain is to lure producers into eating or selling grain which in a normal year would be reserved for seed, then, even if environmental conditions revert to normal in the following year, the harvest will be below average and the price of grain will remain above the norm. This might arise either because a smaller acreage is planted or because grain is less thickly sown, or both. Conversely, presumably an unusually abundant harvest encourages a liberal use of seed with benign results to mirror the malign effects of a bad harvest. The mechanism involved seems *prima facie* less plausible as an explanation of runs of years with low prices than of runs of high prices, since there were conventional seeding densities which were unlikely to be exceeded however cheap grain might be (unless the grain was grown, as in the case of oats sometimes, as a 'smother' crop). A satisfactory explanation, however, needs to be symmetric in this respect since runs of low prices were as conspicuous and pronounced as runs of high prices.[43]

Equally attractive on general grounds, and less vulnerable in relation to the need for an explanation which implies symmetric price behaviour, is an explanation couched in terms of the carry-over of grain from one harvest year to the next. The price of grain is affected by the total supply on offer or in prospect, which at any given point in time will be influenced not only by the scale of the last harvest (and, in the later months of the harvest year, by the prospects of the next), but also by the quantity carried forward into the current year from its predecessor.[44] Here, then, there is also a mechanism that might transmit from one year to the next the price effects of good or bad harvests. Such effects might be felt not simply in the year following the 'shock', but over a more extended period.

The explanation via seed-corn usage implies that the annual output of grain, if known, would reveal runs to match those observed in prices. The explanation via the stock of corn carried forward from one

[42] See above, p. 244.
[43] See tables 7A.3 and 7A.7 below and the accompanying text.
[44] For Davenant's view of the scale of the carry-over from year to year see above, p. 256.

year to the next, on the other hand, would hold good even if output fluctuated randomly. The discovery that price data displayed runs while output data did not would, therefore, be fatal to the former explanation, but would be congenial to the latter. As a contribution to this debate it is instructive to consider price and production data for a period when both are available and then to examine the implications of any findings for earlier data referring to price alone.

France began to collect acreage and output data from as early as 1815.[45] It is therefore possible to discover whether from this date onwards there was any tendency for good or bad harvests to be followed by others of the same type. In table 7A.1 a very simple method has been used to throw light on the subject. The yield of wheat per hectare was expressed as a ratio to its own twenty-five year moving average. Thus a figure of 1.10 for a particular year would indicate that in that year output per hectare was 10 per cent above the twenty-five year moving average centred on the year in question. If a yield in one year tended to be associated with an above-average yield in the following year, then if all years in which, say, yields were between 10 and 15 per cent above average were treated as a set, it would be expected that a set of years consisting of all years next following the years in the first set would also have above-average yields. The nature of the underlying process supposedly at work suggests that the years in the second category on average would be closer to the moving mean than those in the first category. Thus, for example, the average score of years next following years in which the yield was 10 to 15 per cent above average might be, say, 5 per cent above average and so on.

Table 7A.1 shows that there was no clear tendency for the yield in any one year to be affected by the yield in the preceding year, suggesting an absence of serial autocorrelation. The ratios in the third column of table 7A.1 are usually close to 1.00 whether following good, bad or indifferent years. Yields appear to have been randomly distributed around the long-term moving average. Any aberrant values are probably due to the small numbers of years in each category. This point can be crudely tested by considering all below-average harvests *en bloc* (the twenty-seven cases where yields were less than 97 per cent of the long-term moving average) and comparing the value associated with them to those associated with above-average years (the twenty-nine cases where yields were more than 103 per cent of the average). The average yield in year $t + 1$ in the former case was 1.032; in the latter, 0.982. This suggests, if anything, a weak tendency for poor harvests to be followed by good ones, and vice versa, but it is

[45] Yield data are available for the UK only from 1884 onwards.

Table 7A.1 *France 1828–1900: harvest yields in successive years (wheat)*

Number of cases	Yield in year t	Average yield in year $t + 1$
10	<0.85	1.097
4	0.85–0.90	1.014
13	0.91–0.96	0.988
14	0.97–1.02	0.985
14	1.03–1.08	0.946
7	1.09–1.14	1.017
8	≥1.15	1.015
	mean 0.999	s.d. 0.124

Note: The figures in the second column show the harvest yield in any one year; those in the third column the yield in the following year. Both are expressed in relation to a twenty-five-year moving average of the yield. Thus in the period 1828–1900 there were ten instances of years when the harvest yield was less than 85 per cent of the twenty-five-year moving average for the years in question. In the ten years next following them the average yield was almost 10 per cent above average and so on. Note that the series contains two fewer cases than might be expected from the dates beginning and ending the series (seventy rather than seventy-two). This occurs because the series contained no yield figure for 1870.
Source: Annuaire Statistique de la France.

probable that the apparent pattern arises only because of the relatively small number of cases involved. A more searching and systematic test of the same point is to test the extent of the correlation between each value in the series t and its successor $t + 1$. The French yield data enable seventy paired observations to be made. The correlation coefficient $r = 0.185$. This is not a significant level and it would be unsafe to assume that the series was other than random.[46]

The same issue can be tested by another simple method. Assume once more that the yields in successive years are unrelated. If in year t the yield were above average, in year $t + 1$ there would be an equal chance that the yield would again be above average or that it would be below average: if the latter, a run of one year would result; if the former, a run of two or more years would have been established. By parallel reasoning, this run would have an equal chance of extending from two to three years or of ending at two, and so on. Thus, a half of all runs would be one year in length, a quarter two years in length, an eighth three years in length, and so on. In table 7A.2, using the same

---

[46] Bartlett, 'Autocorrelated time series'. The 95 per cent confidence interval would require a reading of 0.239 or greater.

Table 7A.2 *France 1828–1900: the frequency
of runs of above- or below-average yields*

Length of run in years	Number of runs	'Expected' number of runs
1	17	16.5
2	7	8.3
3	5	4.1
4	2	2.1
5	0	1.0
6	1	0.5
7	1	0.3
	33	

Note: See text for derivation of 'expected'
totals
Source: Annuaire Statistique de la France.

data as for table 7A.1, the frequency of runs of varying length in nineteenth-century French wheat yields is set out together with the 'expected' figure given the total number of runs. It is clear at a glance that this test, too, strongly suggests that yields in successive years were not related. The point can be established more formally. A one-sample runs test shows that it is highly probable that the sequence of above- and below-average yields is random.[47]

Price data for the same period, however, tell a different story. In table 7A.3 the same technique has been used as that employed for table 7A.1. The tabulation can either be carried out with the raw French data, or after the price ratios have been converted into yield ratios using the formula of Bouniatian.[48] Both are given in the table. The former produces a less symmetrical pattern than the latter because prices rise proportionately much higher in relation to the long-term moving average in years of low yield than they fall in bumper years.

In studying table 7A.3 it should be remembered that cases which are found at the head of the prices section will be found at the foot of the implied yield section and vice versa. This happens because Bounia-

---

[47] The number of runs is only slightly smaller than the 'expected' figure (33 and 34.4), and $z = 0.3535$. With a one-tailed test $p = 0.36$ and it would clearly be unwise to reject the assumption of randomness. The way in which above- and below-average yields are defined in relation to a moving average might in certain circumstances tend to increase the length of runs. This underscores the strength of the evidence afforded by the test.   [48] See above, p. 252.

Table 7A.3 *France 1828–1900: wheat price ratios and implied yields in successive years*

Price ratio			Implied yields		
Number of cases	Price ratio in year t	Average price ratio in year t + 1	Number of cases	Yield in year t	Average yield in year t + 1
5	<0.75	0.750	2	<0.85	0.955
9	0.75–0.84	0.870	6	0.85–0.90	0.983
16	0.85–0.94	0.962	14	0.91–0.96	0.971
15	0.95–1.04	1.009	24	0.97–1.02	1.004
12	1.05–1.14	1.145	13	1.03–1.08	1.020
5	1.15–1.24	1.033	9	1.09–1.14	1.087
5	1.25–1.34	1.031	2	⩾1.15	1.157
3	⩾1.35	1.185			
	mean 1.000	s.d. 0.179		mean 1.010	s.d. 0.076

Note: Bouniatian's formula by which the implied yield is derived from price data is given above, p. 252. The price ratios refer to harvest years (August–July). They were derived from twenty-five year moving averages of prices in the manner described in the notes to table 7A.1.

Source: Labrousee *et al.*, *Le prix du froment*, pp. 13–14.

tian's formula converts high prices into low implied yields and low prices into high implied yields.

The general implication of table 7A.3 is clear. Allowing for the effect of small numbers in obscuring underlying patterns, it is still evident that years of high prices tended to be followed by similar years. Similarly, low prices in one year were often succeeded by further low prices. There was a drift back towards the mean, of course, but the overall association is pronounced. This effect is, of course, transmitted through to implied yields and they therefore display the same pattern.[49] It is worth noting that the implied yields tend to 'bunch' more closely around the mean than the 'true' yields (table 7A.1), though spanning the same range. This is chiefly because the variability of wheat prices declined sharply in France after the mid century, presumably in large measure because of transport improvements. The standard deviation of physical yields actually rose slightly between 1829–59 (0.119) and 1860–1900 (0.126), but fell relatively sharply for implied yields (from 0.093 to 0.059). In the first half of the period, therefore, the variability of the two series was not greatly dissimilar. As might be expected, given the pattern visible in table 7A.3, price data also produce runs of high and low prices and implied yields which suggest that one year influences the next. In table 7A.4, and in subsequent tables, the runs in implied yields are set out. Using price data would result in a substantially similar pattern but it is convenient to concentrate on the implied yield material because the unequal distribution of prices around the long-term average means that runs of below-average prices are more common than runs of above-average prices (in table 7A.3, for example, there are thirty cases where the price ratio is below 0.95, but only twenty-five where the ratio is above 1.05).

It is immediately obvious from table 7A.4 that one-year runs are more rare than would be expected if the scale of each successive harvest were independent of its predecessor, and that long runs occurred more often than would be expected on this assumption.[50] French nineteenth-century price and yield data, therefore, leave no doubt that patterns may exist in the former which could be taken as suggesting that successive harvests were not independent events, even though there is no matching pattern in the yields themselves.

At this point it is natural to seek to discover whether English wheat

---

[49] The correlation coefficient between implied yields at t and $t + 1$ was 0.551, well above a significant level (0.237).

[50] A one-sample runs test gives $z = 2.7759$. With a one-tailed test $p = 0.0028$. It is therefore highly improbable that the pattern of the 'runs' occurred because of random effects.

Table 7A.4 *France 1828–1900: the frequency of runs of above- or below-average implied yields (wheat)*

Length of run in years	Number of runs	'Expected' number of runs
1	3	10.0
2	5	5.0
3	4	2.5
4	3	1.3
5	1	0.6
6	4	0.3
	20	

Source: Labrousse *et al.*, *Le prix du froment*, pp. 13–14.

price series display the same characteristics as those observable in French nineteenth-century data. Table 7A.5 is based on the Exeter wheat price series.[51] It shows the patterns found in implied yields over a very long period of time, from 1328 to 1789, and in three sub-periods. The first and third of these sub-periods were times of near stability in prices, but in the second sub-period there was a long-sustained rise in wheat prices, which went up more than fivefold during the 140 years in question.

If the overall English pattern is compared with that of nineteenth-century France (table 7A.3), there is a striking parallelism in the readings in the $t + 1$ column in the two cases. Extreme deviations from the average were substantially more common in England than in France, but within each yield category at time t the response in the following year was closely similar. It is easy to appreciate how a single exceptional harvest, producing unusually high or low prices, might produce a run of prices above or below the average.

In the first and last sub-periods, when there was little long-term change in the price level, the patterns in the $t + 1$ year are similar to each other though in the later period there were proportionately far fewer years of extreme prices. In the middle period the pattern is more confused. High implied yields were followed by other 'good' years as at other times, but low yields produced an irregular result. Implied yields only slightly below average appeared to have a more marked

[51] Mitchell and Deane, *British Historical Statistics*, chapter 16, table 9.

Table 7A.5 *England (Exeter prices): implied yields of wheat in successive years*

Yield year t	1328–1519 (1)	1328–1519 (2)	1520–1659 (1)	1520–1659 (2)	1660–1789 (1)	1660–1789 (2)	1328–1789 (1)	1328–1789 (2)
<0.85	11	0.912	7	1.020	6	0.928	24	0.948
0.85–0.90	16	0.995	11	1.041	8	0.975	35	1.005
0.91–0.96	34	1.007	14	0.935	25	0.975	75	0.979
0.97–1.02	35	1.003	29	0.997	26	1.010	90	1.003
1.03–1.08	36	1.011	20	1.018	34	1.024	90	1.017
1.09–1.14	24	1.062	16	1.066	13	1.072	53	1.066
≥1.15	22	1.128	14	1.223	11	1.099	47	1.120
mean	1.023		1.022		1.017		1.021	
s.d.	0.109		0.113		0.092		0.106	

Note: (1) Number of cases.
(2) Average yield in year $t + 1$.
The data refer to harvest years running October–September. See also notes to table 7A.3.
Source: Mitchell and Deane, *British Historical Statistics*, chapter 16, table 9, pp. 484–7.

effect on succeeding years than 'worse' years. Very possibly the comparatively small number of years involved resulted in a deceptive outcome.[52] And it should be noted that the overall mean implied yield for the period was 1.022. This rather than 1.000 should be thought of as the standard by which to judge the average yield. Means greater than 1.000 are found generally with implied yields because the asymmetry of the price data from which they are derived is slightly over-compensated. Very low prices are found nearer to the mean than very high prices (table 7A.3), but although Bouniatian's conversion formula produces broadly 'correct' results, there is a tendency for the mean implied harvest size to be a little above unity.

The frequency of years of very high or low implied yields (which is of course, a reflection of price movements) is a matter of interest in its own right. The information set out in table 7A.6 is the same as that used in tables 7A.3 and 7A.5 but the distributions are re-expressed as percentages, and in the lower panel summary statistics are used covering only the two highest and two lowest categories to highlight gross changes over time. Table 7A.6 also contains additional French data. The nineteenth-century harvest year material has been split into two shorter periods, and calendar year data have been added covering both the nineteenth-century periods given for harvest year distributions and the preceding century.

In England there was no significant change in the percentage distributions before the last sub-period. The middle period was if anything slightly more given to extreme variations than the early period. Thereafter there was a very substantial reduction in extreme variations. Both the rising yield per acre and improved transport probably contributed to the new pattern after 1660.[53] Before then either these changes had yet to make a material difference, or they were offset by factors acting in the opposite sense; for example, the rapid population growth of the middle period may possibly have caused exceptional pressures on supply.

In France there was a marked contrast between the first and second halves of the nineteenth century. In the earlier period the percentage distribution of price variations was very similar to those in England before 1660, but after 1860 there was a radical reduction in extreme

---

[52] The correlation coefficients between values at t and $t + 1$ were as follows (number of observations are given in brackets); 1328–1519, 0.430 (178); 1520–1659, 0.330 (112); 1660–1789, 0.499 (124); 1328–1789, 0.413 (414). All are significant: the related 95 per cent confidence intervals which allowed the assumption of randomness to be rejected are respectively: 0.150, 0.189, 0.180 and 0.098.

[53] The effect of rising gross yields in reducing the variance of net yields is discussed above, pp. 257–9.

Table 7A.6 *Percentage distribution of implied wheat yields*

	England (Exeter prices: harvest year)				France (harvest year)		
Yield	1328–1519	1520–1659	1660–1789	1328–1789	1828–59	1860–1900	1828–1900
<0.85	6.2	6.3	4.9	5.8	6.5	0.0	2.9
0.85–0.90	9.0	9.9	6.5	8.5	9.7	7.9	8.6
0.91–0.96	19.1	12.6	20.3	18.1	22.6	18.4	20.0
0.97–1.02	19.7	26.1	21.1	21.7	25.8	42.1	34.3
1.03–1.08	20.2	18.0	27.6	21.7	9.7	23.7	18.6
1.09–1.14	13.5	14.4	10.6	12.8	19.4	7.9	12.9
≥1.15	12.4	12.6	8.9	11.3	6.5	0.0	2.9
	100	100	100	100	100	100	100
	n = 178	n = 111	n = 123	n = 414	n = 31	n = 38	n = 70

	France (calendar year)			
Yield	1738–1827	1828–59	1860–1900	1828–1900
<0.85	2.4	0.0	0.0	0.0
0.85–0.90	8.5	12.9	0.0	5.7
0.91–0.96	20.7	32.3	28.9	30.0
0.97–1.02	24.4	22.6	39.5	31.4
1.03–1.08	25.6	6.5	26.3	17.1
1.09–1.14	15.9	19.4	2.6	11.4
≥1.15	2.4	6.5	2.6	4.3
	n = 82	n = 31	n = 38	n = 70

Table 7A.6 (*continued*)

	England (Exeter prices: harvest year)				France (harvest year)		
Yield	1328–1519	1520–1659	1660–1789	1328–1789	1828–59	1860–1900	1828–1900
<0.91	15.2	16.2	11.4	14.3	16.2	7.9	11.5
≥1.09	25.9	27.0	19.5	24.1	25.9	7.9	15.8

	France (calendar year)			
Yield	1738–1827	1828–59	1860–1900	1828–1900
<0.91	10.9	12.9	0.0	5.7
≥1.09	18.3	25.9	5.2	15.7

Notes: See notes to table 7A.3 and table 7A.5.
Sources: France: Labrousse *et al.*, *Le prix du froment*, pp. 113–14. The calendar year data were taken from pp. 9–11.
England: Mitchell and Deane, *British Historical Statistics*, chapter 16, table 9, pp. 484–7.

variations, presumably in part a result of railway construction. Rising yields no doubt also played a part. They rose 41 per cent between 1828 and 1900, but the improvement was evenly spread throughout the century.[54]

Calendar year data are available for a much longer period for France. As might be expected, price variations are somewhat less marked for calendar than for harvest years in each period for which the two series are available. It is interesting to note that the calendar year series suggest that eighteenth-century price fluctuations were rather less violent than those in the early nineteenth century, and perhaps not greatly different from those for England at much the same period. The significance of international comparisons is, however, dubious. The English series is for a single market, whereas the French is based on data drawn from all parts of the country.[55] This must tend to reduce the variability of the French series. Moreover, France in any case includes wheat-growing areas with very different climatic regimes whereas such differences are less marked in England, and this also would tend to reduce *national*, though not necessarily *local*, variation in France.

We may turn finally to the pattern of runs in English implied yield data set out in table 7A.7. In general the pattern is similar to that found in nineteenth-century France (table 7A.4). There are always more long, and fewer short, runs than would be expected on the assumption that each successive annual figure was independent of its predecessor. Overall, the picture is both straightforward and clear cut. There are only about half as many one-year runs as expected, but two or three times as many five-year runs or longer. In the sub-periods there is more irregularity, perhaps associated with the relatively small number of cases involved. There is, however, some suggestion that the disparity between actual and expected was less in the first period than in the two subsequent ones. The average length of a 'run' overall was 2.60 years, and in the sub-periods 2.33, 2.83, and 2.89 respectively. The comparable French figure derived from the data in table 7A.4 is 3.30 years, while the figure to be expected if there were no tendency for the length of runs to be affected by anything other than chance is 2.00 years. It is interesting to note that runs above and below the twenty-five year average implied yields were equally common (sixty-six and sixty-seven respectively) and that they were of almost exactly the same average length (2.58 and 2.63 years respectively).

---

[54] The twenty-five year moving average of wheat yields measured in hectolitres per hectare rose from 11.85 in 1828 to 16.75 in 1900.

[55] Labrousse *et al.*, *Le prix du froment*, Introduction, gives details of the sources and methods used in constructing the French national series.

Table 7A.7 *England (Exeter prices): the frequency of runs of above- or below-average implied yields*

Length of run in years	1328–1519 (1)	(2)	1520-1659 (1)	(2)	1660–1789 (1)	(2)	1328–1789 (1)	(2)
1	26	33.0	5	14.5	8	19.0	39	66.5
2	14	16.5	9	7.3	11	9.5	34	33.3
3	14	8.3	9	3.6	8	4.8	31	16.6
4	6	4.1	2	1.8	4	2.4	12	8.3
5	2	2.1	2	0.9	3	1.2	7	4.2
6	4	1.0	0	0.5	3	0.6	7	2.1
7	0	0.5	2	0.2	1	0.3	3	1.0
	66		29		38		133	

Note: (1) Observed.
(2) 'Expected'.
Source: As table 7A.5.

The data of table 7A.7, like those of tables 7A.2 and 7A.4, can also be examined by using a one-sample runs test to establish how probable it is that the observed patterns arose from random influences. The z scores for the three successive sub-periods and for the entire period 1328–1789 were -1.7142, -2.8744, -3.4483 and -4.4105 respectively. With a one-tailed test the corresponding p values were 0.0436, 0.0021, 0.0003 and $< = 0.00003$. The p values are suggestive in that for the earliest period, 1328–1519, the null hypothesis can only just be rejected at the 5 per cent significance level, but in the two subsequent periods it is increasingly and ultimately extremely improbable that the runs were random. If the reason for the runs were to do with trenching upon seed-corn, one might have expected the effect to be most pronounced in medieval times and least in the period after 1660 when yields were much higher and supplies in general comparatively abundant. If, alternatively, the carry-over effect was the chief cause of the phenomenon, the pattern found is that to be expected. As storage capacity and effectiveness increased, and supply more commonly met or exceeded demand, the 'knock-on' effect of one year's good or bad harvest in the subsequent harvest years would become more pronounced. On this assumption, in medieval times each harvest year was, so to speak, largely self-contained, and the price of corn in one year would be comparatively little influenced by anything other than the harvest in that year. In the seventeenth and eighteenth centuries, in contrast, with a larger proportionate buffer of grain in store or accessible through better transport, harvest years were less isolated from one another.

The example of nineteenth-century France shows that runs may occur in wheat price data even though there are no runs in the physical yields per hectare; and comparison of the French data with earlier English data shows that patterns of price behaviour were closely similar. It does not follow, of course, that this similarity was due to the same cause or causes. Nor does it prove that physical yields in England were also free from serial autocorrelation. But it is clear that it is imprudent to assume that, because prices must be strongly affected by supply, they must reflect annual fluctuations in production, and that the existence of price runs necessarily implies parallel runs in yields. The French evidence suggests that fluctuations in the scale of the carry-over from one harvest year to the next is a more plausible mechanism for explaining the generation of price runs than an effect due to the consumption of seed-corn. It remains an open question, however, whether the same is true of medieval or early modern England.[56]

Explanations which involve seed-corn and those related to carry-over are not mutually exclusive. It is possible that a seed-corn effect existed as Hoskins supposed, but the example of France should caution us against accepting his argument *tout court*. Again, the general economic circumstances of the nineteenth century were so different from those of the fourteenth, or even the sixteenth, that to proceed in the manner adopted here begs many questions. My object is simply to re-open an issue of great importance in any pre-industrial society. Much remains to be done, however, before either the general or the particular relationships involved will have been fully teased out.

---

[56] It is worth stressing that French wheat yields were still quite low in the nineteenth century. The twenty-five-year moving average in 1828 was only 11.85 hectolitres per hectare, or 13.2 bushels per acre (using the following conversion factors: 1 hectare = 2.471 acres; 1 hectolitre = 2.75 bushels), a figure similar to that found in England 200 years earlier.

8

Family structure, demographic behaviour, and economic growth

ROGER SCHOFIELD

Historical demography, together with its parent discipline, has been through a long phase of technical abstraction.[1] While this has produced some notable advances both in method and in our understanding of population processes, I believe that the crucial question is still that with which the discipline began, namely to understand the parameters that determine the success or failure of populations to keep in balance with the economic space they inhabit. The process is a complex one, for population change is not only embedded in an economic context, but also itself modifies that context. The outcome of the mutual interaction between population and economy is obviously relevant to many of the issues considered in this volume: societies that outrun their economic space are more likely to experience dearth and famine than are those that can contrive to keep population and economy in balance. Moreover, since Malthus, it has been recognised that the nature of the mutual accommodation that is in practice reached between the processes of demographic and economic change in a specific society is influenced not only by the economic and political power-structures governing the ownership of wealth and the allocation of rewards to labour, but also by value systems affecting inter-personal relations within the family and the wider collectivity.[2]

In this chapter I shall re-examine the nature of the long-term

---

[1] For a discussion of these developments and their consequences, see Schofield and Coleman, 'Introduction'.

[2] Malthus' insight that demographic behaviour is contingent on certain key elements in the social structure has been well appreciated, less so his insistence that economic relationships are conditioned by institutionalised power relations. Since Malthus, many demographers and economists, in the excitement of pursuing tractable theoretical models of the widest possible generality, have lost sight of the importance of institutions as constituting a set of 'initial conditions' that determine the domains in which theories can be expected to apply.

accommodation between population and economy that was reached in England in the past and contrast it with other possible outcomes. In accounting for differences in the historical experiences of pre-industrial societies I shall suggest that value systems regulating inter-personal relationships, more specifically the degree to which they were dominated by 'familistic' principles, constitute a critical institutional variable that profoundly influences not only a society's demographic behaviour, but also its potentiality for economic growth. Since my argument is very much an essay in conjecture, I shall cut a lot of intellectual corners. I shall use concepts, such as 'traditional' and 'peasant' societies, without defining them, and I shall undoubtedly rehearse arguments that I owe to others which I have so completely assimilated that I may fail to acknowledge my debts in due measure.

The set of possible relationships between different aspects of demographic and economic change is a large and complex one. To help us see the wood for the trees, let us begin with a diagrammatic simplification that owes much to Malthus' conceptualisation of the issues involved.[3]

The Malthusian schema

Figure 8.1 summarises in schematic form a hypothetical set of relations between elements of population and economic change. The arrows indicate direction of influence; a positive sign indicates that the second element moves in the same direction as the first, a negative sign that it moves in the opposite direction. So far as the influence of demography on the economic context is concerned, the critical link is the one between 'population size' and 'food price'. It has a positive sign in deference to Malthus' view that agricultural production in long-settled societies will become increasingly subject to diminishing marginal returns to land and labour. Wage rates in a pre-industrial society, in so far as they are influenced by market forces, rather than remaining at customary levels, are likely to move in the opposite direction to population growth, and so are more likely to intensify, than to counteract, the effect of changing food prices on the standard of living. The same point might be made even more firmly with regard to endogenously determined changes in the demand for labour, since pre-industrial societies are usually not well-equipped to expand or

---

[3] The diagram is taken from Wrigley and Schofield, *Population History*, p. 465. It is a distillation of the contributions of many scholars, notably Malthus, *Essay*; Mackenroth, *Bevölkerungslehre*; and Lee, 'Population in pre-industrial England', 'Models of pre-industrial population dynamics'.

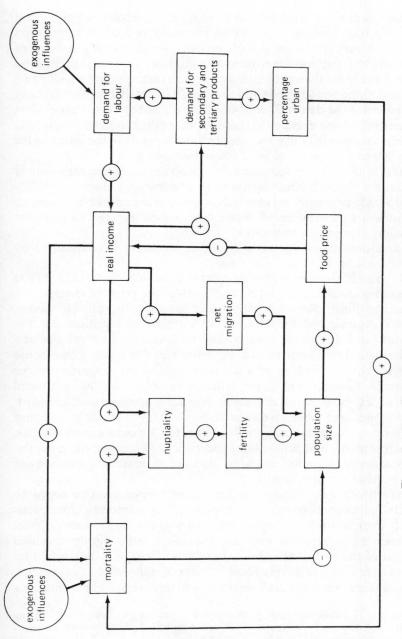

Figure 8.1 Population and economy: a positive feedback system

Note: net migration = immigration less emigration.

Source: Wrigley and Schofield, *Population History*, fig. 11.5, p. 465.

contract capital or land to match changes in labour supply. 'Real income', therefore, is likely to be inversely related to population growth. Moreover, since a high proportion (about 70 per cent) of pre-industrial expenditures normally goes on food, a shift in food prices has a more than proportionate impact on the aggregate effective demand for non-food goods and services.[4] Unless there is an offsetting movement in the demand for labour from distant markets ('exogenous influences'), those engaged in these sectors of the economy are likely to experience especially marked negative movements in the demand for their labour as a result of food price changes.

So far as the effect of economic change on demographic behaviour is concerned, figure 8.1 represents three possible outcomes.

1 Nuptiality may respond inversely to economic circumstances and so counteract movements in population growth through an effect on fertility (the preventive check).
2 Individuals may respond to changing economic circumstances by moving into, or out of, the area.
3 At the limit, the standard of living may fall so low that access to food becomes insufficient, and mortality rises (the positive check).

Each of these outcomes may occur within a 'traditional' demographic regime; but they have very different implications for the standard of living of the society, and for its ability to break out of a pre-industrial economic mould. By definition, the limiting case of the positive check involves immiseration and scant opportunity for economic development. The efficacy of migration as a control mechanism will depend critically on how far movement into, or out of, an economic area is perceived as a desirable, or even possible, response to changing material conditions. In general, I would expect that the more traditional and peasant-like the values of a society, the more the advantages of migration would be discounted, making it a strategy of last, rather than first, resort.

The efficacy of the preventive check clearly depends on the degree to which marriage behaviour is responsive to economic conditions, which in figure 8.1 are represented very generally in terms of real incomes. However, one can also imagine a more tightly specified version of the preventive check, in which marriage is dependent on access to one of a relatively fixed number of units of physical capital, such as a farmstead or a craft workshop. In this version of the check the

---

[4] Shammas, 'Food expenditure', p. 91; Komlos, 'Food Budget'; Lindert and Williamson, 'English workers' living standards', appendix table B1. Food accounts for 80 per cent of expenditure in Phelps Brown and Hopkins' model budgets, but the latter omit payments for accommodation expenses. 'Seven centuries of prices', table 1.

number of reproducing couples is kept fairly constant, since the rate of entry into the reproductive state is governed by the rate at which economic niches are vacated. The relation is represented in the figure by a positive link between mortality and nuptiality. Societies with this version of the preventive check are likely to be relatively undifferentiated economically, and to have value systems which stress the indivisibility of holdings. They will also need to have inheritance rules to determine who will succeed to a holding when more than one child survives, and develop rules for allocating the property of parents who die with no surviving children to the 'surplus' children of other families. Marriage is an important institution for adjusting the allocation of property between families, so family marriage strategies are likely to play an important role constraining the independence and life-chances of young adults. We might, therefore, expect peasant societies operating this version of the preventive check to have familistic ideologies, embracing a kin group wider than the immediate nuclear family.

Clearly any control mechanism that comes into play before the operation of the positive check is likely to alleviate the social and economic strains of accommodating population growth within the existing allocation of resources. But a mechanism, such as the preventive check, which operates through fertility, has the added advantage of enabling the age structure of the population to be considerably older than is the case when fertility is unconstrained. This reduces the dependency burden: typically 30–40 per cent of pre-industrial European populations were under age fifteen, compared to about 50 per cent when the full female reproductive age span is used.[5] *Ceteris paribus* an older age structure also increases both the propensity to save and the proportion of consumption devoted to non-food expenditures. Thus the presence or absence of the preventive check is likely to influence not only the level of economic welfare that a peasant society can attain, but also its ability to develop a significant amount of economic activity beyond subsistence agriculture.

In considering specific peasant economies and demographies,

---

[5] In the absence of contraception and significant levels of illegitimacy, fertility is effectively determined by nuptiality. With a pre-industrial European marriage pattern (i.e. an average age at marriage in the range 25–30, and 5–10 per cent of individuals never marrying) the gross reproduction ratio (GRR) typically lies in the range 2.00–3.00, whereas with a non-European nuptiality pattern the GRR usually exceeds 3.00. The effect of varying the level of nuptiality (and hence of GRR) on the age structure of a population can conveniently be appreciated by comparing the model age structures for stable populations tabulated in Coale and Demeny, *Regional Model Life Tables*.

therefore, it seems to me that a primary distinction that needs to be made is whether the social structure and value system together enable, or disable, the operation of a preventive check. Where entry into the reproductive state for women is universal, and its timing normatively linked to the attainment of physical maturity, the preventive check is disabled and the likelihood of immiseration enhanced. Moreover, in such societies marriage usually involves co-residence in the parental household, so that individuals spend their entire lives within a single multi-generational family economy (women changing families on marriage). This is not only likely to inhibit the development of cross-family social mechanisms of support for individuals, but it also builds in an incentive for early marriage and high fertility to ensure adequate economic support within the family in old age.[6]

Malthus attributed the contrast between the relative affluence of European societies of his day and the economic misery of Asian populations to the presence or absence of the preventive check.[7] European living standards do indeed appear to have been high relative to those of other pre-industrial societies, and historically the European pattern of nuptiality was unusual in that it entailed for both sexes relatively late, and far from universal, marriage. But within this broad distinctiveness of historical Europe, which sets it apart from most peasant societies, there were differences which have important implications for the operation of the preventive check and, more widely, for the nature of the interaction between demographic and economic processes.

One dimension which seems to me to be of crucial importance is the degree to which the prevailing ideology of social relations was predicated on familistic, or individualistic, principles. To be provocative, I will advance the view that familistic ideologies tend to evolve political and legal structures which favour stability, resisting change in the distribution of property, and constraining individual independence and mobility.[8] Thus familistic ideologies are likely to inhibit economic differentiation and the emergence of markets in labour and

[6] These relationships have been perceptively discussed by Lesthaeghe, 'Social control of human reproduction'; and Smith, 'Fertility, economy and household formation'.

[7] *Essay* (1826), vol. 2, pp. 125–8 (China and Japan), pp. 157–278 (various European countries), p. 315 (comparison between 'modern Europe' and 'the more uncivilised parts of the world').

[8] The work of four scholars in particular has alerted me to the ramifications of differences in family ideologies in the past: Lesthaeghe, 'Social control of human reproduction'; Smith, 'Fertility, economy and household formation', and 'Some issues concerning families'; Macfarlane, *Origins of English Individualism* and *Culture of Capitalism* and Todd, *Explanation of Ideology* and *Causes of Progress*.

goods. If, for the purposes of argument, we were to combine the familial and economic dimensions, we might construct a stylised contrast of ideal-types along the following lines.

At one extreme stands the relatively undifferentiated economy of family farms and rural crafts and services. Economic activity is largely a family affair in which labour is applied to capital in the family's control. Access to the means of production is mainly through inheritance (or by marriage to an heir); kinship plays an important role in marriage decisions and other property transactions; and support for the elderly is primarily a family responsibility. Consequently the population is relatively immobile.

At the other extreme stands the more differentiated pre-industrial economy in which a significant proportion of the population sells its labour to be applied to capital over which it has no control. Although some individuals may acquire land or capital through inheritance, inter-generational links are weak: most children are expected to leave home, accumulate their own wealth, choose their own marriage partners, and locate and occupy their own economic niche. Consequently the population is mobile. Since the generations no longer usually live in the same village children cannot easily care for their elderly parents. In pre-industrial conditions, therefore, an individualistic ideology needs to be complemented by a collective responsibility amongst neighbours for the support of the weak and elderly.

At the familistic extreme the preventive check is likely to follow the economic-niche model, with nuptiality being linked to the mortality of the previous generation. In this kind of society, as in the case of societies subject to the positive check, children are valuable for their labour power and as a source of support in old age. At the non-familistic end of the spectrum, the preventive check is likely to operate through the more diffuse mechanisms of markets in goods and labour, and so is open to exogenous, as well as endogenous, influences in the latter domain. For a substantial proportion of the population children have a negative, rather than a positive economic value; for support in old age and at difficult times their significant relations are not with their family, but with the community.

England in the past

England seems to me to have been a pre-industrial society that was located near the individualist–collectivist end of the preventive-check spectrum. First the findings of *The Population History of England* are

Growth
rate

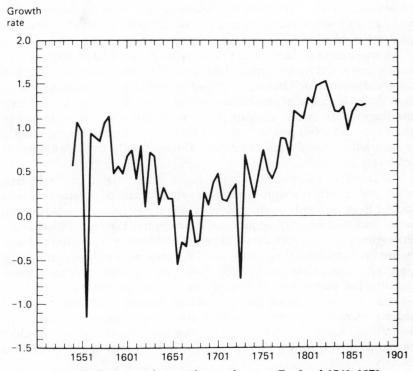

Figure 8.2 Compound annual growth rates, England 1541–1871

Note: each point represents the compound annual growth rate over the five-year period
beginning at the date indicated.
Source: Wrigley and Schofield, *Population History*, fig. 7.2, p. 211.

consistent with the operation of the various elements in the preventive
check cycle.

1 Population growth rates described a smooth cycle, oscillating
between zero and 1.5 per cent per annum (figure 8.2).

2 Rates of change in food prices were closely related to population
growth rates, as were rates of change in real wages (figure 8.3, figure
8.4).

3 Long-run changes in mortality were not systematically related to
changes in real wages (figure 8.5); but long-run changes in a crude
first-marriage rate were (figure 8.6).

Secondly, England was a highly differentiated economy by European standards. Already in the Middle Ages a considerable degree of
occupational specialisation can be found in rural villages; by 1700 it was

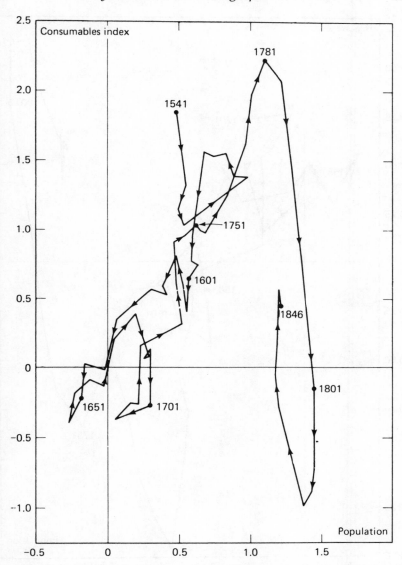

Figure 8.3 Annual rates of growth of population and of a basket of consumables price index

Note: growth rates for twenty-five year periods beginning at the date indicated.
Source: Wrigley and Schofield, *Population History*, fig. 10.2, p. 405.

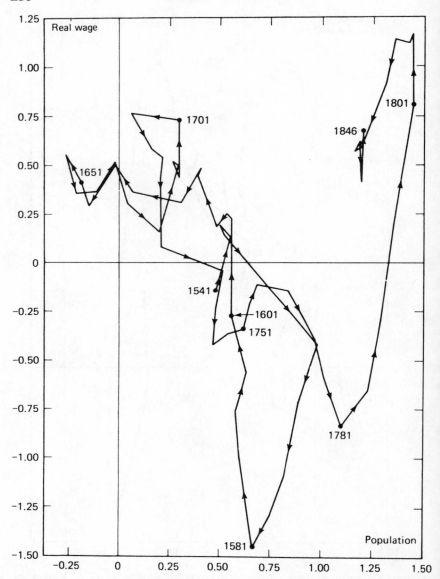

Figure 8.4 Annual rates of growth of population and of a real-wage index

Note: growth rates are for twenty-five year periods beginning at the date indicated.
Source: Wrigley and Schofield, *Population History*, fig. 10.4, p. 410.

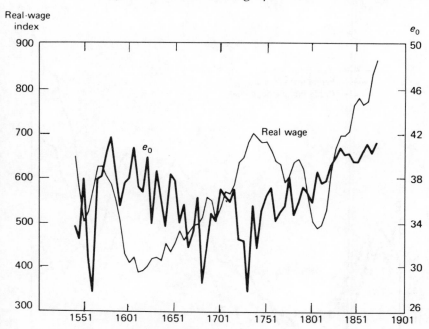

Figure 8.5 Quinquennial expectation of life at birth compared with an eleven-year moving average of a real-wage index

Note: the quinquennial e_0s and the eleven-year real-wage values are plotted for periods centring on the years shown.

Source: Wrigley and Schofield, *Population History*, fig. 10.5, p. 414.

more urbanised than the rest of north-west Europe taken as a whole, though less urban than the Netherlands.[9] Furthermore, proto-industry and an agricultural proletariat, two aspects of economic organisation usually associated with the seventeenth or eighteenth centuries, were already substantially present in England at a much earlier date. From the late fourteenth century several rural areas were involved in the household production of textiles that were ultimately sold in overseas markets;[10] and in the areas of midland England covered by the Hundred Rolls of 1279 at least 29 per cent of villein tenants, and 46 per cent of freehold tenants, held insufficient land to

[9] Occupational specialisation by the end of the fourteenth century is visible in the Poll Tax returns, especially those of 1381. Printed examples can be found for Essex in Oman, *The Great Revolt*, and for the West Riding in *Yorkshire Archaeological Journal*, 5–7 (1879–85). For the sixteenth century see Patten, 'Village and town', and 'Changing occupational structures'. For urbanisation, see Wrigley, 'Urban growth', pp. 148, 152.

[10] Carus-Wilson, 'Industrial revolution of the thirteenth century', 'Evidences of industrial growth'; Thirsk, 'Industries in the countryside'.

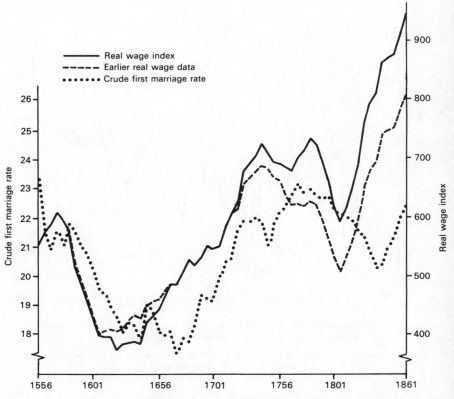

Figure 8.6 Real wage trends and crude first-marriage rates (both twenty-five
year moving averages centred on the dates shown)

Source: Wrigley and Schofield, *Population History*, preface to 1988 reprinted edition,
figure p. 1.

provide subsistence, implying the existence of markets for both labour
and food.[11] This is not to deny that England became more proletarianised and more 'proto-industrialised' over time; but to emphasise the
scale and, above all, the time-depth of the market for labour both in
agriculture and, organised on a household basis, in textile
production.[12]

[11] Kosminsky, *Studies in Agrarian History*, pp. 253–4.
[12] The literature on proletarianisation and on the growth of domestic production is
extensive. For a recent summary of developments in the early modern period,
emphasising their demographic consequences see Levine, *Reproducing Families*,
chapter 2–3.

Thirdly, in many important respects the ideology of English social relations was individualist–collectivist, rather than familist, in its orientation. Apart from the celebrated lack of any family rights in property, which gave descendants no rights until the death of the property holder, in practice a substantial proportion of English children left home in their teens to work in a succession of other households scattered over several communities.[13] In due course they chose their own spouses, and English registers significantly omit the long lists of relatives witnessing the marriage to be found in other countries.[14] After marriage they lived in economically and physically separate households, in three out of four cases in a village other than the one in which they had been brought up and in which their parents still resided.[15]

In such a mobile society the highly abbreviated nuclear family is clearly not the ideal institution for coping with life-cycle dependency. Instead, the task of supporting individuals in sickness and old age was devolved on the community collectively.[16] From 1598 an act of parliament required 'overseers of the poor' to be appointed each year in every parish in the country. The overseers, in turn, had a legal duty to identify and relieve those who were in need, and were empowered to levy sufficient sums for this purpose by way of local taxation.[17] Recent research has shown that in practice relief was given on a temporary basis to the sick, and to families with large numbers of children in years when food prices were high. Regular relief was given to the elderly poor, enabling them to continue to reside in their own homes.[18] Although the overseers could demand reimbursement from

---

[13] For property rights see Macfarlane, *Origins of English Individualism*, chapter 4, especially pp. 82–4; and Smith, 'Families and their property'. For mobility see Hallam, 'Some thirteenth-century censuses'; Schofield, 'Age-specific mobility'; Wall, 'Leaving home'; Kussmaul, *Servants in Husbandry*, chapter 4; Souden, 'Pre-industrial English local migration fields', pp. 286–98.

[14] For the relative freedom of choice of spouse in England, see Smith, 'Marriage processes'. For the relative freedom of women to move, take employment, and choose their spouses in medieval England, see Goldberg, 'Marriage, migration, servanthood'.

[15] For residential independence see Laslett and Wall, *Household and Family*, chapter 4–5. For inter-generational distances see Hallam, 'Some thirteenth-century censuses'; Schofield, 'Age-specific mobility'; Souden, 'Movers and stayers', pp. 1–22.

[16] For poor relief before the Reformation see Tierney, *Medieval Poor Law*. The subsequent development of a compulsory secular system of relief in England is summarised in Clay, *Economic Expansion*, vol. 2., chapter 7.

[17] The overseers comprised the two churchwardens and four substantial householders appointed by two justices of the peace: 39 Elizabeth I, c. 3. The ways in which local entitlement to relief affected the mobility of labour are discussed in Taylor, 'Impact of pauper settlement'.

[18] Wales, 'Poverty, poor relief'. Even under the 'harsh' New Poor Law of early Victorian

the children of those they relieved, the law was very clear that primary responsibility for providing relief lay with the parish. In case of default, suit to compel support could only be brought against the parish community; the law recognised no direct obligation between child and parent.[19]

If both economic development and demographic behaviour are powerfully mediated by social ideology, as I believe to be the case, then the peculiarities of the English position towards the non-familistic end of the spectrum may well have produced a rather different style of interaction between population and economy from what one might expect to have been the case in a more typical 'traditional' or 'peasant' society. In the remainder of this chapter I shall consider two topics, agricultural productivity and the operation of the preventive check, to exemplify the ways in which social ideology may influence demographic and economic outcomes.

Agricultural productivity

To keep the discussion within reasonable bounds, I shall only touch on a few points which emerge from a comparison of the long-run movements in food prices, real wages and population growth, as in figures 3 and 4. I had better begin by acknowledging a number of difficulties in drawing inferences from the series plotted on the graphs.

1 Arguments about agricultural productivity usually refer to arable crops, but the food prices plotted represent a composite basket of consumables, of which grains comprised 42.5 per cent.[20]

2 The prices are for wholesale quantities taken from a few institutional buyers. Individual consumers purchased foodstuffs in smaller quantities, often in processed form. Consequently, the prices shown on the figure are likely to exaggerate the scale of movement in retail prices over the long-run, which would have been dampened by a higher labour component which did not increase in price to the same extent.[21]

3 The nominal wage data used to calculate real wages have an even narrower evidential basis; they refer to building craftsmen and labourers in southern England.[22]

England, old age pensions comprised a higher percentage of a working-class adult's gross income than is the case today. Thomson, 'Decline of social welfare', p. 453.
[19] Thomson, 'I am not my father's keeper', pp. 266–72.
[20] Made up of 20 per cent 'farinaceous' and 22.5 per cent 'drink' (largely malt). Phelps Brown and Hopkins, 'Seven centuries of prices', table 1.
[21] For example, flour prices rose considerably less than wheat prices over the period from the 1490s to the decade 1600–9. See above p. 11.
[22] Phelps Brown and Hopkins, 'Seven centuries of building wages'.

4 Although changes in nominal wage rates in other occupations may not have been very different, given the normative, 'sticky', nature of the rates, occupational differences in shifts in the demand for labour may have produced large differences in earnings.

5 Large, structural changes in the demand for labour, as between the southern agricultural and northern industrial sectors in the late eighteenth century, produced very different trends in wage rates.[23]

Nonetheless, subject to some doubts about the proper representation of the scale of change, and to a caveat about concealed regional and sectoral heterogeneity, I think some reasonable inferences can be made from the series plotted on the figures, particularly with regard to food prices up to '1781'. Before this date, it is evident from the close linear relation in figure 8.3 between the pace of population growth and the rate of change of food prices that agricultural production was not immediately elastic with respect to demand. Yet the resulting long-run movements in prices appear to have provoked increases in supply to a remarkable extent. Indeed, a second conspicuous feature of the figure is the lack of any curvilinearity: the ratio of the rates of increase in prices to the rates of population growth is about 1.5 across the whole range. Either the pace of food-price increases was subject to purchasing power constraints, or English agriculture was capable of rapid expansion in output, or both. Thirdly, the linear relationship held over a period of more than two centuries during which the population more than doubled and food imports were negligible. Indeed, if one were to discount many of the late eighteenth- and early nineteenth-century imports as being more of flavourings, e.g. tea and coffee, than of essential foodstuffs, English agricultural production could be considered to have expanded sufficiently to cope with a fourfold increase in population between the late Middle Ages and the first quarter of the nineteenth century, when it was still able to meet more than 90 per cent of basic food requirements.[24]

Moreover, the challenge posed by population growth in pre-industrial England was exceptionally severe by European standards. As can be seen from figure 8.7, in the sixteenth century only the Netherlands experienced population growth on the same scale as England, and during the period 1650–1820 English population growth was very much greater than in other countries. Even more remarkably, in England during this period there was a substantial increase in the proportion of the population living in an urban environment: in 1600 6 per cent of the population lived in towns of 10,000 or more inhabitants;

[23] Wrigley and Schofield, *Population History of England*, pp. 431–3.
[24] Thomas, 'Escaping from constraints', p. 184.

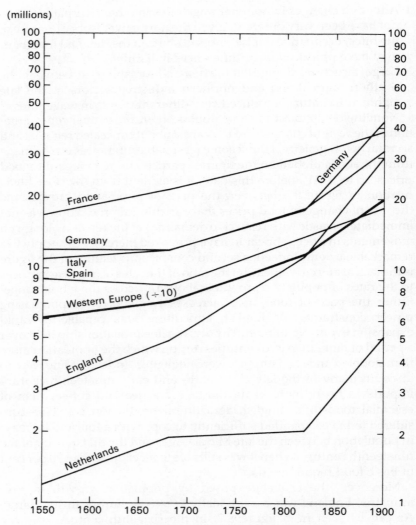

Figure 8.7 Population growth in western Europe
Source: Wrigley, 'Population growth', 123.

by 1700 this figure was 13 per cent, and by 1800 it was 24 per cent. In contrast, elsewhere in Europe there was little urbanisation in this period, even some de-urbanisation in the Netherlands.[25] Thus not only must the increase in agricultural output in England have been

[25] Wrigley, 'Urban growth', pp. 148, 152.

unusually large by European standards, but it must also have gone beyond the traditional response to population pressure of a greater labour intensiveness and involved increases in labour productivity. Indeed, recent estimates of the proportion of the labour force involved in agriculture in early modern England (56 per cent in 1688, 48 per cent in 1759, 37 per cent in 1801) contrast with estimates of 60–80 per cent for other European countries in the same period, the late seventeenth-century English levels only being attained elsewhere in Europe in the late nineteenth century.[26]

In England, therefore, although the pressure of population on food supply could drive up prices and lower the standard of living, in a long-run perspective it is clear that English agriculture was remarkably productive by contemporary European standards. Thus an important part of the English story must be the nexus of land use-rights and economic power-relations that enabled a market-orientated agriculture to emerge, and allowed the organisation of production to respond flexibly and efficiently to the price signals produced by demographically-induced changes in demand.[27] Equally important is the role that agricultural productivity played in enabling a significant development of non-agricultural activities. As has already been noted, in societies in which a high proportion of expenditure normally goes on food, changes in food prices will have had a more than proportional impact on purchasing power for non-agricultural goods and services. In such circumstances there is a danger that population growth will inhibit economic development in the form of specialisation, by choking off demand for labour outside the agricultural sector. However, in the case of England, it would seem that increases in agricultural productivity not only enabled a much greater number of people to be fed, but also released labour so that urbanisation proceeded apace, even during periods of population pressure and rising food prices.

The expansion of the non-agricultural sector seems to have been particularly marked during the century after 1650, when falling cereal prices were accompanied by an increase in the effective demand for non-food goods, as can be seen from the increasing numbers of small manufactured articles listed in probate inventories in that period.[28] To this increase in endogenous demand for non-agricultural goods should

---

[26] Crafts, *British Economic Growth*, pp. 14–15, 57–9.

[27] The importance of these institutional variables for the emergence of an exceptionally productive agriculture in England has been stressed by Brenner, 'Agrarian roots of European capitalism'. For a recent empirical study that raises important theoretical issues, see Glennie, 'In search of agrarian capitalism'.

[28] Weatherill, 'Consumer behaviour'.

be added a rapidly increasing captive exogenous demand for a wide range of manufactured articles from the colonies.[29] Labour could be released to meet this demand for non-agricultural goods, because the cereal farmers' response to falling prices was to increase productivity still further. A more diversified and mature 'traditional' economy, and a higher standard of living, were the economic rewards of a system of social power-relations and values that responded to population pressure not by the hardening of the arteries of a family-based subsistence economy, but by market-induced changes in agricultural practice and landholding structure.

The preventive check

In *The Population History of England* we described the preventive check in terms of nuptiality responding to changes in the standard of living as captured by a real-wage index. Since then work by a number of scholars (notably Weir, Goldstone, and Levine) has considerably advanced our appreciation of the nature of the changes in nuptiality and our understanding of how they might be related to changes in the economic context.[30] Yet some intriguing problems remain.

First, while it remains true that a first-marriage rate tracks a real-wage index quite well from the sixteenth to the nineteenth century, it is clear that the nature of the nuptiality response changed over time.[31] Figure 8.8, based on an ingenious idea by Weir, decomposes shifts in nuptiality into changes in average age at marriage and changes in the proportion ever marrying, and shows their relative impact on legitimate fertility.[32] From the figure it is evident that while both aspects of nuptiality changed over time, amongst those born before 1700 changes in the proportion ever marrying had a much greater impact on fertility than did changes in the age at marriage,

---

[29] Clay, *Economic Expansion*, pp. 152, 153–4, 188–91. Thomas and McCloskey, 'Overseas trade'.

[30] Weir, 'Rather late than never'; Goldstone, 'Demographic revolution'; Levine, *Reproducing Families*.

[31] Improvements that other scholars have made to the series reduce the lag and improve the fit between them. See Wrigley and Schofield, *Population History*, reprinted ed., 1989, preface.

[32] Schofield, 'English marriage patterns revisited', developing an approach pioneered in Weir, 'Rather never than late'. The figures for proportions ever marrying are for both sexes combined, because data to calculate sex-specific proportions were lacking. The age at marriage figures are for women. Although the average age at marriage for men was usually about two years higher, the pattern of movement in marriage age through time was similar for both sexes, so the figure can also be used to read off the scale and direction of changes in marriage age for men. Wrigley and Schofield, 'English population history', p. 162.

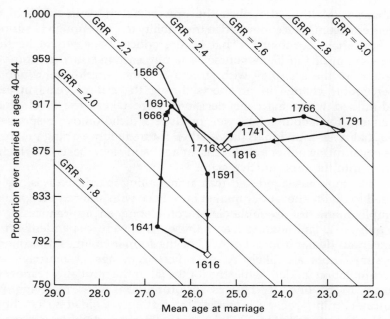

Figure 8.8 Celibacy and age at marriage in English cohort fertility

Note: points refer to data for twenty-five-year birth cohorts and are plotted against the mid-year of the cohort. Add twenty-five years to obtain the centred twenty-five year time-period of marriage.

while for those born during the eighteenth century most of the changes in fertility were due to a sharp fall, then rise, in the age at marriage. Furthermore, at all dates the changes in proportions ever marrying were much more coherently related to changes in real wages than were changes in age at marriage.[33]

The first problem, then, is to explain why in England before 1700 the nuptiality valve operated through changes in the incidence, rather than the timing, of marriage. I think it is a problem only if we conceive of the acquisition of the material basis of marriage *exclusively* in terms of accumulating sufficient capital. If this were indeed the operative process, then changes in real wages should be reflected in changes in the age at marriage, which in fact was the case, but only to a limited extent in the period before 1700. The accumulation model may correctly capture one aspect of the economic dimension of marriage in the past; but it pre-supposes full employment after marriage. For

---

[33] Schofield, 'English marriage patterns revisited', p. 16.

labourers Malthus described the preventive check in terms of the degree of confidence they had in their ability to earn enough to support a household economy.[34] That is, the critical issue would be their perception of the likely course of family earnings in the future. In sectors of the economy with structural under-employment, and no perceptible change in prospects during the critical years in early adulthood when marriage decisions were taken, the level of the demand for labour might well produce a dichotomous response in nuptiality, as individuals judged their future family earning prospects as constituting either a sufficient, or an insufficient, basis on which to enter into the reproductive state.[35]

Goldstone has suggested that in modelling marriage decisions we need to divide the labour market into those with assured prospects of employment (for example, after completing an apprenticeship or acquiring a landholding), and those who were dependent on an uncertain demand for labour.[36] For the former changes in economic circumstances are likely to be reflected in age at marriage (the accumulation model), while the for the latter the nuptiality response is likely to be one of changes in proportions ever marrying (the future-earnings prospects model). Interestingly, Goldstone has shown that in the period before 1700 changes in the proportions ever marrying in fact followed the course of real-wages as experienced in early adulthood.[37] As has been argued elsewhere, the level of real wages is likely to have provided a reasonable guide to the overall demand for labour and so to family earnings prospects.[38]

While a 'future earnings prospect' model of marriage for the poorest element in the population may make it easier to appreciate the operation of the preventive check before 1700, we still have to explain the shift to a dominance of changes in the age at marriage after that date. In tackling this question I think it important not to exaggerate the

[34] Malthus, *Essay* (1798), p. 27.

[35] This argument is asymmetrical, since it implicitly assumes that subsequent improvements in the standard of living would not encourage adults to marry at an advanced age. The assumption would be reasonable if it could be shown that there were strong internalised norms about the inappropriateness of marrying for the first time later in life. Direct information is hard to obtain, and inferences drawn from the age distribution at marriage are hazardous since the latter can be influenced by many factors. Nevertheless, marrying for the first time late in life was a relatively rare event: even in the late seventeenth century, when about 20 per cent never married, and the average age at marriage was 28.1 years for men and 26.2 years for women In this period only 5 per cent of men, and 3 per cent of women, married for the first time after age 35. See figure 8.8; and Wrigley and Schofield, 'English population history', pp. 162, 164.

[36] Goldstone, 'Demographic revolution', pp. 23–6.

[37] *Ibid*, p. 11.   [38] See above pp. 7–15.

phenomenon to be explained. Though the change is striking enough, it is important to remember both that age at marriage did vary before 1700, and that proportions ever marrying changed after that date. Furthermore, in the nineteenth century both components of nuptiality continued to change, though on a much-reduced scale, and with age at marriage only slightly out-distancing proportions ever marrying in its impact on fertility.[39] The problem to be explained, it seems to me, is not a once-and-for-all nuptiality transition occurring in the eighteenth century, as Goldstone has proposed, but rather a temporary interlude in which the age at marriage experienced a secular fluctuation of exceptional magnitude. Moreover, although the substantial fall in age at marriage in the late eighteenth century necessarily entailed a great increase in the proportion marrying at very young ages, unlike Goldstone I do not believe that there was a significant change in the overall shape of the age-distribution of marriages, from which we might deduce that major changes had occurred in the underlying structure of nuptiality.[40]

In searching for an explanation for the eighteenth-century shift in nuptiality patterns, one tempting possibility is to relate it to a major transformation in the structure of the economy, in which a society of peasants and craftsmen became urbanised and proletarianised. Personally, I find the temptation resistable. First, there is a problem of timing: long before 1700 England had acquired a substantial proletariat and a far from insignificant urban economy. It would be difficult, I think, to argue that there was a major transition from a subsistence and craft economy to a wage-labour economy in the early eighteenth century. Secondly, in England in the late sixteenth and seventeenth centuries there is no sign of the systematic inverse relationship between expectation of life and nuptiality, that one would associate with the niche variant of the positive check (compare e_0 in figure 8.5 with the crude first-marriage rate in figure 8.6). This is all the more interesting because just such a systematic relationship existed in France in the eighteenth century, when a long and substantial rise in e_0 was almost perfectly offset by movements in nuptiality, so that the population growth rate remained close to zero.[41] Moreover, the

[39] Wrigley and Schofield, *Population History*, pp. 436–8.
[40] Goldstone finds a *statistically* significant difference between the age-distribution of marriages in the later eighteenth century and that of earlier distributions with their mean shifted to correspond to the late eighteenth century location. But *substantively* the differences are small; for example, there is little difference in the relative position of the quartiles, once one has standardised for changes in the level of the median. Wrigley and Schofield, 'English population history', p. 165.
[41] For the offset between movements in mortality and fertility, see Wrigley and Schofield, *Population History*, fig. 7.13, p. 246. For the attribution of changes in fertility

adjustment in nuptiality in France involved changes in both age at marriage and proportions ever marrying, to an almost equal degree, in terms of their impact on legitimate fertility.[42] Patterns of nuptiality change in England in the same period could scarcely have been more different.

If we may conclude from this that in England since the sixteenth century the preventive check operated through the mechanisms of the wage-economy, rather than through the filling of niches, there may none the less have been important changes in the structure of employment in the eighteenth century which so altered the evaluation of earnings prospects that those who at earlier dates would have foregone marriage altogether now married, and at progressively earlier ages. Levine has argued powerfully for the importance of the development of 'proto-industry' as providing a new and effective framework for family earnings.[43] I find this an attractive argument, providing the demand for labour holds up. Since the household was the unit of production, and since demand for the products often originated obscurely outside the immediate economic context, individuals might well be inclined to take a more optimistic view of prospective family earnings than would be the case with general labouring. And the 'cottage economy' argument gathers more force from the observation that the main growth area in demand for labour in eighteenth-century England lay outside agriculture, in the manufacture of textile and metal goods, activities which were well-suited to household production.[44]

To an increasing demand for labour outside agriculture, from both home and overseas markets, one might add significant changes in the structure of the demand for labour in the agricultural sector itself. The changing ratio of food prices and nominal wage rates in the late eighteenth century was accompanied by a shift in farmers' preferences away from the traditional form of living-in labour on annual contract, which was becoming increasingly expensive to feed, to living-out labour hired by the day.[45] The progressive elimination of service in husbandry removed from the rural economy a structural demand for unmarried labour. Also in the later eighteenth century, under the pressure of population growth, jobs in agriculture became allocated

before the French Revolution to changes in nuptiality, see Weir, 'Life under pressure', p. 33.

[42] Mapping the data provided in *Ibid.* on to figure 8.
[43] Levine, *Reproducing Families*, chapter 3.
[44] Crafts, *British Economic Growth*, pp. 116–21, 137–40.
[45] Kussmaul, *Servants in Husbandry*, chapter 6.

preferentially to males, making it progressively more difficult to secure a dual-income household from labouring alone.[46]

Both the decline in service in husbandry, and the marginalisation of women from the agricultural labour force went much further in the arable zones of the south-east than in the pastoral regions of the north and west.[47] We might, therefore, expect that nuptiality might be more depressed in the rural south-east, especially since the pastoral zones typically contained more opportunities for family-based household economies of a proto-industrial kind.[48] However, with some exceptions, in the late eighteenth century age at marriage fell in villages full of agricultural labourers producing crops for the market as well as in those engaged in pastoral agriculture or in proto-industrial production.[49] Interestingly, among the few places for which family reconstitution results are available, and which record little or no change in age at marriage, are Gainsborough and Banbury, two substantial market towns and regional service centres, each with a wide range of craft occupations. This may suggest that the large movements in age at marriage occurring in other communities in this period were produced not by those in traditional occupations finding that economic circumstances enabled them to accumulate material wealth quicker and so marry earlier, but by those who sold their labour in a variety of sectoral markets finding that the structure of their employment now favoured early marriage.

To help explain how this could be the case even during periods when the prospects for earnings were deteriorating, we need to take into account the impact of contemporaneous changes in welfare policy. Towards the end of the eighteenth century welfare payments not only took account of the size of the dependency burden in the family, but may also have come to be allocated preferentially to married males.[50] If women, therefore, also experienced discrimination in the labour market, and it has been suggested that this occurred in the traditional urban craft sector as well as in the arable countryside, marriage may well have become a more attractive option to them.[51] It is, perhaps,

---

[46] Snell, *Annals of the Labouring Poor*, chapter 1.
[47] Kussmaul, *Servants in Husbandry*, chapter 7; Snell, *Annals of the Labouring Poor*, pp. 40–9.
[48] Levine, *Reproducing Families*, pp. 106–9.
[49] Cambridge Group: unpublished research results.
[50] Snell, *Annals of the Labouring Poor*, pp. 348–52. The extent to which unmarried individuals, or women, were discriminated against in the operation of the poor law needs further research. In Colyton, for example, the rich poor law documentation for the eighteenth and nineteenth century reveals no discrimination in the size or frequency of payments by marital status or sex. Personal communication from Pamela Sharpe. [51] *Ibid.*, chapter 6.

significant that it was during the two periods of slack population pressure, in the late Middle Ages and at the end of the seventeenth century, that there seem to have been both the greatest opportunities for female employment, and the lowest nuptiality.[52] If more women found fewer viable economic alternatives to marriage as the eighteenth century progressed, the linking of welfare payments to prices and to the size of the family would have enabled both sexes to discount the economic consequences of reproduction, and embark upon marriage at a young age. Changes in welfare policy would have removed the fear of the economic consequences of underemployment in the future, and so effectively disabled the traditional operation of the preventive check.[53] Those who at an earlier date would not have married at all, could now do so at a young age.

It seems to me, therefore, that by the eighteenth century a number of changes in structure of the economy had produced a demand for labour that enabled a growing proportion of the population to become employed in activities in which, in the light of contemporary changes in the welfare support system, early marriage was not irrational. But many aspects of these changed conditions continued into the nineteenth century, when age at marriage changed direction and rose substantially. How can we explain the reversal? And does it not cast doubt on the validity of the explanations offered for the sharp fall in age at marriage in the eighteenth century? Unfortunately, there are very few parishes for which data are available on age at marriage in the early nineteenth century, so no clues can be gleaned from a comparison between the pattern of ages at marriage in communities in different economic circumstances. On a general level, however, one might point to a decline in the prevalence of household production in several industries during the first half of the nineteenth century, as it became out-competed by more mechanised forms of production.[54] But shifting people from household production to the wage economy of the factory should have had no implications for age at marriage, if the arguments about the welfare system developed above are correct. Yet the welfare system is one factor that did change radically in the nineteenth

---

[52] *Ibid*. For the late medieval period, see Goldberg, 'Marriage, migration, servanthood'.

[53] As Malthus feared at the time. *Essay* (1798), p. 33. It should be emphasised that Malthus' objection to the poor laws was based on his belief that in practice they did disable the preventive check, and so 'in some measure . . . create the poor they maintain'. *Ibid*. However, he also stated explicitly that if his belief could be shown to be mistaken, his objection would fall. 'Population', p. 238. The relationship between the ethical and economic dimensions of Malthus' views on social security systems is discussed in Smith, 'Transfer incomes'.

[54] Levine, *Reproducing Families*, pp. 143–59.

century. The provisions of the New Poor Law of 1834 were framed with the express intention of reinstating a proper appreciation of the economic consequences of marriage, by abolishing child-related payments, and making financial assistance available only in an institutional context.[55]

Thus two of the factors which in the eighteenth century provided individuals with economic support that enabled them to marry early in life receded in the nineteenth century, one gradually, the other abruptly. In this perspective the eighteenth century appears not so much as a decisive transition from one nuptiality regime to another, but as a temporary aberration in which major structural shifts in the economy combined with a particularly flexible operation of the welfare support system, to induce a 'perverse' movement in the age at marriage, of such a magnitude that it swamped the 'correct' movement in proportions ever marrying, and temporarily disabled the preventive check.

Indeed, one might hazard a general rule that the more the connections between demographic and economic change are mediated through a diffuse and complex network of market relations, the greater the opportunity for confounding, or offsetting, influences to have an effect. Thus in certain circumstances in England in the past the operation of the preventive check may have been less efficient than in more simply structured peasant societies in which the niche mechanism prevailed. For example, we have noted how calculation of individual advantage by farmers could lead them to prefer to dispense with living-in, unmarried labour when food prices were high. Since grain prices moved in step with the rate of population growth, farmers' employment preferences favoured nuptiality just when the logic of the preventive check cycle required nuptiality to be depressed in order to reduce the rate of population growth.

Thus in periods of strongly rising population and food prices, as in the later sixteenth and eighteenth centuries, some market mechanisms could prove dysfunctional to an effective operation of the preventive check.[56] But by symmetry, in the period from the mid seventeenth to the mid eighteenth century, when population was static or growing slowly and food prices were falling, farmers' employment preferences held back nuptiality when the logic of the preventive check cycle

---

[55] Except in cases of the non-able-bodied poor, who could still be relieved at home. However, it should be noted that the strict principles governing the payment of relief in the New Poor Law were often sabotaged by local officials. The implementation of the 1834 Act is discussed by contributors to Fraser, *The New Poor Law*.

[56] This point was first elaborated in the discussion in Kussmaul, *Servants in Husbandry*, pp. 110–16.

required it to rise. In this case, however, the dysfunction proved beneficial, prolonging the period in which real wages remained high. Combined with the unusually strong increase in agricultural productivity in this period by way of response to falling grain prices, the 'dysfunctional' delay in the operation of the preventive check produced a long period in which the inter-sectoral terms of trade favoured the generation of a substantial endogenous demand for non-agricultural goods.

Conclusion

I have argued that a pre-industrial society, like England, in which an ideology of social relations located individual economic activity firmly within a structure of reciprocal collective responsibilities, will be more likely than a society based on a familistic, 'peasant' set of values to evolve flexible markets in goods and labour and to develop a productive agriculture. In a 'peasant' society the familistic structures of social relations through which nuptiality is mediated may well provide a more efficient means of keeping population in balance with its economic space; but that space is unlikely to be well-stocked with a wide range of goods and services. In the individualist–collectivist society, on the other hand, its very success in evolving richer, and more complex, economic and social spaces entails a risk that other variables may intervene to disable, to a greater or lesser degree, the operation of the preventive check. However, that same success furnishes the society with a greater potential for generating increases in productivity with which to meet the challenge of population growth. And it provides an opportunity for intervening variables to enter into a benign interaction with the society's demographic processes that may greatly enhance the quality of its economic space.

Consolidated bibliography

Aaby, P. *et al.* 'Overcrowding and intensive exposure as determinants of measles mortality', *American Journal of Epidemiology*, 120 (1984) 49–63

Aarne, A. and S. Thompson, *The Types of the Folktale: A Classification and Bibliography*, Helsinki, 1961

Abel, W. *Agricultural fluctuations in Europe from the Thirteenth to the Twentieth Centuries*, trans. of third German edn, London, 1980

Airs, M. *The Making of the English Country House 1500–1640*, London, 1975

Amussen, S. 'Governors and governed: class and gender relations in English villages, 1590–1725', unpublished Ph.D. thesis, Brown University, 1982

Anderson, J. A. 'A solid sufficiency: an ethnography of yeoman foodways in Stuart England', unpublished Ph.D. thesis, University of Pennsylvania, 1971

Anon. *Doctor Mead's Short Discourse Explain'd*, second edn, London, 1722

Appleby, A. B. 'Agrarian capitalism or seigneurial reaction? The north west of England, 1500–1700', *American Historical Review*, 80 (1975) 574–94

'Common land and peasant unrest in sixteenth century England', *Peasant Studies Newsletter*, 4 (1975) 20–23

'Crises of mortality: periodicity, intensity, chronology and geographical extent', in H. Charbonneau and A. Larose (eds.), *The Great Mortalities: Methodological Studies of Demographic Crises in the Past*, Liège (1979), pp. 283–94

'Diet in sixteenth century England: sources, problems, possibilities', in C. Webster (ed.), *Health, Medicine and Mortality*, pp. 97–116

'Disease, diet, and history', *Journal of Interdisciplinary History*, 8 (1978) 725–35

'Disease or famine? Mortality in Cumberland and Westmorland, 1580–1640', *Economic History Review*, 26 (1973) 403–31

'Epidemics and famine in the Little Ice Age', *Journal of Interdisciplinary History*, 10 (1980) 643–63

Famine in Tudor and Stuart England, Liverpool and Stanford, 1978

'Famine, mortality, and epidemic disease: a comment', *Economic History Review*, 30 (1977) 508–12

'Grain prices and subsistence crises in England and France 1590–1740', *Journal of Economic History*, 39 (1979) 865–87

'Nutrition and disease: the case of London, 1550–1750', *Journal of Interdisciplinary History*, 6 (1975) 1–22

305

'Population crisis and economic change: Cumberland and Westmorland, 1570–1670', unpublished Ph.D. thesis, University of California, Los Angeles, 1973

'The disappearance of the plague: a continuing puzzle', *Economic History Review*, 33 (1980) 161–73

Archer, I. W. 'Social policy in Elizabethan London', unpublished typescript

Arensberg, C. *The Irish Countryman*, New York, 1968

Aries, P. *The Hour of Our Death*, trans. H. Weaver, London, 1981

Arkell, T. 'Multiplying factors for estimating population totals from the Hearth Tax', *Local Population Studies*, 28 (1982) 51–7

Ashley, W. *The Bread of our Forefathers: An Inquiry in Economic History*, Oxford 1928

Ashton, T. S. *Economic Fluctuations in England 1700–1800*, Oxford, 1959

Atkinson, J. C. (ed.) *North Riding Quarter Session Records*, North Riding Record Society, 1–9, London, 1884–92

Ault, W. O. *Open-Field Farming in Medieval England: A Study of Village By-Laws*, London, 1972

Bacon, F. 'Of seditions and troubles', in J. Spedding, R. L. Ellis, and D. D. Heath (eds.), *The Works of Francis Bacon*, 14 vols., London, 1857–74, 6, pp. 406–12

Baehrel, R. *Une croissance: la Basse-Provence rurale*, Paris, 1961

Bairoch, P. 'Impact des rendements agricoles de la productivité agricole et des coûts des transport sur la croissance urbaine de 1800 à 1910', paper presented to seminar on Urbanization and Population Dynamics in History, IUSSP Committee on Historical Demography, Tokyo, January 1986

Baltazard, M. 'Déclin et destin d'une maladie infectieuse: La Peste', *Bulletin of the World Health Organisation*, 3 (1960) 247–62

Bardet, J-P. *Rouen aux XVIIe et XVIIIe siècles*, Paris, 1983

Barnard, E. A. B. 'Some Beoley parish accounts, 1656–1700', *Transactions of the Worcestershire Archeological Society for 1946*, 22 (1947) 16–40

Bartlett, M. S. 'On the theoretical specification of sampling properties of autocorrelated time series', *Journal of the Royal Statistical Society*, series B (1946) 27–41

Bateson, M. *Records of the Borough of Leicester*, 3 vols., Cambridge, 1899–1905

Batho, G. R. 'The Plague of Eyam: a tercentenary re-evaluation', *Journal of the Derbyshire Archaeological and Natural History Society*, 84 (1964) 81–91

Baulant, M. 'Le prix des grains à Paris de 1431 à 1788', *Annales: E.S.C.*, 23 (3) (1968) 520–40

Baxter, R. *A Christian Directory*, London, 1673

Beckett, J. V. 'English landownership in the seventeenth and eighteenth centuries: the debate and the problems', *Economic History Review*, 30 (1977) 567–81

Beier, A. L. *Masterless Men: The Vagrancy Problem in England 1560–1640*, London, 1985

'The social problems of an Elizabethan county town: Warwick, 1580–90', in P. Slack (ed.), *Country Towns in Pre-Industrial England*, London, 1981, pp. 46–85

Bell, W. G. *The Great Plague in London in 1665*, London, 1951

Benedictow, O. J. 'Disappearance of plague morbidity in historical plague epidemics', *Population Studies*, 41 (1987) 401–31

Bengtsson, T., G. Fridlizius, and R. Ohlsson (eds.). *Pre-Industrial Population Change*, Stockholm, 1984

Bengtsson, T. and R. Ohlsson, 'Age-Specific mortality and short-term changes in the standard of living: Sweden, 1751–1859', *European Journal of Population*, 1 (1985) 309–26

Bennett, M. K. 'British wheat yield per acre for seven centuries', *Economic History* (supplement to *Economic Journal*) 3 (1935) 12–29

Best, H. *The Farming and Memorandum Books of Henry Best of Elmswell 1642*, D. Woodward (ed.), Records of Social and Economic History, new series, 8, London, 1984

Beveridge, W. H., *et al. Prices and Wages in England from the Twelfth to the Nineteenth Century*, London, 1939

Beveridge, W. 'The yield and price of corn in the middle ages', *Economic History* (supplement to *Economic Journal*) 1 (1927) 155–67

Biraben, J-N. *Les Hommes et la peste en France et dans les pays européens et Méditerranéens*, 2 vols., Paris, 1975

Blake, J. B. 'The medieval coal trade of North East England: some fourteenth-century evidence', *Northern History*, 2 (1967) 1–26

Blanchard, M. 'Population change, enclosure and the early Tudor economy', *Economic History Review*, 23 (1970) 427–45

Blayo, Y. 'Le mouvement naturel de la population française de 1740 à 1829', *Population*, 30 (1975) 15–64

Bohstedt, J. *Riots and Community Politics in England and Wales 1790–1810*, Cambridge, Mass. and London, 1983

Bongaarts, J. and M. Cain, 'Demographic responses to famine', Centre for Policy Studies Working Papers, 77 (1981)

Boserup, E. *Conditions of Agricultural Growth*, London, 1965
Population and Technology, Chicago and Oxford, 1981

Bouniatian, M. *La loi de la variation de la valeur et les mouvements généraux des prix*, Paris, 1927

Bourn, W. *Whickham Parish: Its History, Antiquities and Industries*, Carlisle, 1983

Bowden, P. 'Agricultural prices, farm profits and rents', in J. Thirsk (ed.), *The Agrarian History of England and Wales, 1500–1640*, vol. 4, Cambridge, 1967, pp. 593–695
'Statistical appendix', in J. Thirsk (ed.), *The Agrarian History of England and Wales, 1500–1640*, vol. 4, Cambridge, 1967, pp. 814–70

Bradley, L. 'An enquiry into seasonality in baptisms, marriages and burials', *Local Population Studies*, 4 (1970) 21–40
'Some medical aspects of plague', in P. Slack (ed.), *The Plague Reconsidered*, pp. 11–23
'The most famous of all English plagues: a detailed analysis of the Plague of Eyam 1665–6', in P. Slack (ed.), *The Plague Reconsidered*, pp. 63–94

Brenner, R. 'Agrarian class structure and economic development in pre-industrial Europe', *Past and Present*, 70 (1976) 30–75
'The agrarian roots of European capitalism', *Past and Present*, 97 (1982) 16–113

Brent, C. 'Devastating epidemics in the countryside of eastern Sussex between harvest years 1558 and 1640', *Local Population Studies*, 14 (1975) 42–8

Breschi, M. and M. Livi-Bacci, 'Saison et climat comme de la survive des enfants, l'expérience italiénne au XIXe siècle', *Population*, 41 (1986) 9–35

Briggs, K. M. *A Dictionary of British Folk-Tales in the English Language*, 4 vols., London, 1970–71

Brooks, F. W. (ed.). 'Supplementary Stiffkey Papers', *Camden Miscellany 16*, Camden Soc., third series, 52, 1936

Buchan, A. and A. Mitchell, 'The influence of weather on mortality from different diseases and at different ages', *Journal of the Scottish Meteorological Society*, 4 (1875) 187–265

Bulkeley 'The Diary of Bulkeley of Dronwy, Anglesey, 1630–1636', H. Owen (ed.), *Transactions of the Anglesey Antiquarian Society and Field Club 1937* (1937) 26–172

Bushaway, B. *By Rite: Custom, Ceremony and Community in England 1700–1880*, London, 1982

Butlin, R. A. 'Land and people, *c.* 1600', in T. W. Moody, F. X. Martin, and F. J. Byrne (eds.) *A New History of Ireland*, 3, Oxford, 1976, pp. 142–67

Bynum, W. F. (ed.), *Living and Dying in London*, London, 1988

Campbell, B. M. S. 'Agricultural progress in medieval England: some evidence from eastern Norfolk', *Economic History Review*, 36 (1983) pp. 26–46

'Arable productivity in medieval England: some evidence from Norfolk', *Journal of Economic History*, 43 (1983) 379–404

'Population decline in late medieval England: A re-evaluation of the 1522 Muster Rolls and 1524/5 Lay Subsidies', unpublished abstract of paper to Historical Geography Research Group, Cambridge 1978

'Population pressure, inheritance and the land market in a fourteenth-century peasant community', in R. M. Smith, *Land, Kinship and Life-Cycle*, pp. 87–134

Campbell, M. *The English Yeoman under Elizabeth and the Early Stuarts*, London, 1960

Capp, B. *Astrology and the Popular Press*, London, 1979

Carew, R. *The Survey of Cornwall (1602)*, ed. F. E. Halliday, London, 1953

Carmichael, A. G. 'Infection, hidden hunger, and history', in R. I. Rotberg and T. K. Rabb (eds.), *Hunger and History*, pp. 51–66

Carus-Wilson, E. M. 'Evidences of industrial growth on some fifteenth-century manors', *Economic History Review*, 12 (1959) 190–205.

'Industrial revolution of the thirteenth century', *Economic History Review*, 11 (1941) 39–60

Chadwick, S. J. 'Some papers relating to the plague in Yorkshire', *Yorkshire Archaeological and Topographical Journal*, 15 (1900) 467–75

Chalkin, C. W. *Seventeenth Century Kent: A Social and Economic History*, London, 1965

Chambers, J. D. 'The Vale of Trent, 1670–1800: a regional study of economic change', *Economic History Review, Supplement*, 1957

Chanter, J. R. *Sketches of the Literary History of Barnstaple*, Barnstaple, 1886

Chappell, W. and J. W. Ebsworth (eds.). *The Roxburghe Ballads*, 9 vols., Hertford, 1871–99

Charbonneau, H. and A. Larose (eds.). *The Great Mortalities: Methodological Studies of Demographic Crises in the Past*, Liège, 1979

Charles, L. and L. Duffin (eds.). *Women and Work in Pre-Industrial England*, London, 1985

Charlesworth, A. *An Atlas of Rural Protest in Britain 1548–1900*, London, 1983
'The development of the English rural proletariat and social protest, 1700–1850: A comment', *Journal Peasant Studies*, 8 (1980) 101–11

Charlot, E. and J. Dupâquier. 'Mouvement annuel de la population de la ville de Paris de 1670 à 1821', *Annales de Démographie Historique*, (1967) 512–531

Chartres, J. *Inland Trade in England 1500–1700*, London, 1977
'The marketing of agricultural produce', in J. Thirsk (ed.), *The Agrarian History of England and Wales, 1640–1750*, 2 vols., Cambridge, 1985, 2, pp. 406–502

Chaunu, P. *La civilisation de l'Europe classique*, Paris, 1966
'Malthusianisme économique et malthusianisme démographique', *Annales: ESC*, 17 (1972) 1–19

Chaytor, M. 'Household and kinship: Ryton in the late 16th and early 17th centuries', *History Workshop*, 10 (1980) 25–51

Chester, J. A. 'Poor relief in Coventry, 1500–1640', unpublished M.Phil. thesis, University of Reading, 1982

Cipolla, C. M. *Cristofano and the Plague*, 1973
Public Health and the Medical Profession in the Renaissance, Cambridge, 1976

Clark, A. *Working Life of Women in the Seventeenth Century*, London, 1919

Clark, C. 'Household economy, market exchange and the rise of capitalism in the Connecticut Valley, 1800–1860', *Journal of Social History*, 13 (1979) pp. 169–89

Clark, P. *English Provincial Society from the Reformation to the Revolution: Religion, Politics and Society in Kent 1500–1640*, Hassocks, 1977
The English Alehouse: A Social History 1200–1830, London, 1983
'Migration in England during the late seventeenth and early eighteenth centuries', *Past and Present*, 83 (1979) 81–90
'The migrant in Kentish towns 1580–1640', in P. Clark and P. Slack (eds.), *Crisis and Order in English Towns 1500–1700: Essays in Urban History*, London, 1972, pp. 117–63
'"The Ramoth-Gilead of the Good": urban change and political radicalism at Gloucester 1540–1640', in A. G. Clark, R. Smith and N. Tyacke (eds.), *The English Commonwealth, 1547–1640*, London, 1979, pp. 167–87

Clark, P. and P. Slack. *English Towns in Transition 1500–1700*, Oxford, 1976

Clarkson, L. A. *The Pre-Industrial Economy in England 1500–1750*, London, 1971

Clay, C. *Economic Expansion and Social Change: England 1500–1700*, 2 vols., Cambridge, 1984

Cliffe, J. T. *The Puritan Gentry: The Great Puritan Families of Early Stuart England*, London, 1984
The Yorkshire Gentry from the Reformation to the Civil War, London, 1969

Coale, A. J. and P. Demeny. *Regional Model Life Tables and Stable Populations*, Princeton, 1966

Cockburn, J. S. 'The nature and incidence of crime in England 1559–1625: a preliminary survey', in Cockburn (ed.), *Crime in England 1500–1800*, London, 1977, pp. 49–71

Coleman, D. C. and R. S. Schofield. *The State of Population Theory: Forward from Malthus*, Oxford, 1986

Colson, E. 'In good years and bad: food strategies of self-reliant societies', *Journal of Anthropological Research*, 35 (1979) 18–30

Cook, J. *Unum Necessarium: Or, The Poor man's Case: Being An Expedient to make Provision for all poore People in the Kingdome*, London, 1647/8

Cooper, C. H. *Annals of Cambridge*, 3 vols., Cambridge, 1842–53

Coppolani, J. *Toulouse: étude de géographie urbaine*, Paris, 1954

Cornwall, J. *Revolt of the Peasantry 1549*, London, 1977

Cox, J. C. *The Parish Registers of England*, London, 1910

Crafts, N. *British Economic Growth during the Industrial Revolution*, Oxford, 1985

Creighton, C. *A History of Epidemics in Britain*, repr. London, 1965

Cressy, D. 'Kinship and kin interaction in early modern England', *Past and Present*, 113 (1986) 38–69

Croix, A. *Nantes et les pays Nantais au XVIe siècle*, Paris, 1974

Croot, P. The commercial attitudes and activities of small farmers in Somerset in the Seventeenth Century, Paper read to the Early Modern English Economic and Social History Seminar, Cambridge, 1983

Cullen, L. M. *An Economic History of Ireland since 1660*, London, 1972

The Emergence of Modern Ireland 1600–1900, London, 1981

'Population growth and diet, 1600–1850', in J. M. Goldstrom and L. A. Clarkson (eds.), *Irish Population, Economy, And Society*, Oxford, 1981, pp. 89–112

'Population trends in seventeenth century Ireland', *Economic and Social Review*, 6 (1975) 149–65

Culverwell, E. *A Treatise of Faith, wherein is Declared how a man may live by Faith, and find releefe in all his necessities*, London, 1623

Curtis, H. *Biology*, New York, 1978

Darnton, R. *The Great Cat Massacre and Other Episodes in French Cultural History*, London, 1984

Daultrey, S., D. Dickson, and C. Ó Gráda. 'Eighteenth century Irish population: new perspectives from old sources', *Journal of Economic History*, 41 (1981) 601–28

Davenant, C. *An Essay upon the probable Methods of making a People Gainers in the Balance of Trade*, London, 1699

Davies, D. A. 'Plague, death and disease in Herefordshire, 1575–1640', *Transactions of the Woolhope Naturalists' Field Club*, 43 (1981) 307–14

Davis, R. *The Rise of the English Shipping Industry in the Seventeenth and Eighteenth Centuries*, London, 1962

Dendy, F. W. (ed.). *Extracts from the Records of the Company of Hostmen of Newcastle-upon-Tyne*, Surtees Society, 105, 1901

Derouet, B. 'Une démographie différentielle: clés pour un système autorégulateur des populations rurales d'Ancien Régime', *Annales: E.S.C.*, 35 (1980) 3–41

de Vries, J. 'Measuring the impact of climate on history: the search for appropriate methodologies', *Journal of Interdisciplinary History*, 10 (1980) 599–630

D'Ewes, S. *The Journals of All the Parliaments during the reign of Queen Elizabeth*, London, 1682

Deyon, P. *Amiens: capitale provinciale*, Paris, 1967

Dirks, R. 'Social responses during severe food shortages and famine', *Current Anthropology*, 21 (1980) 21–44

Dobson, M. J. 'Population, disease and mortality in South-east England, 1600–1800', unpublished D.Phil thesis, University of Oxford, 1982

Drake, M. *Historical Demography: Problems and Projects*, Open University, Milton Keynes, 1974

'An elementary exercise in parish register demography', *Economic History Review*, 14 (1961/2) 427–45

'The Irish demographic crisis of 1740–41', *Historical Studies*, 6 (1965) 101–24

Drummond, J. C. and A. Wilbraham. *The Englishman's Food: A History of Five Centuries of English Diet*, London, 1939

Dunbabin, J. P. *Rural Discontent in Nineteenth Century Britain*, London, 1974

Dupâquier, J. *La population rurale du Bassin parisien à l'époque de Louis XIV*, Paris, 1979

Dupâquier, J., M. Lachiver, and J. Meuvret. *Mercuriales du Pays de France et du Vexin français (1640–1792)*, Paris, 1968

Durant, D. N. and P. Rider (eds.). *The Building of Hardwick Hall*, 2 vols., Derbyshire Record Society, 4 (1980) and 9 (1984)

Dyer, A. *The City of Worcester in the Sixteenth Century*, Leicester, 1973

Dyer, C. 'Changes in nutrition and standard of living in England, 1200–1500', in R. Fogel (ed.), *Long Term Changes in Nutrition and the Standard of Living* (Papers of the Ninth International Economic History Congress, Bern, 1986: Section B7) pp. 35–43

'English diet in the later Middle Ages', in T. H. Aston, *et al.* (eds.), *Social Relations and Ideas: Essays in Honour of R. H. Hilton*, Cambridge, 1983, pp. 191–216

Dymond, D. 'The famine of 1527 in Essex', *Local Population Studies*, 26 (1981) 29–40

Ebsworth, J. W. (ed.). *The Bagford Ballads Illustrating the Last Years of the Stuarts*, Hertford, 1878

Eckstein, Z., T. P. Schultz, and K. I. Wolpin. 'Short-run fluctuations and mortality in pre-industrial Sweden', *European Economic Review*, 26 (1985) 295–317

Eden, F. M. *The State of the Poor: Or, An History of the Labouring Classes in England*, 3 vols., London, 1797

Ell, S. R. 'Interhuman transmission of medieval plague', *Bulletin of the History of Medicine*, 54 (1980) 497–510

Emmison, F. G. *Elizabethan Life: Morals and the Church Courts*, Chelmsford, 1973

'Poor relief accounts of two rural parishes in Bedfordshire, 1563–1598', *Economic History Review*, 3 (1931–2) 102–16

Everitt, A. *Change in the Provinces: the Seventeenth Century*, University of Leicester Department of English Local History, Occasional Papers, 1, Leicester, 1972

'Farm labourers', in J. Thirsk (ed.), *The Agrarian History of England and Wales, 1500–1640*, 4, Cambridge, 1967, pp. 396–465

'The marketing of agricultural produce', in J. Thirsk (ed.), *The Agrarian History of England and Wales, 1500–1640*, 4, Cambridge, 1967, pp. 466–592

Eversley, D. E. C. 'Epidemiology as social history', in C. Creighton (ed.), *A History of Epidemics in Britain*, London, 1891; reprinted London, 1965, pp. 1–39

Eyre, A. 'A Dyurnall, or catalogue of all my accions and expences from the 1st of January, 1646–[7]', in H. J. Moorehouse (ed.), *Yorkshire Diaries and*

Autobiographies in the Seventeenth and Eighteenth Centuries, Surtees Society, 65, 1875, pp. 1–118

Faraday, M. 'Mortality in the Diocese of Hereford, 1442–1541', *Transactions of the Woolhope Naturalists' Field Club*, 43, part 2 (1977) 163–74

Farmer, D. L. 'Some grain price movements in thirteenth-century England', *Economic History Review*, 10 (1957) 207–20

Federowicz, J. K. *England's Baltic Trade in the Early Seventeenth Century: A Study in Anglo-Polish Commercial Diplomacy*, Cambridge, 1980

Fieldhouse, R. 'Social structure from Tudor lay subsidies and probate inventories: a case study, Richmondshire (Yorkshire)', *Local Population Studies*, 12 (1974) 9–24

Finlay, R. *Population and Metropolis: The Demography of London, 1580–1650*, Cambridge, 1981

Fletcher, A. *A County Community in Peace and War: Sussex, 1600–1660*, London, 1975

Reform in the Provinces: The Government of Stuart England, New Haven and London, 1986

Tudor Rebellions, London, 1973

Flinn, M. W. *The European Demographic System 1500–1820*, Brighton, 1981

'The stabilization of mortality in pre-industrial Western Europe', *Journal of European Economic History*, 3 (1974) 285–318

'Plague in Europe and the Mediterranean Countries', *Journal of European Economic History*, 8 (1979) 139–46

Flinn, M. W. *et al.* (eds.). *Scottish Population History: from the Seventeenth Century to the 1930s*, Cambridge, 1977

Foley, H. (ed.). *Records of the English Province of the Society of Jesus*, 6 vols., Roehampton, 1875–80

Foot, S. *The Effect of the Elizabethan Statute of Artificers on Wages in England*, Exeter Research Group Discussion Papers, 5, Exeter, 1980

Fordyce, W. *The History and Antiquities of the County Palatine of Durham*, 2 vols., Newcastle, 1857

Foster, D. 'Demography in the North-West: the parish of Poulton-le-Fylde', *University of Lancaster Regional Bulletin*, 5 (1976)

Fox, H. S. A. and R. A. Butlin (eds.). *Change in the Countryside*, London, 1978

Fraser, D. *The New Poor Law in the Nineteenth Century*, London, 1976

Frêche, G. and Frêche, G. *Les prix des grains, des vins, et des légumes à Toulouse, 1486–1868*, Paris, 1967

Toulouse et la région Midi-Pyrénées au siècle des lumières (vers 1670–1789), Paris, 1974

Frisch, R. 'Nutrition, fatness and fertility: the effect of food intake on reproductive ability', in W. H. Moseley (ed.), *Nutrition and Human Reproduction*, New York, 1978, pp. 91–122

Fuller, T. *The Holy State*, Cambridge, 1648

Fussell, G. E. (ed.). *Robert Loder's Farm Accounts 1610–1620*, Camden Soc., third series, 53, London, 1936

Galloway, P. R. 'Annual variations in death by age, deaths by cause, prices and weather in London 1670–1830', *Population Studies*, 39 (1985) 487–505

'Basic patterns in annual variations in fertility, nuptiality, mortality and prices in pre-industrial Europe', *Population Studies*, 42 (1988) 275–304

'Differentials in demographic responses to annual price variations in pre-revolutionary France: a comparison of rich and poor areas in Rouen, 1681–1787', *European Journal of Population*, 2 (1986) 269–305

'Long term fluctuations in climate and population in the pre-industrial era', *Population and Development Review*, 12 (1986) 1–24

'Population, prices and weather in pre-industrial Europe', unpublished Ph.D. thesis, University of California, Berkeley, 1987

Garden, M. *Lyon et les Lyonnais au 18e siècle*, Paris, 1970

Gardiner, S. *The Cognizance of a True Christian, or the outward marks whereby he may be the better knowne: Consisting especially in these two duties: Fasting and giving of Almes: verie needfull for these difficult times*, London, 1597

George, J. 'Les mercuriales d'Angoulême, de Cognac et de Jarnac (1595–1797)', *Bulletins et Mémoires de la Société Archéologique et Historique de la Charente*, series 8, vol. 11 (1920) 5–94

Gibbon, E. *The Decline and Fall of the Roman Empire*, 6 vols., London, 1910

Gibson, E. *Codex Juris Ecclesiastici Anglicani*, Oxford, 1761

Gibson, T. E. (ed.). *Crosby Records: A Cavalier Notebook*, London, 1880

Gillespie, R. 'Harvest crises in early seventeenth-century Ireland', *Irish Economic and Social History*, 11 (1984) pp. 5–18

Gittings, C. *Death, Burial and the Individual in Early Modern England*, London, 1984

Glass, D. V. and D. E. C. Eversley (eds.). *Population in History: Essays in Historical Demography*, London, 1965

Glennie, P. 'In search of agrarian capitalism: manorial land markets and the acquisition of land in the Lea valley, c. 1450–c.1560', *Continuity and Change*, 3 (1988) 11–40

Goldberg, P. J. P. 'Marriage, migration, servanthood and life-cycle in Yorkshire towns of the later Middle Ages', *Continuity and Change*, 1 (1986) 141–69

Goldstone, J. 'The demographic revolution in England: a re-examination', *Population Studies*, 40 (1986) 5–33

Gooder, A. 'The population crisis of 1727–30 in Warwickshire', *Midland History*, 1 (1972) 1–22

Goose, N. 'Economic and social aspects of provincial towns: a comparative study of Cambridge, Colchester and Reading, c. 1500–1700', unpublished Ph.D. thesis, University of Cambridge, 1984

Goring, J. and J. Wake (eds.). *Northampton Lieutenancy Papers and other Documents 1580–1614*, Northamptonshire Record Society, 27, Gateshead, 1975

Gottfried, R. S. *Epidemic Disease in Fifteenth Century England: The Medical Response and the Demographic Consequences*, New Brunswick, 1978

Goubert, P. *Beauvais et le Beauvaisis de 1600 à 1730*, Paris, 1960

'En Beauvaisis: problèmes démographiques du XVII siècle', *Annales, E.S.C.*, 7 (1952) 453–68

'La mortalité en France sous l'ancien regime: problèmes et hypothèses', in P. Harsin and E. Helin (eds.), *Actes du Colloque International de Demographie Historique*, Liège, 1965, pp. 79–82

'Recent theories and research in French population between 1500 and 1700', in D. V. Glass and D. E. C. Eversley (eds.), *Population in History: Essays in Historical Demography*, pp. 457–73

Gouge, W. *God's Three Arrowes: Plague, Famine, Sword*, London, 1631

Gough, R. *Human Nature Displayed in the History of Myddle written by Richard Gough*, Fontwell, 1968

Granger, C. W. J. and C. M. Elliott. 'A fresh look at wheat prices and markets in the eighteenth century', *Economic History Review*, 20, 1967, 257–65

Gras, L. J., *Histoire du commerce locale de la région Stéphanoise*, St Etienne, 1910

Gras, N. *The Evolution of the English Corn Market from the Twelfth to the Eighteenth Century*, Cambridge, Mass., 1915

Gray, W. *Chorographia; Or, a Survey of Newcastle upon Tyne in 1649*, Newcastle, 1813

Greaves, R. L. *Society and Religion in Elizabethan England*, Minneapolis, 1981

Griffiths, M. 'Kirtlington: an Oxfordshire community, 1500–1750', unpublished D.Phil. thesis, University of Oxford, 1979

Grigg, D. *The Dynamics of Agricultural Change*, London, 1982

Hajnal, H. J. 'European marriage patterns in perspective', in D. V. Glass and D. E. C. Eversley (eds.), *Population in History*, London, 1965, pp. 101–147

Hallam, H. E. 'Some thirteenth-century censuses', *Economic History Review*, second series, 10, 1958, 349–55

Halliwell, J. O. *A Minute Account of the Social Conditions of the People of Anglesea in the reign of James I*, London, 1860

Halliwell, J. O. and T. Wright (eds.). *A Collection of Seventy-Nine Black Letter Ballads . . . 1559–1597*, London, 1867

Hanauer, A. *Etudes économiques sur l'Alsace ancienne et moderne*, 2 vols., Strasbourg, 1878

Harrison, C. J. 'Elizabethan village surveys: a comment', *Agricultural History Review*, 27 (1979) 82–9

  'Grain price analysis and harvest qualities, 1465–1634', *Agricultural History Review*, 19, 135–55

Harrison, D. J. D. 'A census of households in County Durham, 1563', *Cleveland and Teeside Local History Society Bulletin*, 11 (1970) 14–18

Harrison, W. *The Description of England*, Ithaca, 1968

Hartley, D. *Food in England*, London, 1954

Hatcher, J. *Plague, Population and the English Economy, 1348–1530*, London, 1977

Hauser, H. *L'histoire des prix en France de 1500 à 1800*, Paris, 1936

Heal, F. 'Hospitality and honor in early modern England', *Food and Foodways*, 1 (1987) 321–50

  'The idea of hospitality in early modern England', *Past and Present*, 102 (1984) 66–93

Hendley, W. *Loimologia Sacra*, London, 1721

Henry, P. (ed.). *Diaries and Letters of Philip Henry*, M. H. Lee (ed.), London, 1882

Herlan, R. W. 'Poor relief in London during the English Revolution', *Journal British Studies*, 17 (1979) 30–51

  'Poor relief in the London parish of Dunstan in the West during the English Revolution', *Guildhall Studies in London History*, 3 (1977) 13–36

Hey, D. G. *An English Rural Community: Myddle under the Tudors and Stuarts*, Leicester, 1974

  Rural Metal Workers of Sheffield Region, University of Leicester Department of English Local History, Occasional Papers, second series, 5, Leicester, 1972

Heywood, O. *Autobiography and Diaries of Rev. Oliver Heywood*, J. H. Turner (ed.) 4 vols., Brighouse, 1882–85

Hill, C. *Society and Puritanism in Pre-Revolutionary England*, London, 1966

  'The uses of Sabbatarianism', in *Society and Puritanism in Pre-Revolutionary England*, London, 1966, pp. 145–218

Hinde, W. *A Faithful Remonstrance of the Holy Life and Happy Death of John Bruen of Bruen-Stapleford, in the County of Chester, Esq.*, London, 1641

Hirst, L. F. *The Conquest of Plague*, Oxford, 1953

Hobbes, T. *The Elements of Law*, F. Tonnies (ed.), 1928

Hobbs Pruitt, B. 'Self-sufficiency and the agricultural economy of eighteenth century Massachusetts', *William and Mary Quarterly*, 42 (1984) 333–64

Hodgson, R. I. 'Demographic trends in County Durham, 1560–1801: data sources and preliminary findings, with particular reference to North Durham', University of Manchester School of Geography Research Papers, no. 5, 1978

  'The progress of enclosure in County Durham, 1550–1870', in H. S. A. Fox and R. A. Butlin (eds.), *Change in the Countryside*, London, 1978, pp. 83–102

Hoffman, R. C. 'Medieval origins of the common fields', in W. N. Parker and E. Jones (eds.), *European Peasants and their Markets*, Princeton, 1975, pp. 23–71

Holderness, B. A. *Pre-Industrial England: Economy and Society 1500–1750*, London, 1976

  'Credit in English rural society before the nineteenth century, with special reference to the period 1650–1720', *Agricultural History Review*, 24 (1976) 97–109

  'Widows in pre-industrial society: an essay upon their economic functions', in R. M. Smith (ed.), *Land, Kinship and Life-cycle*, Cambridge, 1985, pp. 423–42

Holmes, M. E. 'Sources for the history of food supplies and marketing during the eighteenth and nineteenth centuries in local record offices', in W. Minchinton (ed.), *Population and Marketing: Two Studies in the History of the Southwest*, Exeter Papers in Economic History, 11, Exeter, 1976

Horton, P. H. 'The administrative social and economic structure of the Durham Bishopric Estates, 1500–1640', unpublished M. Litt. thesis, University of Durham, 1975

Hoskins, W. G. *Provincial England: Essays in Social and Economic History*, London, 1965

  The Midland Peasant: The Economic and Social History of a Leicestershire Village, London, 1965

  'Harvest fluctuations and English economic history, 1480–1619', *Agricultural History Review*, 12 (1964) 28–46

  'Harvest fluctuations and English economic history, 1620–1759', *Agricultural History Review*, 16 (1968) 15–31

  'The Leicestershire farmer in the sixteenth century', in *Essays in Leicestershire History*, Liverpool, 1950, pp. 123–83

Houston R. and R. M. Smith. 'A new approach to family history?', *History Workshop*, 14 (1982) 120–31

Howard, J. *An Account of the Principal Lazarettos in Europe*, Warrington, 1789

Howe, G. M. *Man, Environment and Disease in Britain*, London, 1972

Howell, R. *Newcastle-upon-Tyne and the Puritan Revolution. A Study of the Civil War in North England,* Oxford, 1967

Howson, W. G. 'Plague, poverty and population in parts of north-west England, 1580–1720', *Transactions of the Historical Society of Lancashire and Cheshire,* 112 (1960) 29–55

Hudson, P. 'From manor to the mill: the west Riding in transition', in M. Berg *et al.* (eds.), *Manufacture in Town and Country,* pp. 124–44

Hudson, W. and J. C. Tingey (eds.). *The Records of the City of Norwich,* 2 vols., Norwich, 1910

Hughes, A. L. 'Politics, society and civil war in Warwickshire 1620–50', unpublished Ph.D. thesis, University of Liverpool, 1979

Hull, F. 'Agriculture and rural society in Essex, 1560–1640', unpublished Ph.D. thesis, University of London, 1950

Hunt, W. *The Puritan Moment: The Coming of Revolution in an English County,* Cambridge, Mass., 1983

Husbands, C. 'The Hearth Tax and the structure of the English economy', unpublished Ph.D. thesis, University of Cambridge, 1986

Hutchinson, F. E. (ed.). *The Works of G. Herbert,* Oxford, 1941

Ingram, M. 'Ecclesiastical justice in Wiltshire 1600–1640, with special reference to cases concerning sex and marriage', unpublished D.Phil. thesis, University of Oxford, 1976

'Religion, communities and moral discipline in late sixteenth- and early seventeenth-century England: case studies', in K. von Greyerz (ed.), *Religion and Society in Early Modern England 1500–1800,* London, 1984

Jackson, J. 'Mortality and Disease in eighteenth-century Somerset and Wiltshire', unpublished paper to Institute of British Geographers' Symposium, 1979

James, M. *Family, Lineage and Civil Society. A Study of Society, Politics and Mentality in the Durham Region, 1500–1640,* Oxford, 1974

Janetta, A. B. *Epidemics and Mortality in Early Modern Japan,* Princeton, 1987

Jenkins, P. *The Making of a Ruling Class: The Glamorgan Gentry 1640–1790,* Cambridge, 1983

Jevons, W. S. *The Theory of Political Economy,* Harmondsworth, 1970

Johnston, J. A. 'The impact of the epidemics of 1727–30 in South-west Worcestershire', *Medical History,* 15 (1971) 278–92

Jones, E. L. *Seasons and Prices: The Role of the Weather in English Agricultural History,* London, 1964

(ed.). *Agriculture and Economic Growth in England 1660–1750,* London, 1967

Jones, E. L. and M. J. R. Healy. 'Wheat yields in England 1815–59', in E. L. Jones (ed.), *Agriculture and the Industrial Revolution,* Oxford, 1974

Jones, J. G. 'The Wynn Estates of Gwydir: aspects of its growth and development c. 1500–1580', *The National Library of Wales Journal,* 22 (1981–2) 141–69

Jones, W. R. D. *The Tudor Commonwealth 1529–1559: A Study of the Impact of the Social and Economic Developments of Mid-Tudor England upon Contemporary Concepts of the Nature and Duties of the Commonwealth,* London, 1970

Jupp, E. B. and R. Hovenden. *The Registers of the Parish of Allhallows London Wall,* London, 1878

Kaplan, S. L. *Bread, Politics and Political Economy in the reign of Louis XV,* 2 vols., The Hague, 1976

Kempe, A. J. *Historical Notices of the Collegiate Church of St. Martin-le-Grand*, London, 1825

Kent, J. R. 'Population mobility and alms: poor migrants in the Midlands during the early seventeenth century', *Local Population Studies*, 27 (1981) 35–51

Kerridge, E. *The Farmers of Old England*, London, 1973
'The movement of rent 1540–1640', *Economic History Review*, 4 (1951) 16–34

Kershaw, I. 'The Great Famine and Agrarian Crisis in England 1315–1322', *Past and Present*, 59 (1973) 3–50

Keys, A. et al. *The Biology of Human Starvation*, Minneapolis, 1950

King, P. 'Crime, law and society in Essex, 1740–1820', unpublished Ph.D. thesis, University of Cambridge, 1984

Kingsman, M. J. 'Markets and marketing in Tudor Warwickshire: the evidence of John Fisher of Warwick and the crises of 1586–7', *Warwickshire History*, 4 (1978) 16–28

Kirby, D. A. 'Population density and land values in County Durham during the mid-seventeenth century', *Institute of British Geographers Transactions*, 57 (1972) 83–98

(ed.) *Parliamentary Surveys of the Bishopric of Durham*, Surtees Society, 185

Komlos, J. 'The food budget of English workers: a comment on Shammas', *Journal of Economic History*, 48 (1988), 149

Kosminsky, E. A. *Studies in the Agrarian History of England in the Thirteenth Century*, Oxford, 1956

Kunitz, S. J. 'Speculations on the European mortality decline', *Economic History Review*, second series 36 (1983) 349–64

Kussmaul, A. *Servants in Husbandry in Early Modern England*, Cambridge, 1981
'Agrarian change in seventeenth century England: the economic historian as palaeontologist', *Journal of Economic History*, 45 (1985) 1–30

Labrousse, C. E. *Esquisse du mouvement des prix et des revenus en France au 1798 à 1820*, Paris, 1932
La crise de l'économie Française à la fin de l'Ancien Régime et au debut de la Révolution, Paris, 1944

Labrousse, E., R. Romano, and F. G. Dreyfus. *Le prix du froment en France au temps de la monnaie stable (1726–1913)*, Paris, 1970

Lacqueur, T. 'Bodies, death and pauper funerals', *Representations*, I (1983) 109–31

Laforce, F. M. 'Clinical and epidemiological observations on an outbreak of plague in Nepal', *Bulletin of the World Health Organisation*, 45 (1971) 693–706

Lamb, H. H. *Climate: Present, Past and Future*, 2 vols., London, 1972 and 1977

Landers, J. 'Mortality and metropolis: the case of London 1625–1825', *Population Studies*, 41 (1987) 59–76
'Mortality, weather and prices in London 1675–1825: a study of short-term fluctuations', *Journal of Historical Geography*, 12 (1986) 347–64

Landers, J. and A. Mouzas. 'Burial seasonality and cause of death in London 1670–1819', *Population Studies*, 42 (1988) 59–83

Large, P. 'Urban growth and agrarian change in the West Midlands during the seventeenth and eighteenth centuries', in P. Clark (ed.), *The Transformation of English Provincial Towns 1600–1800*, pp. 169–89

Larkin, J. F. and P. L. Hughes (eds.). *Stuart Royal Proclamations*, 2 vols., and *Tudor Royal Proclamations*, Oxford, 1973, 1983, 1964–9.
Lasker, G. W. and D. F. Roberts. 'Secular trends in relationship as estimated by surnames: a study of a Tyneside parish', *Annals of Human Biology*, 9 (1982) 299–307
Laslett, P. *The World We Have Lost*, London, 1965
The World We Have Lost Further Explored, London, 1983
'Family, kinship and the collectivity: systems of support in pre-industrial Europe – a consideration of the nuclear hypothesis', unpublished paper to the conference on 'Struttere e rapporti familiari in epoca moderna', Trieste, 1983
(ed.). *The Earliest Classics: John Graunt and Gregory King*, London 1973
Laslett, P. and R. Wall. *Household and Family in Past Time*, Cambridge, 1972
Latimer, J. *Annals of Bristol in the Seventeenth Century*, Bristol, 1908
Lebrun, F. 'Les crises démographiques en France aux XVIIe et XVIIIe siècles', *Annales: ESC*, 35 (1980) 205–34
Ledermann, S. *Nouvelles tables-types de mortalité*, Paris, 1969
Lee, J. J. 'Irish economic history since 1500', in J. J. Lee (ed.), *Irish Historiography, 1970–79*, Cork, 1981
Lee, R. D. 'Methods and models for analyzing historical series of births, deaths and marriages', in R. D. Lee, (ed.), *Population Patterns in the Past*, Princeton, 1977, pp. 337–70
'Models of pre-industrial population dynamics, with applications to England', in C. Tilly (ed.), *Historical Studies of Changing Fertility*, Princeton, 1978, pp. 155–207
'Population in pre-industrial England: an econometric analysis', *Quarterly Journal of Economics*, 87 (1973) 581–607
'Short-term variations in vital rates, prices, and weather', in E. A. Wrigley and R. Schofield (eds.), *The Population History of England, 1541–1871: a reconstruction*, London, 1981, pp. 356–410
Lee, W. *Daniel Defoe: His Life and Recently Discovered Writings 1716–29*, London, 1869
Lefebvre-Teillard, A. *La population de Dôle au XVIIIe siècle*, Paris, 1969
Leighton, W. A. 'Early chronicles of Shrewsbury, 1372–1603', *Transactions of the Shropshire Archaeological and Natural History Society*, 3 (1880) 239–352
Lennard, R. 'Statistics of corn yields in medieval England', *Economic History* (supplement to *Economic Journal*), 3 (1936) 172–92; and 3 (1937) 325–49
Leonard, E. M. *The Early History of English Poor Relief*, Cambridge, 1900
Le Roy Ladurie, E. 'L' aménorrhée de famine (XVIIe–XXe siècles)', *Annales: ESC*, 24–6 (1969) 1589–1601
Lesthaeghe, R. 'On the social control of human reproduction', *Population and Development Review*, 6 (1980) 527–48
Levine, D. *Reproducing Families: The Political Economy of English Population History*, Cambridge, 1987
'The Demographic implications of rural industrialisation, a family reconstitution study of two Leicestershire villages, 1600–1851', unpublished Ph.D. thesis, University of Cambridge, 1974
Lindert, P. H. and J. G. Williamson. 'English workers' living standards during the industrial revolution: a new look', *Economic History Review*, 36 (1983) 1–25

'English workers' living standards during the industrial revolution: a new look', Department of Economics, University of California, Working Paper Series, no. 156 (1980)

'Revising England's social tables, 1688–1812', *Explorations in Economic History*, 19 (1982) 387–91

Ling, N. *Politeuphia, Wit's Common-wealth*, London, 1661

Livi-Bacci, M. *Population and Nutrition: Antagonism and Adaptation*, Cambridge, 1989

Lodge, E. (ed.). *The Account Book of a Kentish Estate, 1616–1704*, British Academy Records of the Social and Economic History of England and Wales, 6, London 1927

Lucas, A. T. 'Nettles and charlock as famine food', *Breifne*, 1 (1959) 137–46

Mabey, R. *Food for Free: A Guide to the Edible Wild Plants of Britain*, London, 1972

MacCaffrey, W. T. *Exeter 1540–1640*, Cambridge, Mass, 1958

Macfarlane, A. *The Culture of Capitalism*, Oxford, 1987

  The Family Life of Ralph Josselin, a Seventeenth-Century Clergyman: An Essay in Historical Anthropology, Cambridge, 1970

  The Origins of English Individualism: the Family, Property and Social Transition, Oxford, 1978

  Witchcraft in Tudor and Stuart England: a Regional and Comparative Study, London, 1970

  (ed.), *The Diary of Ralph Josselin 1616–1683*, British Academy, Records of Social and Economic History, new ser. 3, London, 1976

Mackenroth, G. *Bevölkerungslehre. Theorie, Soziologie und Statistik der Bevölkerung*, Berlin, 1953

Malcomson, R. W. '"A set of ungovernable people": the Kingswood colliers in the eighteenth century', in J. Brewer and J. Styles, (eds.), *An Ungovernable People: The English and their Law in the Seventeenth and Eighteenth Centuries*, London, 1980, pp. 85–127

Malthus, T. R. *An Essay on the Principle of Population*, first edn, London, 1798; reprinted in Wrigley and Souden, *Works of Malthus*, vol. 1

  An Essay on the Principle of Population, sixth edn, London, 1826; reprinted in Wrigley and Souden, *Works of Malthus*, vols. 2 and 3

  An Investigation of the Cause of the Present High Price of Provisions, London, 1800; reprinted in Wrigley and Souden, *Works of Malthus*, vol. 7, pp. 5–18

  'Population', in *Encyclopaedia Britannica*, 6, 1824, pp. 307–33; reprinted in Wrigley and Souden, *Works of Malthus*, vol. 4, pp. 179–243

Manley, G. 'Central England temperatures: monthly means 1659–1973', *Quarterly Journal of the Royal Meteorological Society*, 100 (1974) 389–405

Marshall, J. *Mortality in the Metropolis*, London, 1932

Marshall, J. D. *The Autobiography of William Stout of Lancaster, 1665–1752*, Chetham Society, third series, 14, Manchester, 1967

  'The domestic economy of the Lakeland yeoman, 1660–1749', *Transactions of the Cumberland and Westmorland Antiquarian and Archaeological Society*, 73 (1973) 190–219

Martin, M. 'The parish register and history', *Warwickshire History*, 2 (1973–4) 3–15

Matthews, W. *British Dairies*, Cambridge, 1950

Mauss, M. *The Gift: Form and Function of Exchange in Archaic Societies*, London, 1954 edn

Mayo, C. H. (ed.). *The Municipal Records of the Borough of Dorchester, Dorset*, Exeter, 1908

McCloskey, D. N. and J. Nash. 'Corn at interest: the extent and cost of grain storage in medieval England', *American Economic Review*, 74 (1984) 174–87

'English open fields as behaviour towards risk', *Research in Economic History*, 1 (1976) 124–70

'The persistence of the English common fields', in W. N. Parker and E. Jones (eds.), *European Peasants and their Markets*, Princeton, 1975, pp. 73–119

McGrath, P. V. 'The marketing of food, fodder and livestock in the London area in the seventeenth century, with some reference to the sources of supply', unpublished MA thesis, University of London, 1948

McIntosh, M. K. 'Responses to the poor in late medieval and Tudor England', unpublished typescript of paper to Seminar on Charity and Welfare, Shelby Cullom Davis Center, Princeton University, 1984–86

McNeill, W. H. *Plagues and Peoples*, Oxford, 1976

Meeke, R. *Extracts from the Diary of the Rev. Robert Meeke*, H. J. Morehouse (ed.), London, 1874

Mennell, S. *All Manners of Food: Eating and Taste in England and France from the Middle Ages to the Present*, Oxford, 1985

Mercer, A. J. 'Smallpox and epidemiological–demographic change in Europe: the role of vaccination', *Population Studies*, 39 (1985) 287–307

Mestayer, M. 'Les prix du blé et de l'avoine à Douai de 1329 à 1793, *Revue du Nord*, 178 (1963) 157–76

Meuvret, J. 'Demographic crisis in France from the sixteenth to the eighteenth century', in D. V. Glass and D. E. C. Eversley (eds.), *Population in History*, pp. 507–22

'Les crises de subsistances et la démographie de la France de l'Ancien Régime', *Population*, 1 (4) (1946) 643–50

Miller, E. and J. Hatcher. *Medieval England: Rural Society and Economic Change 1086–1348*, London, 1978

Mingay, G. E. 'The agricultural depression, 1730–1750', *Economic History Review*, 8 (1955/6) 324–9

Mintz, S. 'Internal market systems as mechanisms of social articulation', *Annual Proceedings American Ethnological Society* (1959) pp. 20–30

Mitchell, B. R. and P. Deane. *Abstract of British Historical Statistics*, Cambridge, 1962

European Historical Statistics, 1750–1975, second edn, London, 1981

Mitchinson, R. 'Local and central agencies in the control of famine in pre-industrial Scotland', in M. Flinn (ed.), *Proceedings of the Seventh International Economic History Congress*, 2 vols., Edinburgh, 1978, 2, pp. 395–404

Mokyr, J. and C. Ó Gráda. 'New developments in Irish population history, 1700–1850', unpublished paper to the Conference on British Population History, Asiloma, California, 1982

Morris, R. H. *Chester in the Plantagenet and Tudor Regions*, Chester, 1983

Mullett, C. F. *The Bubonic Plague and England*, Lexington, 1956

'A century of English quarantine (1709–1825)', *Bulletin of the History of Medicine*, 23 (1949) 527–45

'Plague policy in Scotland, 16th-17th Centuries', *Osiris*, 9 (1950) 435–56

Nef, J. U. *The Rise of the British Coal Industry*, 2 vols., London, 1932

Newcome, H. *The Autobiography of Henry Newcome*, R. Parkinson (ed.), 2 vols.,
  Chetham Society, old series, 26–27, 1852
  The Diary of Rev. Henry Newcome, T. Heywood (ed.), Chetham Society, 18,
  1849
Newman Brown, W. 'The receipt of poor relief and family situation:
  Aldenham, Hertfordshire 1630–90', in R. M. Smith (ed.), *Land, Kinship and
  Life-Cycle*, pp. 405–22
Noake, J. *Worcester in Olden Times*, London, 1849
Norris, J. 'East or west? the geographic origin of the Black Death', *Bulletin of the
  History of Medicine*, 51 (1977) 1–24
  'Geographic origin of the Black Death: a response', *Bulletin of the History of
  Medicine*, 52 (1978) 117–19
Oddy, D. J. 'Urban famine in nineteenth century Britain: the effect of the
  Lancashire cotton famine on working-class diet and health', *Economic
  History Review*, 36 (1983) 68–86
Oglander, J. *A Royalist's Notebook: The Commonplace Book of Sir John Oglander Kt.
  of Nunwell, 1585–1655*, F. Bamford (ed.), London, 1936
Ó Gráda, C. 'Malthus and the pre-famine economy', Irish Economy from the
  18th Century to the Present Day series, Working paper, no. 8, 1983
  'The population of Ireland 1700–1900', *Annales de Démographie Historique*,
  (1979) 281–99
Oman, C. *The Great Revolt of 1381*, second edn, Oxford, 1906
Ortiz, S. 'Reflections on the concept of "Peasant Culture" and peasant
  "Cognitive Systems"', in T. Shanin (ed.), *Peasants and Peasant Societies*,
  Harmondsworth, 1971, pp. 322–36
Outhwaite, R. B. 'Dearth and government intervention in English grain
  markets, 1590–1700', *Economic History Review*, 33 (1981) 389–406
  'Dearth, the English crown and the crisis of the 1590s', in P. Clark (ed.), *The
  European Crisis of the 1590s: Essays in Comparative History*, London, 1985, pp.
  23–43
  'Progress and backwardness in English agriculture, 1500–1650', *Economic
  History Review*, 39 (1986) 1–18
Overall, W. H. and H. C. Overall (eds.) *Analytical Index to the Remembrancia of
  the City of London 1579–1664*, London, 1878
Overton, M. 'Agricultural revolution?' England, 1540–1850', *ReFresh*, 3 (1986)
  pp. 1–4
  'English probate inventories and the measurement of agricultural change',
  A. A. G. Bijdragen, 22 (1979) 205–15
  'Estimating crop yields from probate inventories: an example from East
  Anglia, 1585–1735', *Journal of Economic History*, 39 (1979) 363–78
Palliser, D. M. *The Age of Elizabeth: England under the later Tudors 1547–1603*,
  London, 1983
  'Dearth and disease in Staffordshire, 1540–1670', in C. W. Chalkin and
  M. A. Havinden (eds.), *Rural Change and Urban Growth 1500–1800:
  Essays in Regional History in Honour of W. G. Hoskins*, London, 1974,
  pp. 54–74.
  'Tawney's century: brave new world or Malthusian trap', *Economic History
  Review*, 35 (1982) 339–53
Patten, J. *Rural–Urban Migration in Pre-Industrial England*, University of Oxford
  School of Geography, Research Papers, 6, Oxford, 1973

Patten, J. H. C. 'Changing occupational structures in the East Anglian countryside', in H.S.A. Fox and R. A. Butlin (eds.), *Change in the Countryside*, London, 1979, pp. 103–21

'Village and town: an occupational study', *Agricultural History Review*, 20 (1974) 1–16

Pearl, V. 'Social policy in early modern London', in H. Lloyd-Jones, Pearl and B. Worden (eds.) *History and Imagination: Essays in Honour of H. R. Trevor-Roper*, London, 1981, pp. 115–31

Pendlebury, G. *Aspects of the English Civil War in Bolton and its Neighbourhood 1640–1660*, Manchester, 1983

Penry, J. *Three Treatises Concerning Wales*, D. Williams (ed.), Cardiff, 1960

Perkins, W. *A Golden Chaine, or the Description of Theology Containing the Order of the Causes of Salvation and Damnation*, Cambridge, 1597

Perrenoud, A. *La population de Genève du seizième au début du dix-neuvième siècle*, Geneva, 1979

'Mortality decline in its secular setting', in T. Bengtsson *et al.* (eds.), *Pre-industrial Population Change*, pp. 41–69

Perrot, J-C. *Genèse d'une ville moderne: Caen au XVIIIe siècle*, 2 vols., Paris, 1975

Pettit, P. A. J. *The Royal Forests of Northamptonshire: A Study in their Economy, 1558–1714*, Northampton, 1968

Phelps Brown, H. and S. V. Hopkins. *A Perspective of Wages and Prices*, London, 1981

'Seven centuries of building wages', *Economica*, 22 (1955) 195–206

'Seven centuries of the prices of consumables compared with builders' wage-rates', *Economica*, 23 (1956) 296–314

'Wage-rates and prices; evidence for population pressures in the sixteenth century', *Economica*, 24 (1957) 289–305

Phillips, C. B. *The Lowther Family Estate Books 1617–1675*, Surtees Society, 191, Gateshead, 1979

Phillips, C. J. *History of the Sackville Family*, 2 vols., London, 1930

Phythian-Adams, C. *Desolation of a City: Coventry and the Urban Crisis of the late Middle Ages*, Cambridge, 1979

Pickard, R. *The Population and Epidemics of Exeter in Pre-Census Times*, Exeter, 1947

Pilkington, J. *The Works of James Pilkington*, J. Scholefield (ed.), Cambridge, 1842

Platt, H. *Sundry new and Artificiall remedies against Famine. Written by H. P. Esq. uppon thoccasion of this present Dearth*, London, 1596

Pollitzer, R. *Plague* Geneva, 1954

Polwhele, R. *History of Devonshire*, 3 vols., Exeter, 1793

Poos, L. 'The rural population of Essex in the later middle ages', *Economic History Review*, 38 (1985) 515–30

Porter, R. 'Cleaning up the Great Wen', in W. F. Bynum (ed.), *Living and Dying in London*

Post, J. D. *Food Shortage, Climatic Variability and Epidemic Disease in Pre-Industrial Europe: The Mortality Peak in the early 1740s*, Ithaca and London, 1985

'Famine, mortality and epidemic disease in the process of modernization', *Economic History Review*, 29 (1976) 14–37

Postan, M. *The Medieval Economy and Society*, Harmondsworth, 1975

Pound, J. *Poverty and Vagrancy in Tudor England*, London, 1971

Pound, J. F. 'An Elizabethan census of the poor', *University of Birmingham Historical Journal*, 8 (1962) 135–61 (ed.). *The Norwich Census of the Poor 1570*, Norfolk Record Society, 40, 1971

Pounds, N. J. G. 'Food production and distribution in pre-industrial Cornwall', in W. Minchinton (ed.), *Population and Marketing: Two Studies in the History of the Southwest*, Exeter papers in Economic History, 11 (1976)

Powell, R. *Depopulation Arraigned, Convicted and Condemned, By The Lawes of God and Man*, London, 1636

Pye, G. *A Discourse of the Plague*, London, 1721

Raine, A. (ed.), *York Civil Records, V*, Yorkshire Archaeological Society Record Series, 60, 1946

Rappaport, S. *Social Structure and Mobility in Sixteenth Century London*, Cambridge, 1989

Raveau, P. 'Essai sur la situation économique et l'état social en Poitou au 16e siècle', *Revue d'Histoire Economique et Sociale*, 18 (1930) 314–65

Razi, Z. *Life, Marriage and Death in a Medieval Parish: Economy, Society and Demography in Halesowen, 1270–1400*, Cambridge, 1980

Rebaudo, D. 'Le mouvement annuel de la population Française rural de 1670 à 1740', *Population*, 34 (1979) 589–606

Richards, T. 'Weather, nutrition and the economy: the analysis of short-run fluctuations in births, deaths and marriages, France 1740–1909', in T. Bengtsson, *et al.* (eds.), *Pre-industrial Population Change*, pp. 357–89

Richardson, M. A. *The Local Historian's Table Book of Remarkable Occurrences*, 2 vols., Newcastle, 1841

Richardson, T. L. 'The agricultural labourer's standard of living in Kent 1790–1840', in D. Oddy and D. Miller, (eds.), *The Making of the Modern British Diet*, London, 1976, pp. 103–16

Riley, J. C. *The Eighteenth-Century Campaign to Avoid Disease*, London, 1987

Rives, J. 'L'évolution démographique de Toulouse, 1750–1789', *Bulletin d'Histoire Economique et Sociale de la Révolution Française* (1968) 85–146

Roberts, M. 'Sickles and scythes: women's work and men's work at harvest time', *History Workshop*, 7 (1969) 3–28

Roberts, M. F. 'Wages and wage-earners in England: the evidence of the wage assessments 1563–1725', unpublished D.Phil. thesis, University of Oxford, 1981

Robinson, G. W. *et al. Winthrop Papers*, 5 vols., Massachusetts Historical Society, Boston, 1929–37

Rogers, C. D. *The Lancashire Population Crisis of 1623*, Manchester, 1975

Rogers, J. E. T. *A History of Agriculture and Prices in England from 1259 to 1793*, 7 vols., Oxford, 1866–1902

Six Centuries of Work and Wages, London, 1884

The Economic Interpretation of History, London, 1888

Rollins, H. E. *The Pack of Autolycus or Strange and Terrible News of Ghosts, Apparitions, Monstrous Births, Showes of What Judgements of God, and other Prodigious and Fearful happenings as told in Broadside Ballads of the Years 1624–1693*, Cambridge, Mass., 1927

The Pepys Ballads, 8 vols., Cambridge, Mass., 1929–32

'An analytical index to the ballad-entries in the registers of the Company of Stationers of London', *Studies in Philology*, 21 (1924) 1–324

Rose, A. 'Winchester in transition, 1580–1700', in P. Clark (ed.), *Country Towns in Pre-industrial England*, London, 1981, pp. 144–95

Rotberg, R. I. and T. K. Rabb. (eds.). *Hunger and History: The Impact of Changing Food Production and Consumption Patterns on Society*, Cambridge, 1985

Population and Economy: Population and History from the Traditional to the Modern World, Cambridge, 1986

Rowlands, M. B. *Masters and Men in the West Midlands Metalware Trades before the Industrial Revolution*, Manchester, 1975

Rule, J. *The Labouring Classes in Early Industrial England 1750–1850*, London, 1986

Sachse, W. L. (ed.). *Minutes of the Norwich Court of Mayoralty 1630–1631*, Norfolk Record Society, 15, 1942

Salter, E. G. *Tudor England Through Venetian Eyes*, London, 1930

Salter, H. E. (ed.). *Oxford Council Acts 1583–1626*, Oxford Historical Society, 87, Oxford, 1928

Sampson, M. 'Property and poverty in mid-seventeenth-century England: an intellectual history with particular reference to doctrines permitting theft in the case of extreme necessity', unpublished typescript

Sayce, R. V. 'Need years and need foods', *The Montgomeryshire Collections*, 53 (1953/4), 55–80

Schofield, R. S. 'Age-specific mobility in an eighteenth century rural English parish', *Annales de Démographie Historique* (1970) 261–74

'An anatomy of an epidemic: Colyton, November 1645 to November 1646', in P. Slack (ed.), *The Plague Reconsidered* 1985, pp. 95–126

'Did the mothers really die? Three centuries of maternal mortality in "The world we have lost"', in L. Bonfield *et al.* (eds.), *The World We Have Gained. Histories of Population and Social Structure*, Oxford, 1986, pp. 231–60

'English marriage patterns revisited', *Journal of Family History*, 10 (1985) 2–20

'The impact of scarcity and plenty on population change in England, 1541–1871', in R. I. Rotberg and T. K. Rabb (eds.), *Hunger and History*, pp. 67–93

'Population growth in the century after 1750: the role of mortality decline', in T. Bengtsson *et al.* (eds.), *Pre-industrial Population Change*, pp. 17–39

'Representativeness and family reconstitution', *Annales de Démographie Historique* (1972) 121–5

'Through a glass darkly: *The Population History of England* as an experiment in history', in R. I. Rotberg and T. K. Rabb (eds.), *Population and Economy*, pp. 11–13

Schofield, R. S. and D. C. Coleman. 'Introduction: the state of population theory' in Coleman and Schofield, *The State of Population Theory*, pp. 1–13

Schofield, R. S. and E. A. Wrigley. 'Infant and child mortality in England in the late Tudor and early Stuart period', in C. Webster (ed.), *Health, Medicine and Mortality*, pp. 61–95

Scott, J. C. *The Moral Economy of the Peasant: Rebellion and Subsistence in Southeast Asia*, New Haven and London, 1976

Scrimshaw, N. S. 'Functional consequences of malnutrition for human populations: a comment', in R. I. Rotberg and T. K. Rabb (eds.), *Hunger and History*, pp. 211–13

'The value of contemporary food and nutrition studies for historians', in R. I. Rotberg and T. K. Rabb (eds.), *Hunger and History*, pp. 331–6

Seavoy, R.E. *Famine in Peasant Societies*, New York and London, 1986

Sen, A. *Poverty and Famines: An Essay on Entitlement and Deprivation*, Oxford, 1981

Seyer, S. *Memoirs Historical and Topographical of Bristol and its Neighbourhood*, 2 vols., Bristol, 1823

Shammas, C. 'Food expenditure and well-being', *Journal of Economic History*, 43 (1983), 89–100
'The eighteenth-century English diet and economic change', *Explorations in Economic History*, 21 (1984) 254–69
Sharpe, J. A. *Crime in Early Modern England 1550–1750*, London, 1984
Crime in Seventeenth-Century England: A County Study, Cambridge, 1983
Shirley, E. P. *Stemmata Shirleiana, or the Annals of the Shirley family*, Westminster, 1873
Short, T. *New Observations on City, Town and Country Bills of Mortality*, London, 1750, repr. with introduction by R. Wall, London, 1973
Shrewsbury, J. F. D. *A History of Bubonic Plague in the British Isles*, Cambridge, 1971
Simiand, F. *Le salaire, l'évolution sociale et la monaie*, Paris, 1932
Simpkinson, J. N. *The Washingtons: A Tale of a Country Parish in the Seventeenth Century*, London, 1860
Simpson, A. *The Wealth of the Gentry, 1540–1660: East Anglian Studies*, Cambridge, 1961
Skinner, J. 'Crisis mortality in Buckinghamshire 1600–1750', *Local Population Studies*, 28 (1982) 67–72
Skipp, V. *Crisis and Development: An Ecological Case Study of the Forest of Arden 1570–1674*, Cambridge, 1978
Slack, P. *The Impact of Plague in Tudor and Stuart England*, London, 1985
'Books of Orders: the making of English social policy, 1577–1631', *Transactions of the Royal History Society*, fifth series, 30 (1980) 1–22
'The disappearance of plague: an alternative view', *Economic History Review*, second series, 34 (1981) 409–76
'The local incidence of epidemic disease: the case of Bristol 1540–1650', in P. Slack (ed.), *The Plague Reconsidered*, 1985, pp. 49–62
'Mortality crises and epidemic disease in England 1485–1610', in C. Webster (ed.), *Health, Medicine and Mortality in the Sixteenth Century*, Cambridge, 1979, pp. 9–59
'Poverty and politics in Salisbury 1597–1666', in P. Clark and Slack (eds.), *Crisis and Order in English Towns 1500–1700: Essays in Urban History*, London, 1972, pp. 164–203
'Poverty and social regulation in Elizabethan England', in C. Haigh (ed.), *The Reign of Elizabeth I*, London, 1984
'Some aspects of epidemics in England 1485–1640', unpublished D. Phil. thesis, University of Oxford, 1972
'Vagrants and vagrancy in England, 1598–1664', *Economic History Review*, 27 (1974) 369–70
(ed.). *Poverty in Early-Stuart Salisbury*, Wiltshire Record Society, 31, 1975
The Plague Reconsidered, Local Population Studies, supplement, 1977
Slicher van Bath, B. H. *The Agrarian History of Western Europe, A.D. 500–1850*, London, 1963
Smailes, A. E. *North England*, London and Edinburgh, 1960
Smith, C. T. *An Historical Geography of Western Europe before 1800*, London, 1967
Smith, R. M. 'Fertility, economy and household formation in England over three centuries', *Population Development Review*, 7 (1981) 595–622
'Human resources in rural England', in G. Astill and A. Grant (eds.), *The Medieval Countryside*, Oxford, 1988, 188–212
'Marriages processes in the English past: some continuities', in L. Bonfield,

et al. (eds.), *The World We Have Gained: Histories of Population and Social Structure*, Oxford, 1987, pp. 43–99

'Some issues concerning families and their property in rural England 1250–1800', in Smith (ed.), *Land, Kinship and Life-Cycle*, pp. 1–86

'Transfer incomes, risk and security: the roles of the family and the collectivity in recent theories of fertility change', in D. C. Coleman and R. S. Schofield (eds.), *The State of Population Theory*, pp. 188–211

(ed.) *Land, Kinship and Life-cycle*, Cambridge, 1984

Smout, T. C. 'Diet and Scottish history, 1400–1800', unpublished typescript

'Famine and famine-relief in Scotland', in L. M. Cullen and Smout (eds.), *Comparative Aspects of Scottish and Irish Economic and Social History 1600–1900*, Edinburgh, 1977

Smyth, J. *The Berkeley Manuscripts*, J. Maclean (ed.), 3 vols., Gloucester, 1883–85

Sogner, S. 'A demographic crisis averted?', *Scandinavian Economic History Review*, 24 (1976) 114–28

Sonnescher, M. 'Work and wages in Paris in the eighteenth century', in M. Berg *et al.* (eds.), *Manufacture in Town and Country before the Factory*, Cambridge, 1983, pp. 147–72

Souden, D. C. 'Movers and stayers in family reconstitution populations', *Local Population History*, 33 (1984) 11–28.

'Pre-industrial English local migration fields', unpublished Ph.D. thesis, University of Cambridge, 1981

'"Rogues, whores and vagabonds"? Indentured servant emigrants to North America, and the case of mid-seventeenth-century Bristol', *Social History*, 3 (1978) 23–41

Spufford, M. *Contrasting Communities: English Villagers in the Sixteenth and Seventeenth Centuries*, Cambridge, 1974

Standish, A. *The Commons Complaints*, London, 1611

Stevenson, J. *Popular Disturbances in England, 1700–1870*, London, 1979

'Food riots in England, 1792–1818', in Stevenson and R. Quinault (eds.), *Popular Protest and Public Order, Six Studies in British History 1790–1920*, London, 1974

Stirling, P. *Turkish Village*, London, 1965

Stocks, H. (ed.). *Leicester Borough Records, 1603–1688*, Cambridge, 1923

Stone, L. *Family and Fortune: Studies in Aristocratic Finance in the Sixteenth and Seventeenth Centuries*, Oxford, 1973

The Crisis of the Aristocracy 1558–1641, Oxford, 1965

Stone, L. and J. C. Fawtier Stone. *An Open Elite? England 1540–1880*, Oxford 1984

Stone, R. 'Some seventeenth-century econometrics: consumers' behaviour', *Revue Européene des Sciences Sociales*, 81 (1988) 19–41

Strype, J. *The Life and Acts of John Whitgift*, 3 vols., Oxford, 1822

Styles, P. 'The evolution of the Law of Settlement', *University of Birmingham Historical Journal*, 9 (1963) 33–63

Supple, B. *Commercial Crisis and Change in England 1600–1642: A Study in the Instability of a Mercantile Economy*, Cambridge, 1959

Surtees, R. *The History of Antiquities of the County Palatine of Durham*, 4 vols., London, 1816–40

Swinburne, H. *A Treatise of Testaments and Last Wills (1635)*, Facsimile reprint, Amsterdam and Norwood, N. J., 1979

Taylor, C. E. 'Synergy among mass infections, famines, and poverty', in R. I. Rotberg and T. K. Rabb (eds.), *Hunger and History*, pp. 285–304

Taylor, J. R. 'Population, disease and family structure in early modern Hampshire', with special reference to the towns', unpublished Ph.D. thesis, University of Southampton, 1980

Taylor, J. S. 'The impact of pauper settlement, 1691–1834', *Past and Present*, 73 (1976) 42–74

Teall, E. 'The seigneur of Renaissance France: advocate or oppressor?', *Journal of Modern History*, 37 (1965) 131–50

Thirsk, J. *English Peasant Farming*, London, 1957
    'Industries in the countryside', in F. J. Fisher (ed.), *Essays in the Economic and Social History of Tudor and Stuart England*, Cambridge, 1961, pp. 70–88
    'Seventeenth century agriculture and social change', *Agricultural History Review*, 18 (1970) 148–77
    (ed.). *The Agrarian History of England and Wales, 1500–1640*, 4, Cambridge, 1967
    (ed.) *The Agrarian History of England and Wales, 1640–1750* 5, 2 vols., Cambridge, 1985

Thirsk, J. and J. P. Cooper. (eds.) *Seventeenth-Century Economic Documents*, Oxford, 1972

Thomas, B. 'Escaping from constraints: the industrial revolution in a Malthusian context', in R. I. Rotberg and T. K. Rabb (eds.), *Population and Economy*, pp. 169–93
    'Feeding England during the Industrial Revolution: a view from the Celtic Fringe', *Agricultural History*, 56 (1982) 328–42

Thomas, K. *Man And The Natural World*, London, 1983
    Religion and the Decline of Magic: Studies in Popular Belief in Sixteenth- and Seventeenth-Century England, Harmondsworth, 1971
    'Work and leisure in pre-industrial society', *Past and Present*, 29 (1964) 50–66

Thomas, R. P. and D. McCloskey. 'Overseas trade and empire, 1700–1860' in R. Floud and McCloskey (eds.), *The Economic History of Britain since 1700*, 1, Cambridge, 1981

Thompson, E. P. 'Eighteenth-century English society: class struggle without class?', *Social History*, 3 (1978) 133–65
    'Patrician society, plebeian culture', *Journal of Social History*, 7 (1974) 382–405

Thomson, D. '"I am not my father's keeper": families and the elderly in nineteenth-century England', *Law and History Review*, 2 (1984) 265–86
    'The decline of social welfare: falling state support for the elderly since early Victorian times' *Ageing and Society*, 4 (1984) 451–82

Tierney, B. *Medieval Poor Law: A Sketch of Canonical Theory and its Application in England*, Berkeley and Los Angeles, 1959

Tighe, R. R. and J. E. Davis, *Annals of Windsor*, 2 vols., London, 1858

Tilly, C. 'Food supply and public order in modern Europe', in Tilly (ed.), *The Formation of National States in Western Europe*, Princeton, 1975, pp. 380–455

Tilly, L. A. 'The food riot as a form of political conflict in France', *Journal of Interdisciplinary History*, 2 (1971) 23–57

Tinker, P. *Worcester's Affliction*, Worcester [n.d.]

Titow, J. Z. *Winchester Yields: A Study in Medieval Agricultural Productivity*, Cambridge, 1972

Todd, E. *The Causes of Progress: Culture, Authority and Change*, Oxford, 1987.
    The Explanation of Ideology: Family Structures and Social Systems, Oxford, 1985
Tooke, T. *A History of Prices and of the State of the Circulation, from 1793–1837*,
    6 vols., London, 1838–57
Toulmin Smith, L. (ed.). *The Maire of Bristowe Is Kalendar*, Camden Society.,
    new series 5, 1872
Trevor-Roper, H. R. 'The Bishopric of Durham and the capitalistic refor-
    mation', *Durham University Journal*, new series, 7 (1945–6) 45–85
Trigge, F. *The Humble Petition of Two Sisters; The Church and Common-wealth*,
    London, 1604
Trotter, E. *Seventeenth Century Life in the Country Parish with Special Reference to
    Local Government*, Cambridge, 1919
Turner, M. 'Agricultural productivity in England in the eighteenth century:
    evidence from yields', *Economic History Review*, 35 (1982) 489–510
Tusser, T. *Five Hundred Points of Good Husbandry*, 1580; reprinted Oxford, 1984
Tyson, R. E. 'Famine in Aberdeenshire, 1695–1699: anatomy of a crisis', in D.
    Stevenson (ed.), *From Lairds to Lords: County and Burgh Life in Aberdeen
    1600–1800*, Aberdeen, 1986
Usher, A. P. *The History of the Grain Trade in France, 1400–1710*, Cambridge,
    Mass., 1913
Van Andel, M. A. 'Plague Regulations in the Netherlands', *Janus*, 21 (1916)
    410–44
Van Zwanenberg, D. 'The last epidemic of plague in England? Suffolk,
    1906–18', *Medical History*, 14 (1970) 63–74
Vaughan, M. 'Famine analysis and family relations: 1949 in Nyasaland', *Past
    and Present*, 108 (1985) 177–205
Vaughan, W. *The Golden-groue moralized in three Bookes*, second edn, London,
    1608
Von Thünen, J. H. *The Isolated State*, English edn of *Der isolierte Staat in
    Beziehung auf Landwirtschaft und Nationalökonomie*, P. Hall (ed.), London,
    1966
Wales, T. C. 'Poverty and parish relief in seventeenth century Norfolk',
    unpublished typescript
    'Poverty, poor relief and the life-cycle: some evidence from seventeenth-
    century Norfolk', in R. M. Smith (ed.), *Land, Kinship and Life-Cycle*,
    pp. 369–80
Wall, R. 'Leaving home and the process of household formation in pre-
    industrial England', *Continuity and Change* 2 (1) (1987) 77–101
Walter, J. 'A "Rising of the People"? The Oxfordshire Rising of 1596', *Past and
    Present*, 107 (1985) 90–143
    'The geography of food riots 1585–1649', in A. Charlesworth (ed.), *An Atlas of
    Rural Protest in Britain 1548–1900*, London, 1983, pp. 72–80
Walter, J. and K. Wrightson. 'Dearth and the social order in early modern
    England', *Past and Present*, 71 (1976) 22–42
Watkins, S. C. and J. Menken. 'Famine in historical perspective', *Population and
    Development Review*, 11 (1985) 647–75
Watts, M. *Silent Violence: Food, Famine and Peasantry in Northern Nigeria*,
    Berkeley and Los Angeles, 1983
Watts, S. J. *A Social History of Western Europe 1450–1720: Tensions and Solidarities
    Among Rural People*, London, 1984
    From Border to Middle Shire: Northumberland 1586–1625, Leicester, 1975

Weatherill, L. 'Consumer behaviour and social status in England, 1660–1750', *Continuity and Change*, 1 (1986) 191–216

Webster, C. (ed.). *Health, Medicine and Mortality in the Sixteenth Century*, Cambridge, 1979

Weigall, R. 'An Elizabethan gentlewoman: the journal of Lady Mildmay *c.* 1570–1617', *Quarterly Review*, 215 (1911) 119–38

Weir, D. R. 'Life under pressure: France and England, 1670–1870', *Journal of Economic History*, 44 (1984) 27–47

'Rather never than late: celibacy and age at marriage in English cohort fertility, 1541–1871', *Journal of Family History*, 9 (1984) 340–54

Welford, R. *History of Newcastle and Gateshead*, 3 vols., London, 1883–87

Wells, R. A. E. *Dearth and Distress in Yorkshire 1723–1802*, University of York Borthwick Institute, Borthwick Papers 52 (1977)

Whaley, J. (ed.). *Mirrors of Mortality: Studies in the Social History of Death*, London, 1981

Whetter, J. *Cornwall in the Seventeenth Century: an Economic History of Kernow*, Padstow, 1974

Whiteway, W. 'The Diary of William Whiteway', *Proceedings Dorset Natural History and Antiquarian Field Club*, 13, Dorchester, (1892) 57–81

Widén, L. 'Mortality and cause of death in Sweden during the eighteenth century', *Statistisk Tidskrift*, 23 (1970) 93–104

Williams, R. *The Country and the City*, St. Albans, 1975 edn

Willis, T. *The Remaining Medical Works*, trans. S. Pordage, London, 1681

Wilson, F. P. *The Plague in Shakespeare's London*, Oxford, 1963

(ed.). *The Plague Pamphlets of Thomas Dekker*, Oxford, 1925

Winchester, A. J. L., 'Responses to the 1623 famine in two Lancashire manors'. *Local Population Studies*, 36 (1986) 47–8

Wood, H. M. *Durham Protestations*, Surtees Society, 135, 1922

(ed.) *Wills and Inventories from the Registry at Durham, Part 4*, Surtees Society, 142, 1929

Wood, W. *The History and Antiquities of Eyam*, sixth edn, Derby, 1865

Woodward, D. M. *The Trade of Elizabethan Chester*, University of Hull Occasional Papers in Economic and Social History, 4, 1970

'Wages rates and living standards in pre-industrial England', *Past and Present*, 91 (1981) 28–45

Wrightson, K. *English Society*, London, 1982

'Household and kinship in sixteenth-century England', *History Workshop*, 12 (1981) 151–8

'The Nadir of English illegitimacy in the seventeenth century', in P. Laslett, K. Oosterveen and R. M. Smith (eds.), *Bastardy and its Comparative History*, London, 1980, pp. 176–91

'The Puritan reformation of manners with special reference to the counties of Lancashire and Essex, 1640–1660', unpublished Ph.D. thesis, University of Cambridge, 1973

Wrightson, K. and D. Levine. *Poverty and Piety in an English Village: Terling 1525–1700*, London and New York, 1979

Wrigley, E. A. 'Fertility strategy for the individual and the group', in C. Tilly (ed.), *Historical Studies of Changing Fertility*, Princeton, 1978, pp. 135–54

'Urban growth and agricultural change: England and the Continent in the early modern period', in R. I. Rotberg and T. K. Rabb (eds.), *Population and Economy*, pp. 123–68

Wrigley, E. A. and R. S. Schofield. *The Population History of England, 1541–1871: A Reconstruction,* London, 1981
  'English population history from family reconstitution: summary results 1600–1799', *Population Studies,* 37 (1983) 157–84
Wrigley, E. A. and D. C. Souden (eds.). *The Works of Thomas Robert Malthus,* 8 vols., London, 1986
Wynn, *Calendar of Wynn (of Gwydir) Papers,* Aberystwyth, 1926
Wynne-Edwards, V. C. 'Self-regulation in populations of red grouse', in J. Dupâquier *et al.* (eds.), *Malthus Past and Present,* London, 1983, pp. 379–91
Wyot, P. 'The diary of Philip Wyot, Town Clerk of Barnstaple 1586–1608', in J. R. Chanter (ed.), *Sketches of the Literary History of Barnstaple,* Barnstaple 1866, pp. 91–121
Yonge, W. *The Diary of Walter Yonge,* G. Roberts (ed.), Camden Society, old series, 41, London, 1848
Youings, J. *Sixteenth-century England,* Harmondsworth, 1984
Zins, H. *England and the Baltic in the Elizabethan Era,* Manchester, 1972

Index

331